Is Fashion a Woman's Right?

For Irene,
who first suggested this would make a book,
and for the memory of my father.

Is Fashion a Woman's Right?

Carolyn Beckingham

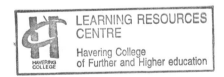
sussex
ACADEMIC
PRESS

BRIGHTON • PORTLAND

2 4 6 8 10 9 7 5 3 1

First published in 2005 in Great Britain by
SUSSEX ACADEMIC PRESS
P.O. Box 2950
Brighton BN2 5SP

and in the United States of America by
SUSSEX ACADEMIC PRESS
920 NE 58th Ave.   Suite 300
Portland, Oregon 97213–3786

British Library Cataloguing in Publication Data
A CIP catalogue record for this book is available from the British Library.

Library of Congress Cataloging-in-Publication Data
Beckingham, Carolyn.
  Is fashion a woman's right? / Carolyn Beckingham.
    p. cm.
  Includes bibliographical references and index.
  ISBN 1–84519–077–7 (hardcover : alk. paper)
  1. Fashion—Social aspects. 2. Women's clothing—Social aspects.
3. Feminism—Social aspects. 4. Women's rights—Social aspects. I. Title.
GT525.B43 2005
  391—dc22
                                                        2004026129
                                                        CIP

Typeset and designed by G&G Editorial, Brighton.
Printed by The Cromwell Press, Trowbridge, Wiltshire
This book is printed on acid-free paper.

CONTENTS

ACKNOWLEDGEMENTS AND AUTHOR'S NOTE

My thanks are due above all to Michael Shaw, Irene Gilchrist and Christine Nuttall, for reading the earlier versions of the manuscript and suggesting much-needed revisions, and to my father, the late Charles Beckingham, for unfailing support. Also to all the other people who made helpful suggestions: Wendy Harman, Colin Harris, the late Magdalene Hewson, Antonia Owen, Dr Patricia W. Romero, Ron Redfern, the late Philip Samuel and some friends of his who wish to remain anonymous, and Professor Edward Ullendorff.

I would also like to acknowledge Margaret Sherry Rich, Reference Librarian/Archivist, Rare Books and Special Collections, Princeton University Library, for assistance in searching for particular images; VGI Entertainment, Gt. Missenden, and Alister Keith for assistance in obtaining the Alex Graham cartoons; and The Cartoon Art Trust for their help (unsuccessful to date) in attempting to track down the copyright holder of the Osbert Lancaster cartoon.

Thanks are also due to my publisher, Anthony Grahame, and Simon Vincent, whose help with the computer narrowly avoided disaster.

The author and publisher gratefully acknowledge the following for permission to reproduce copyright material:

Punch Cartoon Library for Alex Graham, "I fear we must have missed the invitation"(23 January 1963) and "Don't tell me they've lowered the damn waistline again" (7 November 1962); and Sir George du Maurier, "Masculine Inconsistency" (2 April 1885).

The British Museum for 'The old wail about woman's dress'; original publication – *Daily Mirror*, Reflections, 1917.

Hal Leonard Corporation for an excerpt from *Wives and Lovers* (Hey, Little Girl), from the Paramount Picture *Wives and Lovers*. Words by Hal David. Music by Burt Bacharach. Copyright © 1963 (Renewed 1991) by Famous Music Corporation. International Copyright Secured. All rights reserved.

Mike Flanagan for permission to reproduce, 'You said wear anything you like!'

The publishers apologize for any errors or omissions in the above list and would be grateful to be notified of any corrections that should be incorporated in the next edition or reprint of this book.

Author's Note

Unless otherwise indicated, translations from French are my own, italics in quotations are the author's, and the place of publication of books is London. All quotations from the Bible are from the Authorised Version.

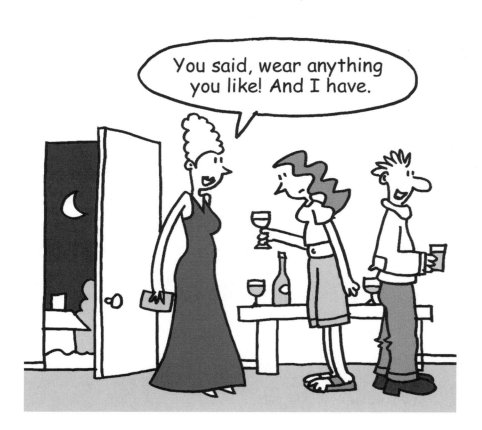

Woman is fine for her own satisfaction alone.
Jane Austen, *Northanger Abbey*

I

THE CASE AGAINST FASHION

Women dress irrationally.
Mrs Humphry ("Madge" of Truth)   Manners for Women (1897)

"Rather degrading, isn't it?"
"How?"
"Chopping and changing shape and hair and all that."
"Good for trade. We consent to be in the hands of men in order that they may be in ours. Philosophy of vamping."
John Galsworthy   Maid in Waiting (1931)

Every wave of feminism has foundered on the question of dress reform. I suppose it is asking too much of women to give up their chief outward expression of feminine difference, their continuing reassurance to men and to themselves that a male is a male because a female dresses and looks and acts like another sort of creature.
Susan Brownmiller   Femininity (1984)

Who needs another feminist book on fashion? Surely the subject has been covered from every possible angle? Not quite. There is one group whose views on fashion have not been adequately dealt with: the feminists who love it. And if your response is either "feminists don't love fashion" or "that's a dead issue", that is what this book is about.

I am a feminist and I love fashion. Must this lead to conflict and if so, can it be resolved? I began asking myself this when I first heard of the women's liberation movement as a schoolgirl in the sixties, and have still not been satisfactorily answered. If I had, what follows need never have been written.

In 1966, I was casually reading a page of interviews with feminists in a colour supplement. I have long since forgotten who they were, and almost all the details of the interviews except that they were asked: "Do you wear make-up? Do you use perfume?" Why shouldn't they? What had that to do with being a feminist? I had just begun to discover make-up, had loved perfume for years and could hardly remember a time when I didn't enjoy dressing up. It was one of the things that made my life worth living. Were these women saying I had to give it up? It was as if they had said "feminists don't enjoy flowers" or "feminists don't read for pleasure." If that was what being a feminist meant, how could I possibly be one? Believing as I did in women's rights, how could I not?

I had to find out. If I hadn't seen those interviews, my first reaction to the news of a mass movement for women's rights would have been "I want to join it", or at least "I want to investigate it." But how could I, if joining that meant allying myself with those who wanted to destroy something I loved? It would be small comfort that I had been able to enjoy it for a while before it vanished. What about the rest of my life, and what about future generations of women? If this was liberation it wasn't good enough, and I was not prepared to accept it unless and until I was convinced that there was no alternative.

If there was something fundamentally wrong with my point of view, however, I wanted to know what it was. I didn't want to stay in a fool's paradise or waste my life trying to run in two directions at once, so I started reading all the feminist literature I could find. The more I read the more puzzled I grew. Here were people who believed, as I did, that women should be able to shape their own lives. The same phrases appeared again and again: we should make our own decisions, develop our capacities, fulfil our potential, be active rather than passive, take what we wanted rather than resigning ourselves to our lot. So why were we being discouraged from taking action in one of the few fields where we were traditionally allowed to? Because it was seen as a tradition for women only, and undervalued for that reason? If so, wasn't that the sort of judgment that feminists, of all people, should be challenging? Practically every feminist book referred to our right to control our own bodies. Yet wasn't the power to alter our appearance part of that? Why was it different from any other power? Was such adornment wrong in itself, and if so, why? Should it be seen as part of our supposed feminine weakness, or as part of the strength which the anti-feminists wanted to deny? If we went on practising it, were we submitting to our wrongs or claiming our rights? The most far-reaching question of all was what this movement was fighting for: was it the right to have high standards, or to feel comfortably smug about low ones?

To me it looked like a flat contradiction. Excellence was excellence; either we should be trying to achieve it, or we should not. Was pretending you didn't understand, say, maths or science when you did so different from pretending you were not interested in what you wore or how you looked when you were? Why should hiding your figure be more liberating than hiding your ability? Was being told, "You don't have to dress up, I like you just as much in an old pair of trousers" so different from being told "You don't need a career, I respect you just as much as a house-wife," or any less irritating? Not to me. Every time somebody tells me I don't have to dress up I long to answer, "Do I have to dress down?" and over twenty years of feminism haven't changed that in the least. According to Jane Austen, "Half the world does not understand the plea-sures of the other," and from my point of view it was the wrong half that was running the movement.

Feminists stressed the importance of every woman telling her own story. I read innumerable women's stories, told in the form of autobiographies, diaries, novels, poems and summaries in books of feminist philosophy. None of them seemed to tell more than half the truth as I saw it. Authors with whom I entirely agreed on every other subject would be totally opposed to me on this one. The phrase "speaking bitterness", borrowed from Chinese revolutionary groups, was more apt than they knew. Where was the woman who dared to speak joy? In Betty Friedan's *The Feminine Mystique*, a woman journalist, at the height of the post-war rebellion against career women, said: "When I remember how I worked to learn this job and loved it – were we all crazy then?"[1] I know it's a much smaller issue, but when I hurried to my favourite shops to buy new clothes and loved them, was I crazy? In no way was that joy less real than any other. When I delighted in wearing clothes that were not chosen for practical reasons but for their looks, when I longed for more occasions to wear them, was I crazy? If so, at least some other women were crazy too. Were there none in the movement and if not, wasn't it perhaps because they, like me, had been put off joining it? How many of them were standing on the sidelines, saying "I'm not a feminist, but . . ." or even "A plague on both your houses!"?

I came to two conclusions. First, no woman in the feminist movement seemed willing to admit that she or any other woman actually enjoyed fashion. It was always a means to an end, something we forced ourselves to put up with to please men or male-dominated society or gain an advantage over other women, to obtain something, such as a job or a husband, or compensate for the lack of something else. Never was it seen as intrinsically good. I lost count of the number of times I read the words "we don't want to be sex objects for men." I could understand and sympathise with this, but it was a description not of adornment as such but of a particular motive for using it, and that motive was not mine. Why was it seen as the only one possible? Why did no-one mention what mattered to me, which was my own aesthetic sense?

This led me to the second point, which was something I had noticed long before I had even heard of feminism (except in connection with suffragettes): that people who were otherwise concerned with aesthetics believed that dress and personal appearance don't matter; and not even that they matter less than the fine arts or natural scenery, but that they simply don't matter at all. They were not supposed to be a legitimate outlet for the aesthetic impulse, but why not? I wasn't expecting anyone to think that the loss of high standards in dress was as important as the destruction of a work of art or architecture, or forests being felled, or wild flowers becoming extinct. Those losses are on a far greater scale and they are irreparable. Nor was I trying to claim that clothing can express ideas in the same way or to the same extent as, say, a book or a piece of music. But that didn't explain why people who cared passionately about the preservation of churches even if they were atheists, who shuddered at the attitude expressed by the City Architect of Bath who said "When the economic life of a building is over, there is no good reason for preserving it",[2] and who extended their concern to the design of everyday objects, did not extend it to the objects that we wear. Why did people who would be ashamed of never reading a book say "I never notice how anybody dresses" as if they were proud of it? Yet isn't there a parallel between "just wearing whatever's comfortable" and just opening a road or building an office block wherever it's convenient to put it? Why was it acceptable to grieve at the prospect of a generation which had never sung in a choir or walked through a meadow full of cowslips, and not at the prospect of one which had never worn any but utilitarian clothes?

This also applied to other arguments against fashion, of which there are two: humanitarian (the money should have been spent on doing good) and ecological (fashions wastes the world's scarce resources). In the last resort they are unanswerable. There is no adequate reply to the question: "How can you spend money on luxuries while millions starve?" If you are prepared to live on bare necessities and spend all you save by doing so on helping those in need, you are beyond praise, but then I doubt if you are reading this book. (If you are, I can't imagine why, and can only urge you to stop wasting time on it.) It is, however, possible to ask another question: doesn't that apply to all luxuries, including art and sport? Do starving people care whether the money that might have saved their lives was spent on dress rather than building a football stadium or running a film festival? I doubt it. Yet ecologists who wouldn't dream of simply saying "abolish art" don't hesitate to say, "resist fashion". With other luxuries, they suggest ways round the problem (printing books on recycled paper, not giving up reading); hardly anybody suggests a way round the problem of clothes which lose their appeal before they wear out, or even of having more clothes than are strictly necessary. For instance, could not materials be recycled, and if the fast turnover of modern fashion could still not be sustained without environmental damage, would it be possible to find some form of decorative clothing whose appeal did last? I read a few years ago of a notice in what was described as a fashionable shop, Fred Segal of Los Angeles: "Buying only what you need helps save the planet." That doesn't allow for what Colette called the need for something useless. The *Friends of the Earth Handbook* warns consumers: "It's hard for parents to refuse their child what others seem to take for granted: . . . the apparent delights of . . . clothes and fashion". What about the real ones? Sir Jonathon Porritt, the editor, wrote in his foreword to *A Green Manifesto*[3] that we did not need to give up all the good things of life, so one must conclude he doesn't think fashion is one.

When male environmentalists ignored women's points of view in other fields, claiming for example that one way of lessening demands on energy would be to abandon labour-saving domestic devices, feminists protested. But not only did they not protest at men who said fashion was trivial – they went further: to them it was positively bad for women, and any woman who claimed to like it didn't know what was good for her.

This argument is different in kind from the green and humanitarian ones, just as believing in vegetarianism is different from believing it is wrong to care about the taste of food, and in a way poses more of a threat. The other attacks are directed not so much at fashion itself as the conditions under which it is produced. The same applies to criticism of particular aspects of it, such as furs, cosmetics tested on animals or the exploitation of workers in the industry. If the conditions changed, these objections would disappear, but the contention that fashion degrades women would not. If it is true, it would still be true even if poverty were abolished, resources were renewed as fast as they were consumed, no animal products were ever used and working conditions were ideal. This is the case I propose to answer.

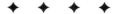

Until I understand a man's ignorance, I deem myself ignorant of his understanding.

Samuel Taylor Coleridge

To rescue a man lost in the woods, you must get to where he is.

John Holt

It is common knowledge that feminists picketed the Miss America contest in 1968 and the Miss World contest in London the following year. Kathie Sarachild, a member of the American radical feminist group the Redstockings, wrote: "Our group's first public action after putting out a journal was an attempt to reach the masses with our ideas on one of those so-called petty topics: the issue of appearance. We protested and picketed the Miss America Contest, throwing high heels, girdles and other objects of female torture into a freedom trash can."[4] (This was the event that gave rise to the rumour of women burning bras.) Yvonne Roberts writes that an American group, Cell 16, "the first of the sisters to move into short hair, combat boots and khaki pants . . . held that women, by having children, marrying, having sex with men, wearing attractive clothes and using make-up, identified themselves as collaborators." She describes the British Women's Liberation Conference in 1970: "a hierarchy was already developing; there was a certain look, a vocabulary, a credo which indicated you were more 'right-on' than the next person. No make-up, no men, no myths about finding true love."[5]

I could easily fill seven or eight pages with quotations showing the same attitude, but let one suffice, from Andrea Dworkin's *Woman Hating* (1974):

> The argument is not simply that some women are not beautiful, therefore it is not fair to judge women on the basis of physical beauty; or that men are not judged on that basis, therefore women also should not be judged on that basis; or that men should look for character in women; or that our standards of beauty are too parochial in and of themselves; or even that judging women according to their conformity to a standard of beauty serves to make them products, chattels, differing from the farmer's favorite cow only in terms of literal form. The issue at stake is different and crucial. Standards of beauty describe in precise terms the relationship that an individual will have to her own body. They prescribe her mobility, spontaneity, posture, gait, the uses

to which she can put her body. *They define precisely the dimensions of her physical freedom.* And, of course, the relationship between physical freedom and psychological development, intellectual possibility and creative potential is an umbilical one.

In our culture not one part of a woman's body is left unretouched, unaltered. No feature, or extremity, is spared the art, or pain, of improvement. Hair is dyed, lacquered, straightened, permanented; eyebrows are plucked, penciled, dyed; eyes are lined, mascaraed, shadowed; lashes are curled, or false – from head to toe, every feature of a woman's face, every section of her body is subject to modification, alteration . . .

Pain is an essential part of the grooming process, and this is not accidental. Plucking the eyebrows, shaving under the arms, wearing a girdle, learning to walk in high-heeled shoes, having one's nose fixed, straightening or curling one's hair – these things *hurt*. . . The body must be freed, liberated, quite literally: from paint and girdles and all varieties of crap. Women must stop mutilating their bodies and start living in them. Perhaps the notion of beauty which will then organically emerge will be truly democratic and demonstrate a respect for human life in its most infinite, and honorable, variety.[6]

When I spoke to friends, most of whom were broadly sympathetic to feminism but, like me, were not active in the movement, I found them anxious to reassure me: only a minority held views proffered by Dworkin, or they were more typical of feminism in America than in Britain or it was just a phase which the movement was outgrowing. My reading showed a different picture. Simone de Beauvoir's attack on fashion in *The Second Sex* was published in 1949, the year I was born, and had never been seriously challenged since. I found the same views expressed in books by American, English, French, Italian and Australian feminists; by those who called themselves radicals, those who called themselves socialists and those who did not call themselves either; in books for parents, books for teenagers and books by them. Mothers asked whether they had failed because their daughters didn't reject fashion. I should have been only too pleased to write their authors off as extremists, but the facts didn't fit. The only alternative to outright condemnation seemed to be a more moderate and less clear-cut version: extremism and water.

One anthology contains an essay by Joan Smith asking: "How feminists ever got a blanket reputation for hating sex and decorative clothes is something I've never managed to figure out. Did anyone ever look at what we were wearing?" but Sarah Dreher writes elsewhere in the same book: "We agonized over the politics, the economics, 'fashion' as a class issue . . . The solution, we knew, was to adopt the universal uniform of Revolution – jeans, blue work shirts, and boots."[7] Caroline Evans and Minna Thornton, among many others, confirm that "By the mid 1970s, feminist dress exemplified de Beauvoir's position, signifying both practicality and indifference . . . Women wore dungarees and jeans; hair might be long or short but it was never 'styled' in any way; adornment was avoided – except in the form of badges – as were high heels. The only accessories were large holdall bags." This was called "a challenge to prescriptive dress codes"[8]! One American writer, Joan Cassell, drew a parallel between the way women dressed and the depth of their involvement in the movement: the more committed they were to women's rights and the more independent were the lives they led, the more plainly they dressed. Members of the reformist National Organisation of Women wore cosmetics and had "attractively styled" hair, while the radicals had hair that was "not so much styled as there".[9] Stylish dressing meant lukewarm feminism.

So much for the prosecution: where was the defence? On other issues there were genuine differences between different strands of feminism. Some feminists reject the idea of God as an invention of an oppressive society (as some non-feminists do); others have fought for women's equal participation in religious rites. Some reject marriage and the family, some reject all sex with men and some reject all sex (Cell 16 did). Others have no objection to men or even marriage as such but only to unequal rights and divisions of labour between the partners. These disputes are outside the scope of this book. But where was the fashion-lover's equivalent to the books on feminist spirituality and egalitarian families? Almost the only one was Janet Radcliffe Richards' *The Sceptical Feminist* (1980), and even that based part of its argument on whether feminists' attitudes to dress put other women off feminism. I can vouch for that, being one of those women, but that wasn't the point. Even Richards didn't strike me either as offering a sufficiently whole-hearted defence or as going deeply enough into the causes of the attack. In spite of some recent developments which seem to give hope, I am still looking.

Why did so many different viewpoints produce such unanimity? To answer this question thoroughly would take another book, because it would mean listing all the overlapping subdivisions within feminism, but one thing was clear: women who agreed in thinking their lot unsatisfactory might disagree as to both the cause and the remedy, but whatever any group identified as the enemy, fashion always seemed to be part of it.

A book by Olive M. Banks identified three types of feminist reaction to the traditional division between men's and women's *rôles*. One was "masculine equalitarianism" (which I prefer, for linguistic reasons, to call egalitarianism): the adoption of "masculine" behaviour by women. The second was the reclamation of traditional "feminine" behaviour, which a pro-male society has allegedly belittled. The third (which she favoured) was androgyny, combining the two.[10] It is easy to see why supporters of the first point of view rejected so-called feminine dressing, and even preoccupation with dress. But that did not explain the supporters of the others. Where was the attempt to reclaim women's adornments? Why did women who protested at the male art world undervaluing women's traditional skills of embroidery and quilting, for example, not say a word about the art of dress? I could only suppose that it was because they didn't see it as women's art at all, but as a result of perverting women's true nature in order to attract men: sex objects again. This is the point of view of those feminists who regard true womanhood as something which can only be achieved in isolation from men. For them, anything which attracts men sexually is automatically suspect, or even forbidden.

But where does that leave supporters of androgyny? Judging androgynously means neither accepting nor rejecting something because it is supposedly female (or male) but trying to assess its merits. Like Banks, I favoured this, but still failed to find any attempt to assess the way we dressed from this point of view.

Fashion-lovers were accused of swallowing male definitions of femininity whole, but weren't their detractors swallowing male denigration whole? I saw two examples quoted over and over again, reminding me of religious fundamentalists quoting a sacred text. The first was Inge and Donald Broverman's study, made in 1972, in which a group of psychotherapists listed the characteristics of a healthy adult female, a healthy adult male and a healthy person of undefined sex. The last two lists were almost identical, leading to the conclusion that you couldn't be a healthy woman and a healthy person. Personal characteristics were assessed on a scale of seven points, the average man's tending more towards one extreme and the average woman's towards the other. Not surprisingly "very interested in own appearance" was a female trait. To be fair, this is one of the twelve items of which the authors say "the feminine pole is more desirable" (the opposite is true of twenty-nine) but this interest was still supposed to be characteristic of the less mentally healthy sex. Should smart clothes and cosmetics carry a Government health warning?

I have seen the obvious pro-male bias of this study challenged in two books,[11] but no feminist to my knowledge has performed the same task with my other example. This is from John Berger's *Ways of Seeing*: *"men act* and *women appear*. Men look at women. Women watch themselves being looked at."[12]

Berger also writes as a Marxist, which raises the issue of class. Again, the relationship between feminism and socialism is too involved to deal with here, but it is certain that many feminists analyse the causes of women's inferior position from a socialist angle. Fashion is traditionally regarded as a symbol of upper-class privilege; for some socialists that is all it is, and their reaction against it is as automatic as that of the type of feminist whose slogan is "men are the enemy". The premises are different but the conclusion is the same: for the latter it symbolises the enslaved sex, for the former the enslaving class.

One writer who has analysed socialist and feminist objections to fashion is Elizabeth Wilson. Her book *Adorned in Dreams* (1985) poses the question I have already noted: why should fashion arouse more moral indignation than other luxuries, when most of the arguments against it could also apply to them? Why the "quite special rage reserved for fashionable dressing"? She adds:

> This relates also to an attitude of persistent hostility to the fine arts that has been evident in certain veins of progressive thought. A 'progressive' condemnation of fashion can extend to a general denigration of 'bourgeois art'. Aesthetes are then equated with the degenerate upper classes, and their preoccupations become suspect. To care or know about traditional art, classical music or 'high culture' generally is often to be convicted of pretentiousness and a damaging involvement with the norms of bourgeois culture. The ultimate example of such an attitude is the radical feminist who dismisses Tintoretto and Rubens as 'all tits and bums' or as 'pornography'.[13]

Similarly, Michelene Wandor recalled that in the seventies "art could only be validated if it was instrumentally harnessed in the interest of some correct political cause, and performed only to working-class audiences. Otherwise it was mere bourgeois cop-out."[14] In January 1987 *New Socialist* printed a letter signed Jonathan Kitching urging that in this time of "terrible want" socialists should reject "high-brow art-forms, fashion . . . and other allied crap."

If terrible want is the issue, it is hard to see why low-brow art should be preferable. Mr Kitching appears to be arguing on the same level as the schoolboy who told my mother that nobody really likes classical music and everybody who claims to is a liar. For him fashion was too high-brow, but it wasn't high-brow enough for some socialists who, as Elizabeth Wilson put it in an article published in the *Guardian* on 26 July 1982, "bemoaned the vulgar tastes of the masses" whom "socialist culture was to guide . . . towards 'great art'." It doesn't have the status of high art (nor, I have argued, does it deserve to) so that defenders and opponents of traditional cultural standards both attack it. It has always been associated with social élites but not so much with intellectual ones, so that it annoys both the straight and the inverted intellectual snob.

Adorned in Dreams sums up:

> Caught between the addicts and the puritans . . . many, perhaps most, indi-viduals experience above all an intense ambivalence about fashion and a love of fine dressing . . . two different ways of understanding culture emerged within feminism. The first of these was a whole-hearted condemnation of every aspect of culture that reproduced sexist ideas of women and femininity, all of which came to seem in some sense 'violent' and 'pornographic'; the other, by contrast, was a populist liberalism which argued that it would be élitist to criticize any popular pastime which the majority of women enjoyed, whether it were reading pulp romances or dressing in smart clothes, an approach that was an offshoot of a general interest in popular culture . . . the thesis is that fashion is oppressive, the antithesis that we find it pleasurable; again no synthesis is possible. In all these arguments the alternatives posed are between moralism and hedonism; either doing your own thing is okay, or else it convicts you of false consciousness. Either the products of popular culture are the supports of a monolithic male ideology, or they are there to be enjoyed and justified.
>
> A slightly different version of these arguments acknowleges that desires for the 'unworthier' artefacts of the consumer society have been somehow implanted in us, and that we must try to resolve the resulting guilt by steering some moderate middle way. To care about dress and our appearance *is* oppressive, so the argument goes, and our love of clothes *is* a form of false consciousness – yet, since we *do* love them we are locked in a contradiction. The best we can then do, according to this scenario, is to try to find some form of reasonably attractive dress that will avoid the worst pitfalls of extrav-agance, self-objectification and snobbery, while avoiding also becoming 'platform women in dingy black'.

This Wilson rejects as "false logic" and cites Susan Brownmiller's *Femininity*, which I quoted at the beginning of this chapter, as an example of it. Brownmiller "defines the erotically appealing as being in direct conflict with the serious and the functional, and offers feminists only the choice between the two", although she "longs for the gracefulness and pretty colours of her discarded gowns . . . Neither a puritanical moralism, nor a hedonism that supports *any* practice in the name of 'freedom' is an adequate politics of popular culture." What is? Brownmiller was not alone in failing to solve the problem. (When her book was published in England, she told an interviewer on the BBC Radio 4 programme *Woman's Hour* that professional women dressed fashionably because they lacked confidence in their ability.) Simone de Beauvoir, who could not be clearer about her hatred of narcissism in all its forms, never gave up "feminine" dressing. Perhaps it would have been socially impossible when *The Second Sex* was first published, but why did she not take up jeans and a scrubbed face in the seventies? Every photograph I have seen of her as an adult shows her wearing strongly coloured lipstick and nail varnish (which, according to her, deprived women of the use of their hands), and this includes those taken on the day of Denunciation of Crimes Committed Against Women in 1972 which is reproduced in the Redstockings' *Feminist Revolution*; hardly an occasion when she wanted to placate men. "It suggests the area is one of unresolved conflict",[15] write Evans and Thornton of her attitude to "femininity". It certainly does.

I met Minna Thornton in 1983 when she taught a course at the City Literary Institute in London on Women and Design, the first of at least two. It will not surprise the reader that she had been criticised for the triviality of the subject. She described one suggestion for solving the problem of feminist dress that I would not have believed: it was all right to buy smart clothes provided they were second-hand. "That's a cop-out", I said. "Doesn't it occur to you that everything has to be first-hand first?" Apparently not: every woman present just looked blank.

For a time it did seem that some feminists were changing their minds, much to the indignation of those who hadn't changed theirs. Julia Penelope wrote in *Gossip, a journal of lesbian feminist ethics* published by Onlywomen Press in 1986: "The wearing of make-up, high heels, and dresses, the shaving of leg and armpit hair, all once regarded as the outer distinguishing features between feminist and non-feminist, are reclaimed, and the women who might've been challenged for 'buying into' male definitions previously can now assert their 'right' to choose how they look. Well, yes, of course, one can 'choose' to embrace her oppression, one can 'choose' to display the external signs of her bondage, and, perhaps, one can even speak of her 'right' to remain in her oppressed state, but is that ALL that feminism was about?"

She seemed to be fighting a losing battle, but so in some ways was the movement. Were these decoratively dressed women really feminists or so-called post-feminists (a term first coined in 1919),[16] who believed that fighting for our rights was no longer necessary because we already had them? The signs were ominous. Once again I found myself looking at superficial reassurances, wishing I could believe them and finding it impossible. I read, and still do, that young women were reluctant to use the word "feminist" about themselves: why? Even those who did use it worried me. For instance, among the names of "new-style" feminists, one that kept recurring was that of Camille Paglia, who said: "Women enjoy colour and fabric and fashion, and we should not have to apologise for that."[17] She also said that if women had been running the world we should still be living in grass huts. When women's magazines cited her as proof that the war between fashion and feminism was over, I wasn't so sure.

Hardly had the alleged post-feminist era begun than there were signs that the years of feminist activity were being followed not by a period when we had achieved our rights, but one in which we were losing them. From saying that feminism did not need to go any farther, popular opinion moved rapidly to saying it had gone too far already. There was a spate of books to that effect, and a spate of feminist protests against them. How does "reclaiming fashion" look to their authors?

Susan Faludi's *Backlash* (1992) has a chapter called "Dressing the Dolls", devoted to attempts by fashion designers to make women wear clothes that were not only impractical but designed to make them look as frivolous as possible: "If High Femininity was supposed to accent womanly curves, its frenetic baroque excrescences succeeded only in obscuring the female figure. It was hard to see body shape at all through the thicket of flounces and floral sprays." No wonder feminists opposed this. Faludi, however, quotes a survey according to which "the more independent women became, the less they liked to shop; and the more they enjoyed their work, the less they cared about their clothes".[18] Is this a comment on "High Femininity" or on all fashion? Holly Brubach commented in the *New Yorker* on 6 July 1992: "Faludi views fashion as something foisted on women. The sensuous pleasure to be found in the slide of fabric along the skin or in the line of a seam drawn along the body's contour seems lost on her. If she makes backhanded acknowledgment of the way in which women look to fashion as a mirror, it is only to condemn it." I wish I could find evidence to the contrary.

13

Rosalind Coward's *Our Treacherous Hearts* (1992) has an alternative theory: women collude in their own oppression. Here too there is a chapter on fashion and beauty culture, entitled "Slim and Sexy: modern woman's Holy Grail". This refers to

> ways of making women's preoccupation with sexual attraction less central; women were to concentrate more on their 'sisters', or were to give less time to make-up and trivia . . . Even among the most ardent of feminists, there has been a resurgence of personal adornment, but always justified as 'doing it for myself, not for men' . . . Accompanying the backlash against feminist puritanism was a belief that fashion and sexual imagery could be seen as a form of play and pastiche . . . Drawing on the belief in a new era of post-feminist equality, these ideas seem attractive, but they disguise the reality of women's relationship to their image. Play and parody may have entered the fashion arena, but they have failed to dislodge a fundamental unevenness between men's and women's relationship to sexual display and adornment . . . The female obsession with rendering oneself the aesthetic sex, with making oneself sexually attractive, remains as strong as ever . . . current female concerns with body image are a long way away from offering self-satisfaction and personal pleasure. As always, measuring yourself up to a prevailing ideal and finding yourself lacking is a source of discontent and unhappiness.[18]

Germaine Greer's *The Whole Woman* denounces the evils of beautification just as vehemently as *The Female Eunuch*, published nearly thirty years earlier.[20] Even Natasha Walter, whose much more positive views on fashion I shall return to later, suggests in *The New Feminism*[21] that the famous slogan "the personal is political" is out of date and women should concentrate wholly on the public sphere; this comes dangerously close to post-feminism.

In 1998 an article in the first issue of a feminist magazine, *Sibyl*, declared: "We've come a long way since the days of policing dress codes." The second issue had one asking "have we swapped one orthodoxy for another? . . . You mustn't let the side down by looking poor, or chaotic, or ugly . . . There are some encouraging signs from the margins, however . . . the teenage 'bag lady' look – all loose, casual clothing, army trousers, trainers and no make-up . . . Do you remember the freedom and sense of empowerment that came with dressing unacceptably? Maybe it's time for a new movement. One gloriously, irreverently christened The New Ugly."[22]

So must the whole cycle of rejection start all over again? Is this the best we can do?

My answer is that pleasures, like people, should be innocent until proved guilty. Those of us for whom dress is a pleasure must admit it, and then thoroughly investigate the arguments of those who refuse to believe us. If we don't stand up and be counted, we shall only have ourselves to thank if their case goes by default.

The first question is: how did this situation arise?

2

HOW DID WE GET HERE?

When men pain themselves to alter the body to make it seem fairer than God made it, they do great sin. For men should not devise nor ask greater beauty than God hath ordained to be at his birth.

Sir John Mandeville

Now, the more primitive a society is, the more the need of conforming real life to an ideal standard overflows beyond literature into the sphere of the actual. Modern man is a worker. To work is his ideal. The modern male costume since the end of the eighteenth century is essentially a workman's dress . . . Without leisure or wealth one does not succeed in giving life an epic or idyllic colour. The aspiration to realize a dream of beauty in the forms of social life bears as a *vitium originis* the stamp of aristocratic exclusiveness.

Johan Huizinga   The Waning of the Middle Ages

Voltaire said that the best way to find how human institutions worked was not to invent theories about them, but first to observe the behaviour of our contemporaries and then to study history. How do feminist theories of fashion oppressing women measure up to this standard?

The short answer is that they don't. If being the decorated sex were at the root of women's oppression, it would not have started until the beginning of the nineteenth century in the West, and in other parts of the world only when they came under Western influence. As it is, there is evidence that women were the subordinate sex in every society of which we have any precise historical records, but it is only recently that they were the only sex to be decoratively dressed. That is why we have to examine the history of both sexes, however briefly: what can we know of women who only women know? Neglecting men's dress and their attitude to it is making the same mistake as the schools which refused to teach German during the First

World War, thus depriving their pupils of the advantages of knowing the enemy's language.

The way men's and women's dress indicates their sex in modern Western and Westernised society is not universal either in humanity or any other species; peacocks and peahens are a well-known example of the reverse, but by no means the only one. (It might be asked what other species have to do with us, and the answer is nothing, but the point has to be made in order to counteract assertions that drab males and ornamental females are part of an eternal natural law.) Almost every item which now seems "feminine" has been worn by men at some time somewhere; to quote one writer, Margaret Leroy, "Prehistoric graves have been found to contain bracelets and necklaces, and both men and women in Sumer, the earliest known civilisation, are known to have painted their faces."[1] I have seen both feminist and antifeminist writing which implies that there is something intrinsically feminine about skirts and masculine about trousers, but in the Chinese and Ottoman empires, women wore trousers and were in subjection to men who wore long robes, and among the Bhekhtiari people of Iran (not a sexually equal or matriarchal society, so far as I know) women wore trousers and men wore skirts. Traditionally dressed Sikh women still wear trousers, and have not achieved equality; the same pattern repeats itself with other aspects of dress, such as whether the body is concealed or displayed (among the Tuareg, for instance, it is men who wear veils). There is no hard and fast rule.

We do have evidence that the sexes have always dressed differently, that male dress has been seen as a sign of privilege (this may well have been why the difference in dress originated, just as differences in "men's work" and "women's work" may have done), and that men have always told women what to wear. Since they have had the power to give us orders, however they acquired it, this was only to be expected; but they haven't always been the same orders. Men have sometimes told us to make ourselves sexually attractive to them (when sexuality was seen as worthy of celebration) and sometimes to avoid exciting their sinful passions (when it wasn't) but one practice is new: that of making us dress up while they dress down. If Susan Brownmiller were right in thinking that what attracts men about "feminine finery" is its difference from what they wear themselves, then for most of history women would have stood a better chance of attracting men by dressing as hardline feminists (or men) do now.

Some kinds of ornament might have been seen as "feminine" but not ornamentation as a whole; as Lisa Tickner has pointed out in the now defunct feminist magazine *Spare Rib*,[2] decoration was a sign of social as opposed to sex distinction, and the higher people were in the class structure, the more of it they wore. This was a matter not only of having more money but of custom and sometimes even of law (as we shall see, laws were passed at various times to prevent the lower classes wearing types of clothing reserved for their social superiors). After what J. C. Flugel called the Great Masculine Renunciation, this still applied, but only to women. What had been the sign of the ruling class was now also that of being female; whereas choosing clothes on aesthetic rather than practical grounds had previously indicated that the wearer could afford to delegate menial work to servants, it now meant feminine dependence on the male. As class distinctions have become increasingly blurred (at least in dress) while sex distinctions have not, this has come more and more to seem like its only meaning, with results we already know. Sheila Jeffreys, who describes herself as a revolutionary feminist, gives a particularly clear example in her book *The Lesbian Heresy*: "Women's clothing represents powerlessness whilst men's clothing represents the opposite. Lesbians, like many heterosexual women presently, routinely dress in what were historically seen as men's clothes because they offer all the comforts and advantages which might be expected of clothes traditionally adopted by the ruling class."[3] Among the articles of clothing she mentions with admiration, in this and her earlier book *Anticlimax*, are work shirts.

Some history! I can only assume she uses "ruling class" loosely to mean "ruling sex", but even so this statement is seriously misleading. If she means "class" literally it is the equivalent of confusing a mayor's chain of office with a slave's neck-ring: men of the ruling class treated men in work shirts, and even comparatively plainly dressed business and professional men, like servants. Can she, and many others like her, really be so ignorant of the way those men used to dress? It hardly seems possible, which suggests they have simply shut the knowledge out of their minds. This explains why believers in social equality (whether explicitly pro-feminist or not) have failed to ask the question about dress that they have asked about other aspects of life which were formerly seen as upper-class or middle-class privileges, from higher education to private transport: is this good or bad? Should it be available to all who want it, or failing that to as many as possible, or should it be abolished? They don't ask if the care which women take of their appearance should be abandoned or encouraged in men. The only reason I can find is that it has become so thoroughly identified with women's inferior status.

To return for a moment to my own experience, I vividly remember how

I became aware of the subject. I had seen pictures of the dress of other periods and some original clothes in museums, but what really struck me was my first visit (at the age of about eight) to a Shakespeare play. The curtain rose, and a man walked on stage wearing scarlet tights, a purple doublet and a white ruff round his neck. "Men used to dress like that!" I thought. "Why ever did they stop?" I decided without hesitation that men had made a stupid mistake. This confirmed the feminist views I had just started forming: I wasn't going to call people who had thrown away their chance to dress beautifully my superiors.

A couple of years later, two boys in my class at school circulated some verses beginning:

Down with girls
With silly old curls
And pleated skirts
They cry at hurts!

(The punctuation is that of the original.) When I was afraid to wear a pleated skirt to school in case of being teased, my mother said: "Tell them the Scottish highlanders and the Greek evzones were very brave male soldiers who wore pleated skirts for going into battle." After that, I knew what to think of expressions like "wearing the trousers", not to mention the remark quoted by Betty Friedan: "feminine women, with truly feminine attitudes, admired by men for their miraculous, God-given, sensationally unique ability to wear skirts, with all the implications of that fact".[4]

The first human beings wore no clothes. Why they started to wear them is anybody's guess, and so is whether this played any part in the development of women's subjection to men. This forms part of a much larger question, the origin of the subjection itself, most of which is outside the scope of this book and which I am not qualified to discuss. Even a brief glance at the various theories on the subject, however, is enough to show that they reveal more about their inventors than they do about the problem, which is why Voltaire was so critical of theorists. The trouble with remote antiquity is that we have so few facts; most of our evidence comes from paintings or sculptures, whose meanings are far from clear. Do cave paintings depict what people hoped or feared would happen or what did happen and if so, is it in a realistic, idealised or caricatured way? If the last, did the caricaturist make the point by exaggerating reality or reversing it (like the cartoonists who, because most men are bigger than most women, draw enormous women and tiny men)?

Some statues appear to show goddesses. Some feminists regard this as evidence of a golden age for women, which Rebecca West called "a period of alleged matriarchy, the surrender of which (if it ever existed) argues such weakness on the part of women that feminists really ought to keep quiet about it".[5] Elizabeth Gould Davis expounds this in *The First Sex* (1973), subtitled "The book that proves woman's contribution to civilization has been greater than man's." (According to her, male outcasts from matriarchy banded together to destroy it, which seems to confirm West's view of the wisdom of casting them out.) But even if we could be certain that all those statues are of goddesses, which we can't, that need not mean women were equal or superior to men on earth. Many modern Catholics use the Virgin Mary's example as an argument for restricting women's lives, saying in effect "If being a submissive wife and mother was good enough for her . . ." Many husbands call their wives angels or queens and treat them like slaves. Probably every reader knows examples. I also seem to remember a book by the sworn enemy of feminism, Dame Barbara Cartland, using these statues as "proof" that men will adore women providing they stay in their traditional *rôles*.

One deduction can be made: ever since people have believed in deities, they have dressed up to serve them. Several historians have noted that male priests dressed like women, as they still do; but this only brings us back to the question of why men and women dressed differently. Thorstein Veblen's *The Theory of the Leisure Class* provides one explanation: his well-known theory of "conspicuous leisure" and "conspicuous consumption", accumulating unnecessary objects to show one can afford the time and money to do so. Men, he claimed, forced women to display such objects on themselves, and worshippers believed gods wished their priests to do likewise. This implies that if we behaved rationally, we should do no such thing and all clothing would be strictly functional. Whatever the truth of this, the "need for something useless" seems to go back a long way.

Evelyn Reed, a member of the Socialist Workers' Party of the United States and also a believer in primitive matriarchy, provides an alternative theory in *Cosmetics, Fashions and the Exploitation of Women*: "In primitive society, where there were no classes, no economic and social competition, the bodies of *both* women and men were painted and 'decorated', and it was *not* for the sake of beauty . . . It was necessary at that time for each individual who belonged to the kinship group to be 'marked' as such . . . These marks identified the kindred member of the group or labor collective. Since primitive society was socialist, these marks also expressed *social equality* . .

20

. Then came class society. The marks that signified, among other things, *social equality* under primitive socialism, became transformed into their opposite."[6] How does she know?

If this matriarchy did exist (I am doubtful) we know too little about it to draw any worthwhile conclusions as to how it might influence us now. Let the Redstockings have the last word: "It's as true as ever that nothing can really be proved about 'pre-history.' (Someone a thousand years from now digging up the remains of New York City and finding the Statue of Liberty, not to mention all the nude ikons of women could deduce – incorrectly – that women ruled.)"[7]

Even when studying societies about which we know far more, we have some of the same problems. We can examine the artefacts in the Egyptians' tombs, but that doesn't mean we know what they thought. One fact is clear, however: both men and women in Egypt wore decorative clothing (although, as the historian Gay Robins points out,[8] that of women was more restrictive) and used scents and cosmetics. Hatshepsut, celebrated for having been Queen in her own right, dressed like a man and wore a false beard.[9]

Was any of this criticised? I suspect that, for as long as there have been people wanting to dress up, there have been others trying to stop them, and if we had access to Stone Age thought, we should find comments like "What do you want to bother with ornaments for? Why not put on any old skin?" Some Greeks used ornaments, though it is tempting for admirers of their aesthetic ideals to forget it. To quote Elizabeth Wilson: "One reason for what is perceived – whether correctly or not – as the difference between the harmonious stability of classical Graeco-Roman dress and the bizarreries of late medieval fashions is often attributed to Christianity and the changed attitude it brought towards the human body. We feel that the Greeks and Romans accepted and celebrated the body, and that their dress reflected this. In art the unclothed body appeared glorious, and, when clad, it was often merely veiled by liquid draperies that clung to and outlined the limbs."[10] This theory is far more wrong than right, as it is grossly oversimplified. Graeco-Roman forms of self-decoration may have been closer to nature than mediæval ones, but they still didn't leave the body alone, though some thought they should; whereas in the Middle Ages, as we shall see, the thinkers who were most hostile to the unadorned body were also hostile to the decorated one.

Referring to the Greeks' and Romans' attitude to "the body" might suggest that they regarded any and every body as acceptable. Aline

Rousselle's book *Porneia* explains how "physical beauty, the beauty of both the male and the female body, which was so important to the Greeks, and which they adored in others if they did not possess it themselves, became such an intolerable obstacle to the accomplishment of God's will." This alone is enough to indicate that they believed some physical types were better than others, and we also know that they were willing to interfere with nature in attempts to produce them. Rousselle describes the "moulding"of a Roman baby by his nurse, as recommended by Soranus of Ephesus: "to satisfy the aesthetic fashion of the time, or perhaps rather to satisfy the desire to dictate, while his body remained pliable, the physique the child would have in later life . . . the head should be round. Long heads would be reshaped, indeed all babies' heads would be reshaped to make them conform to the desired shape. The nurse would lift up flat noses, and press down aquiline noses, bringing out the nostrils."[11]

I do not know what Socrates would have made of these particular practices, but according to Plato he disapproved of some aspects of women's adornments. Xenophon's *The Economist* quotes a dialogue between Socrates and a young man who asks for his opinion on the qualities to look for in a wife. Socrates describes, with approval, a man he knew who reproached his wife for reddening and whitening her skin, saying he preferred her face as it was. Phintys, a follower of Pythagoras, forbade not only cosmetics but scents, jewels, clothes of thin fabric or of any colour but white and frequent baths. If a place ever existed where there was universal agreement on whether or how much to improve on nature, it was neither Greece nor Rome.

The Romans may not have painted their skin blue like the Britons, but they were not so dissimilar from the Gauls, who bleached it with chalk. As the empire grew, philosophers and moralists felt nostalgia for the customs of the Republic, when a woman could be divorced for going out with her face uncovered. The historian Jérôme Carcopino quotes comments, often highly critical, by the elder and younger Pliny, Juvenal, Macrobius, Martial, Petronius and Suetonius on the adornments of both sexes in the second century after Christ. Roman men lavished care on their hair, which was often artificially curled and sometimes dyed (Pliny gives a recipe for black dye) and on having their beards shaved. (Even some slaves were shaved by others.) Unlike the twentieth-century American art collector Edward Perry Warren, who chose to wear a toga, Roman men seem to have found theirs uncomfortable and reserved them as far as possible for formal occasions (women only wore them if they were actresses, prostitutes or disgraced). Men painted their faces (Nero was well-known for it) and wore patches; so did women. Thin-haired men wore wigs,[12] which would have appealed to Julius Caesar, known for his anxiety to cover his baldness with a laurel wreath. It is also said he shaved his body hair. Although it is the received opinion among historians that fashion as we know it, meaning the rapid turnover of styles, began in the fourteenth century, I find it hard to imagine these people wearing out their clothes. Juvenal, who devoted his sixth Satire entirely to women, condemned their bizarre forms of dress in similar terms to critics of modern fads, as well as such "masculine" behaviour as taking part in competitive games and understanding all they read.

It is clear that moralistic attitudes to dress did not start with either the Hebrews or the Christians. Then, as now, there were conflicting views. For proof of this, we need look no further than popular religious books of the "how to be a good Christian in the modern world" school. To quote one: "I know more than one Christian girl who has been rebuked for wearing scarlet because it was 'un-Christian and unsuitable'."[13] The author, Shelagh Brown, points out that though the harlot in the Book of Revelation wore scarlet ("And the woman was arrayed in purple and scarlet colour, and decked with gold and precious stones and pearls", 17: 4) so does the virtuous woman in the Book of Proverbs ("She is not afraid of the snow for her household: for all her household are clothed with scarlet. She maketh herself coverings of tapestry; her clothing is silk and purple" (31: 21, 22). One difference between Jews and Christians was the symbolic meaning ascribed to the length of men's hair. Samson's hair was the secret of his strength; Delilah "called for a man, and she caused him to shave off the seven locks of his head; and she began to afflict him, and his strength went from him" (Judges 16: 19). Yet St Paul wrote to the Corinthians: "Doth not even nature itself teach you, that, if a man have long hair, it is a shame unto him? But if a woman have long hair, it is a glory to her: for her hair is given her for a covering" (I Corinthians 11: 14, 15). What he meant by "nature" is a mystery, since men's hair can, if uncut, grow just as long as women's. It is also a mystery that all the earliest portraits of Jesus Christ (admittedly made long after his lifetime) show him with long hair. The saint's attitude towards women's hair is more understandable when one remembers that prostitutes then had cropped or shaved heads ("Every man praying or prophesying, having his head covered, dishonoureth his head. But every woman that prayeth or prophesieth with her head uncovered dishonoureth her head: for that is even all one as if she were shaven. For if the woman be not covered, let her also be shorn: but if it be a shame for a woman to be shorn or shaven, let her be covered" (I Corinthians 11: 4, 5, 6). Christians evidently wished to distance themselves from the Jewish practice, according to which all men were, and still are, required to cover their heads in the presence of God, which in the opinion of many orthodox Jews means all the time.

Yet it is certainly true that among the early Christians there was a profound change in attitudes to the human body and, above all, to the sexual desire it could arouse. For the first time this was seen not just as something to be kept within certain limits, but as intrinsically evil. Everything which could cause it was therefore evil too, part of "the world, the flesh and the devil" which had to be renounced. The Christians broke with both Roman and Jewish practice in repudiating not only adornment but cleanliness and the desire to maintain good health, no doubt partly in order to distance themselves from the pagan Romans with their frequent baths. The "odour of sanctity" is a metaphor now, but not then. To quote from the life of the Byzantine St Theodore of Sykeon:

> Theodore was eighteen and living in a cave as a hermit for two years. His kinsfolk found out where he was. 'With joy they went to the mountain and brought Theodore out looking like a corpse . . . When he came into the air he fainted and did not speak for a long time. His head was covered with sores and pus, his hair was matted and an indescribable number of worms were lodged in it; his bones were all but through the flesh and the stench was such that no one could stand near him. In a word people looked on him as a second Job. His relations besought him when he had regained consciousness to come home with them to be looked after, but he would not be persuaded.
>
> When Theodosius, the holy Bishop of Anastasioupolis, heard how Theodore had been carried half-dead out of his cave, he immediately went to him in the chapel. And when he saw him, he shuddered at the sores on his head, kissed him and ordained him 'lector' . . . And on the following day he ordained him sub-deacon and then priest.[14]

In the fourth century, St Jerome said that a clean body meant a dirty soul, and St Benedict, in the sixth, believed that bathing should be rare (presumably for both sexes). In the early church not all clergy wore special clothes to indicate their office, and opinion was divided among the Fathers as to whether they should.[15] Christians had another reason for disapproving of women, in particular, looking attractive: Eve tempted Adam. This meant that all women should do penance by abasing themselves as much as possible. Clement of Alexandria and Tertullian wrote that women, both by exposing and adorning their bodies, tempted men to sexual sin. Tertullian even objected to dyeing fabric, on the grounds that it was against nature. This probably started the view that adornment could be a form of witch-craft (the original meaning of the word "glamour") which was ungodly by definition. Juvenal died in AD 140, while Clement was born in about AD 150 and Tertullian in about AD 160. Such beliefs continued throughout the Middle Ages. St Bernard in the twelfth century and Savonarola in the fifteenth preached against all decoration and art of any kind, and the latter was responsible for mass burnings of works of art; it has been suggested that this is the reason for the shortage of nude paintings by Giotto.

In attitudes both to women and dress, there seems to have been less difference between Romans and Christians than between the ascetics and their opponents on both sides of the religious barrier. From this we can conclude that the Christian tendency to regard the physical self as bad was responsible not so much for mediæval fashions as for their rejection. The mere fact that people like Savonarola found it necessary to argue against self-adornment shows that it existed, even if there were not plenty of other evidence. Styles for both sexes were often highly elaborate, with bright colours and much decoration. Some used large quantities of material to cover the body, others revealed it to an extent which caused the passing of laws to restrict the amount which could be shown. The historian Diana de Marly writes of English society: "The court may well have felt that there was no pleasing some people; whether it promoted a semi-naked or a covered-up style somebody would criticize it on moral grounds."[15] Langland disapproved of luxury, but Chaucer apparently did not. It is true that the protagonist of his Parson's Tale denounced "the wast of clooth in vanitee", the costly decoration of clothes and the way they trailed in the mud, and the Monk's Tale describes Nero:

> Of rubies, saphires, and of perles whyte
> Were alle his clothes brouded up and down;
> For he in gemmes greetly gan delyte.
>
> More delicat, more pompous of array,
> More proud was never emperour than he;
> That ilke cloth, that he had wered o day,
> After that tyme he nolde it never see.

On the other hand the young teller of the Squire's Tale had curled hair (like the poet Petrarch) and

Embrouded was he, as it were a mede
Al ful of fresshe floures, whyte and rede . . .
Short was his goune, with sleves longe and wyde.

Chaucer was evidently more sympathetic to at least some of the fashionable dressers than his parson, as he clearly meant the squire to be likeable, and he also makes the Wife of Bath complain of men:

Thou seyst also, that if we make us gay
With clothing and with precious array
That it is peril of our chastitee;
And yet, with sorwe, thou most enforce thee,
And seye thise wordes in the apostles name,
'In habit, maad with chastitee and shame,
Ye wommen shul apparaille yow', quod he,
'And noght in tressed heer and gay perree,
As perles, ne with gold, ne clothes riche'.

She appreciated beauty in men, and chose her fifth and most-loved husband (who was twenty when she was forty), among other reasons, because:

me thoughte he hadde a paire
Of legges and of feet so clene and faire.

It was not only an age of lavish clothing but of rigid rules governing what was to be worn when, where and above all by whom. Huizinga explains the philosophy behind this: "All terrestrial beauty bore the stain of sin. Even where art and piety succeeded in hallowing it by placing it in the service of religion, the artist or the lover of art had to take care not to surrender to the charms of colour and line . . . To be admitted as elements of higher culture all these things had to be ennobled and raised to the rank of virtue . . . Through all the ranks of society a severe hierarchy of material and colour kept classes apart, and gave to each estate or rank an outward distinction, which preserved and exalted the feeling of dignity . . . In the domain of costume art and fashion were still inextricably blended, style in dress stood nearer to artistic style than later, and the function of costume in social life, that of accentuating the strict order of society itself, almost partook of the liturgic."[17] Not only men believed in this: Christine de Pisan (*c.* 1363–1431) established a strict hierarchy of dress, based on colour, for the inhabitants of her "City of Ladies". She could be seen as a precursor of the founders of modern women's communes and centres; it would be interesting to see how feminists today would react to a similar dress code.

This is the reason for the so-called sumptuary laws which sought to prevent the lower classes imitating the clothes of the upper, which began in the fourteenth century. De Marly points out that, given the absence of modern means of transport and communication, they were unenforceable; I suspect there was another reason, which was that many of the poor had to rely on richer people's cast-offs. The other way in which the upper class kept ahead was to change their own style as soon as they saw it being adopted by others, a process which has continued until modern times (though the fashionable and the aristocracy are no longer so closely identified). There was a legal aspect to this process too. Laws were made not only against styles which subverted the social hierarchy or codes of sexual morality, but which were imported from a foreign country or were simply unfamiliar; the City Council of Nuremberg in the fifteenth and sixteenth centuries forbade all deviation from a narrowly defined range of standard patterns.

Mediæval women's clothing was probably more cumbersome and impractical than men's (short gowns were not an option for them). According to popular belief, armour (worn only by men) was an exception, but this is mistaken. Moving in armour was not nearly as difficult as might be thought. When it was made to fit the wearer, as it was, movement was much easier than someone who tries on armour made for someone else could imagine: a fifteenth-century manuscript "depicts a knight in full plate armour doing cartwheels".[18]

The tendency for women's clothes to be less practical than men's appears to have continued throughout Western culture. Whether it is universal is a vexed question, and to settle it would require an encyclopaedic knowledge of dress at all times and places throughout history. It does seem true, however, that forms of dress requiring actual mutilation (in the strict sense of the word) have all been female. The most notorious example of this is Chinese foot-binding, which continued into the twentieth century and to which I shall return later. There was no male equivalent; Chinese mandarins used to grow their fingernails to an impractical length, but no permanent damage was done (nails can always be cut) and no pain involved.

Islam, like Judaism, is a legalistic religion, based on unalterable rules founded on Muhammad's actual or presumed behaviour and covering every possible aspect of life, naturally including dress. The insistence on women covering their bodies and faces when going out is too well known to need comment, but men's dress and appearance are regulated too. A mediæval compilation of the rules, the *Mishkat al-Masabih* ("Niche of Lamps") which includes instructions on which foot to put first when going to the lavatory and whether or not to face Mecca while inside it, devotes the first chapter of Book XXI to clothing: It was wrong to wear silk (except in small quantities or if one had "an itch" caused by bugs), good to wear old clothes (if clean), wrong for women to wear bells and for anyone to wear gold rings (the Prophet had a silver one). Chapter 4, *Combing the Hair*, continues:

> 'Ibn 'Umar reported God's messenger as saying, 'Do the opposite of what the polytheists do; let the beard grow long and clip the moustache' . . .
>
> 'Anas said they were told not to let more than forty days elapse between the times they clipped the moustache, pared the nails, plucked out hairs under the armpits, and shaved the pubes . . .
>
> 'Abu Haraira reported the Prophet as saying, 'Jews and Christians do not dye [their beards], so act differently from them.' . . .
>
> 'Ibn 'Abbas . . . reported the Prophet as saying, 'God has cursed men who imitate women and women who imitate men.' . . .
>
> 'Ibn 'Umar reported the Prophet as saying, 'God has cursed the woman who adds some false hair and the woman who asks for it, the woman who tattoos and the woman who asks for it.' . . .
>
> 'Abdallah b. Mas'ud said: 'God has cursed the women who tattoo and the women who have themselves tattooed, the women who pluck hairs from their faces and who make spaces between their teeth for beauty, changing what God has created.' . . .
>
> 'Ibn 'Umar said he had seen God's messenger with matted hair . . .'

According to the same sources, men's white hair could be dyed but not dyed black, their heads should be shaved entirely or not at all (only the latter was permissible for women), and hair should not be dishevelled. There is conflicting evidence on henna: its colours, used on hands and nails, was good but its smell was bad. The use of scent was allowed, as was antimony, which made hair grow.[19] The fourteenth-century Arab traveller Ibn Battuta noted that in some parts of Africa people used antimony on their eyelids; he was shocked by nudity in West African women, but does not mention men.[20] Another work describing the appropriate behaviour for an Islamic ruler shows women behaving in a manner reminiscent of Hatshepsut: "The most important office was that of the princess (*asarbi*) as the office holder was called in Zamfara, or the mother (*inna*) in Gumi or Gobir. The incumbent had to be a sister to the king. She dressed in male attire assuming that she was possessed by an invisible male spirit which made her act like a man. She was highly respected."[21]

The Muslims evidently wanted to distance themselves from Jews, just as Christians did from Romans; no doubt this reinforced the antipathy of some Christians to washing, which could now be called Muslim just as it had been called pagan.

The European Renaissance was a time of lavish dress, at least for the upper classes. At the court of François I of France, every activity demanded a change of clothes. As in the Middle Ages, life was treated as a fine art, with the collaboration of the most famous artists: Holbein painted a ceiling, which was broken up immediately afterwards, for a ball given by Henry VIII, and in Italy Michelangelo made a statue of snow, and Paolo Uccello one of cheese. At one ball in Florence, all guests were to wear what they pleased, but if any two were dressed alike they were fined.[22] There were, however, attempts to limit this lavishness, and they did not come only from religious extremists. Baldessar Castiglione in his *Il Cortigiano* (*Book of the Courtier*) of 1528, a discussion about the ideal courtier's behaviour, recommended the dark colours (principally black) which prevailed at the Spanish court, except for masquerades, jousting and the theatre. One of the male characters, who denounces women's cosmetics, seems generally misogynistic and is several times reproved for this by one of the women. Castiglione also approved of personal cleanliness, and his advice on taste reads rather like that given by women's magazines today: when breeches were being worn short, he advised, men who did not have well-shaped legs should wear the longest permissible rather than the shortest. It was understandable that men were worried: their breeches showed their legs up to the knee and sometimes much higher, giving them freedom of movement and at the same time putting their legs on show, in exactly the same way as modern women's mini-skirts.

It would be over-simplifying to divide the Renaissance world's attitudes to luxury along religious lines. The Reformation cannot have been responsible (except by exercising an unconscious influence) for advocates of sober dress in Catholic Spain or Italy, such as Antonio de Guevara and Tommaso Campanella, whose books describe their visions of Utopia. In his *Libro des Emperador Marco Aurelio* (1527), Guevara condemns women's spending on dress, and in his *La Città del Sole* (1602) Campanella declares that adornment and persistent sodomy would both be punishable by death (making adornment a worse sin than sodomy that was not persistent). The population of St Thomas More's *Utopia* of 1516 wore a uniform.[23] On the other hand, any portrait of the protestant Queen Elizabeth I of England or her courtiers is enough to show their taste for richness in dress (Sir Walter Raleigh, for instance, went to court in clothes sewn with pearls). Men's beards were regarded as a symbol of their authority, and having them pulled or cut off was a punishment (this seems also to have been true of contemporary Italy, judging from a reference to beard-pulling in one of Monteverdi's operas). The Queen's envoy to Russia, George Killingworth, wore one five feet long. They were cut to improve the shape of the wearer's face, which could easily involve spending four hours at the barber's; a spiral cut called the "screw" was only one example of the possible styles.[24]

Montaigne, whose essays were published posthumously in 1595, pointed out the uselessness of sumptuary laws: saying that only kings were allowed to wear something automatically made everyone else want it. If he really wished to discourage finery, a king should refuse to wear it himself, or even make it compulsory for the most despised members of society. (Kemal Atatürk allegedly brought about the wearing of Western dress in modern Turkey by issuing a law that all prostitutes must wear veils, with the result that they disappeared overnight.) This, Montaigne said, would be the way to banish "ce lourd grossissement de pourpoins . . . ces longues tresses efféminées." He quoted Plato's opinion that letting young people pursue new trends in dress, dances, music and other pastimes encouraged disrespect for tradition, and consequently civil disturbances; he also noted the way that one fashion would be supplanted almost overnight by another, which would in turn be driven away, a short while afterwards, by the return of the first.[25]

Protestants did encourage the view that luxury and pride of any kind were sinful, which reached its climax in Britain with Cromwell's puritans. An essay by "T. T." called *Of Painting the Face*, published in *New Essays* in 1614, begins: "If that which is most ancient be best, then the face that one is borne with, is better than it that is borrowed . . . artificiall facing doth corrupt the naturall colour of it . . . What a miserable vanity is it a man or woman beholding in a glasse their borrowed face, their bought complexion, to please themselves with a face that is not their owne?" It must be "pride of heart, disdaining to bee behind their neighbour, discontentment with the worke of God, and vaine glory, or a foolish affectation of the praise of men . . . will any man out of a well informed judgement say, that this kinde of painting is worthy love, or that a painted face is worthy to be fancied? . . . A painted face is the devils looking-glasse . . . And indeed how unworthy are they to bee credited in things of moment, that are so false in their haire, or colour, over which age, and sicknesse, and many accidents doe tyrannize; yea and where their deceipt is easily discerned?" Yet apparently it was not always easily discerned, for "these artificial creatures steal away the praise from the naturall beauty by reason of their Art, when it is not espyed".[26]

The "Roundheads" did not extend their espousal of short hair to women, but echoed St Paul's views on the subject. One of them, William Prynne, wrote that if a woman had short hair "this is all one as if she should take upon her the forme or person of a man, to whom short cut haire is proper, it being naturall and comly to women to nourish their haire, which even God and nature have given them for a covering, a token of their subjection, and a natural badge to distinguish them from men." His own hair, however, came nearly to his shoulders (to hide the fact that his ears had been cut off), and Diana de Marly points out that he wore his beard trimmed to a point like that of King Charles I, the fashions of whose court he strongly criticised.[27] Cromwell himself, according to his biographer Roy Sherwood, copied royal pageantry on state occasions, to the extent of carrying a sceptre (though not wearing a crown) and wore grey velvet, silk and gold-laced garters to his youngest daughter's wedding.

John Bunyan was certainly not an extreme Puritan (he loved music and did not altogether disapprove of dancing) but in his *Life and Death of Mr Badman* (1680), a dialogue between Mr Wiseman and Mr Attentive concerning the fate of the protagonist, Wiseman quotes Isaiah's condemnation of bodily pride, and concludes:

> The putting on of gold, and pearls, and costly array; the plaiting of the hair, the following of fashions, the seeking by gestures to imitate the proud, either by speech, looks, dresses, goings, or other fools' baubles, of which at this time the world is full, all these, and many more, are signs of a proud heart, so of bodily pride also (I Tim. ii. 9; I Pet. iii. 3–5).
>
> But Mr Badman would not allow, by any means, that this should be called pride, but rather neatness, handsomeness, comeliness, cleanliness, etc., neither would he allow that following of fashions was anything else, but because he would not be proud, singular, and esteemed fantastical by his neighbours . . . For my own part, I have seen many myself, and those church members too, so decked and bedaubed with their fangles and toys, and that when they have been at the solemn appointments of God in the way of his worship, that I have wondered with what face such painted persons could sit in the place where they were without swooning.
>
> [Mr Attentive objects]: "It is whispered that some good ministers have countenanced their people in their light and wanton apparel, yea, have

pleaded for their gold and pearls, and costly array, etc.", [Mr Wiseman admits it]: "it is a shame, it is a reproach, it is a stumbling-block to the blind; for though men be as blind as Mr Badman himself, yet they can see the foolish lightness that must needs be the bottom of all these apish and wanton extravagancies . . . But what can be the end of those that are proud in the decking of themselves after their antic manner? Why are they for going with their bull's foretops, with their naked shoulders, and paps hanging out like a cow's bag? Why are they for painting their faces, for stretching out their neck, and for putting themselves unto all the formalities which proud fancy leads them to? Is it because they would honour God? because they would adorn the gospel? because they would beautify religion, and make sinners to fall in love with their own salvation? No, no, it is rather to please their lusts, to satisfy their wild and extravagant fancies; and I wish none doth it to stir up lust in others, to the end they may commit uncleanness with them. I believe, whatever is their end, this is one of the great designs of the devil; and I believe also that Satan has drawn more into the sin of uncleanness by the spangling show of fine cloths, than he could possibly have drawn into it without them. I wonder what it was that of old was called the attire of a harlot; certainly it could not be more bewitching and tempting than are the garments of many professors this day."

The holy women he approved of were all "in subjection to their own husbands" as enjoined by St Peter.[28]

Bunyan wrote this after the Puritans' defeat, at a time when fashion was certainly extravagant. It was set by France, where the Protestants never took over. Doublets had shrunk and hose expanded, producing the so-called "petticoat breeches". Pepys' diary mentions a man who put both legs into the same half of his breeches and did not notice he had until he undressed at night. (In the "classical" costume used by actors in tragedies set in Greece and Rome, men wore a short skirt called a *tonnelet*, or little barrel, rather like that now worn by women in ballet.)

In Molière's play *Les Précieuses Ridicules* (1659) the pseudo-aristocrat Mascarille boasts that his breeches were wider by a quarter than anyone else's, to the admiration of the ladies who are taken in by his pose. Molière was not, however, altogether anti-fashion. The clearest statement of his attitude is in *L'Ecole des Maris* (1661), in which two sisters are courted by two brothers, their guardians, both much older than themselves: Ariste, who is sixty, is successful and Sganarelle, though only forty, is not. (Their names show the author's opinion of them: Ariste is from the Greek for ("best") and Sganarelle the standard name for ridiculous old men in the theatre of the time). Ariste dresses fashionably; Sganarelle refuses to, claiming that fashion would force him to wear a tiny hat, a huge amount of hair, a doublet which would be lost under his arm and a collar hanging down to his navel, sleeves which would dip into his food at table, beribboned shoes

Et de ces grands canons où, comme en des entraves,
On met tous les matins ses deux jambes esclaves,
Et par qui nous voyons ces messieurs les galants
Marcher écarquillés ainsi que des volants?

Ariste answers that one should defer to the majority and not be conspicuous; he would not wish to be the sort of man who exaggerates the fashion and is annoyed to find someone else has gone farther, but he would rather be foolish in the same way as everyone else than the only wise man. When Sganarelle accuses him of trying to hide his age, he says he doesn't want it thrown in his face, and he feels that old age is unattractive enough "sans se tenir encor malpropre et rechignée." Sganarelle insists that:

Je veux une coiffure, en dépit de la mode,
Sous qui toute ma tête ait un abri commode;
Un beau pourpoint bien long, et fermé comme il faut,
Qui, pour bien digérer, tienne l'estomac chaud;
Un haut-de-chausses fait justement pour ma cuisse,
Des souliers où mes pieds ne soient point au supplice,
Ainsi qu'en ont usé sagement nos aïeux:
Et qui me trouve mal n'a qu'à fermer les yeux.

Sganarelle is also against finery for women, wishing his ward and future wife to dress in serge and wear black only "aux bons jours" (presumably when in mourning, and not for reasons of fashion), whereas Ariste lets his enjoy spending as much on dress as she likes. Again, in *L'Ecole des Femmes* (1662), elderly Arnolphe loses Agnès, whom he has kept in complete ignorance of all worldly matters (including sex) to a young man. He gives her a series of maxims on a wife's duties, among which are:

Elle ne se doit parer
Qu'autant que peut désirer
Le mari qui la possède:
C'est lui que touche seul le soin de sa beauté;
Et pour rien doit être compté
Que les autres la trouvent laide.

Loin ces études d'œillades,
Ces eaux, ces blancs, ces pommades
Et mille ingrédients qui font les teints fleuris:
A l'honneur, tous les jours, ce sont drogues mortelles
Et les soins de paraître belles
Se prennent peu pour les maris.[29]

She is also supposed to hide her eyes under her headdress whenever she goes out (which must have caused practical difficulties). Other characters in his plays who disapprove of fine dressing are the hypocrite Tartuffe, who condemns ribbons, paint and patches and claims to wear a hair-shirt, and the miser Harpagon, whose breeches are fastened with ribbonless metal clasps. Even Alceste, protagonist of *Le Misanthrope*, wears ribbons, merely choosing an eccentric colour (green).

Molière's most famous example of an over-dressed man is M. Jourdain in *Le Bourgeois Gentilhomme* (1670), whose maid is overcome with laughter at the sight of him in his new clothes. I suspect, however, that the author sympathised more with excess in that direction than in the other. M. Jourdain, though a foolish snob, is good-natured and generous; Arnolphe, Tartuffe and Harpagon are not. In *Les Caractères*, Jean de La Bruyère creates his own version of Tartuffe: he dresses plainly but, unlike a genuine ascetic, always takes care to wear light fabrics in summer and warm ones in winter. Though, like Molière, La Bruyère deprecated excessive emphasis on fashion, he also deprecated excessive determination to avoid it: "Un homme fat et ridicule . . . rêve la veille par où et comment il pourra se faire remarquer le jour qui suit. Un philosophe se laisse habiller par son tailleur; il y a autant de faiblesse à fuir la mode qu'à l'affecter." He describes the affectations of a fashion-obsessed man in far more detail than those of a woman, saying that "il met du rouge, mais rarement, il n'en fait pas habitude: il est vrai aussi qu'il porte des chausses et un chapeau, et qu'il n'a ni boucles d'oreilles ni collier de perles: aussi ne l'ai-je pas mis dans le chapitre des femmes."[30] This reflects the contemporary ideal of "l'honnête homme", meaning not an honest but a reasonable man. He noted that when sitting for portraits or statues, people took care to avoid fashionable dress in case it would date, preferring something arbitrary. He claimed to have consulted men on women's cosmetics, and to have drawn the conclusion that most or all men felt that whitening and reddening made them look hideous and disgusting, and was no more attractive than false teeth and the wax balls with which they sometimes plumped out sunken cheeks (also mentioned by Jonathan

Swift). He considered it a kind of lie, not as serious as a verbal or written one, but not as innocent as a masquerade where no deceit was intended. Here he would have agreed with Defoe's Moll Flanders (1683): "I omitted nothing that might set me out to advantage, except painting, for that I never stooped to, and had pride enough to think I did not want it".

As one might expect, since France set the fashions, other countries present a similar picture. A Neapolitan surgeon named Fioravanti was practising plastic surgery in Italy in the late sixteenth century, replacing a man's nose after it had been cut off in a duel, and in 1597 Gaspare Tagliacozzi published a book on the subject, *De Cirurgia Curtorum*. This was condemned by the church, and the French surgeon Ambroise Paré advised against the practice.[31] In England, the Restoration dramatists described the French courtiers' imitators, such as Etherege's Sir Fopling Flutter ("He wears nothing but what are originals of the most famous hands in Paris"), and Vanbrugh's Sir Novelty Fashion, Baron of Foppington, for whom "the business of the morning" was getting dressed. These examples, being fictional, may be exaggerated; as Sir Edmund Gosse put it, "Comedy has always forced the note, and is a very unsafe (though picturesque) guide to historic manners." As a source of information about "the ordinary woman of the world in the reign of Charles II" he recommended a pamphlet, *The Ladies' Calling*, by an anonymous clergyman: "In the frontispiece to this work a doleful dame, seated on what seems to be a bare altar in an open landscape, is raising one hand to grasp a crown dangled out of her reach in the clouds, and in the other, with an air of great affectation is lifting her skirt between finger and thumb. A purse, a coronet, a fan, a mirror, rings, dice, coins, and other useful articles lie strewn at her naked feet; she spurns them, and lifts her streaming eyes to heaven. This is the sort of picture which does its best to prevent the reader from opening the book", he admits, but claims that the author is less moralistic than it suggests. "The ladies came to listen to him bedizened with jewels . . . He does not scream to them to rend them off. He only remonstrates at their costliness . . . our divine tells his auditors that 'any one of the baubles, the loosest appendage of the dress, a fan, a busk, perhaps a black patch, bears a price that would warm the empty bowels of a poor starving wretch.'"[32]

The fops and their extravagances, however, are not entirely the invention of comic writers, as Pepys and others show; Congreve allegedly based Lord Foppington on himself. Can one seriously believe that these men needed to dress as they did in order to attract women? A pamphlet of 1614, *Ester hath hang'd Haman*, suggests otherwise. It was written in answer to another one called *The Arraignment of Women*, by Joseph Swetnam, and was published under the name of Ester Sowernam. In reply to his accusation that "women's dressings and attire are provocations to wantonness and baits to allure men", she accuses men of blaming women for their own propensity to lust, adding:

> Do not men exceed in apparel and therein set themselves out to the view?
> ... Women are so far off from being in any sort provoked to love upon the view of men's apparel and setting forth themselves, that no one thing can more draw them from love than their vanity in apparel. Women make difference betwixt colours and conditions, betwixt a fair show and a foul substance. It shows a levity in man to furnish himself more with trim colours than manlike qualities; beside that, how can we love at whom we laugh? We see him gallant it at the court one day and brave it in the counter the next day; we see him wear that on his back one week which we hear is in the broker's shop the next. Furthermore, we see divers wear apparel and colours made of a lordship, lined with farms and granges, embroidered with all the plate, gold and wealth their friends and fathers left them. Are these motives to love or to laughter?[33]

Yet not all intellectual women were against fashion: Mme de Sévigné loved it.

Nor were all male writers opposed, in spite of their satire on foppishness, as Wycherley shows in *The Plain Dealer* (1676). The characters are the hypocritical Olivia, her servant Lettice, and Eliza, who only appears as a contrast to Olivia:

> *Eliza.* What d'ye think of Dressing, and fine Cloaths?
>
> *Olivia.* Fie, fie, 'tis of all things my aversion. But, come hither, you Dowdy, methinks you might have opened this Toure better: O hideous! I cannot suffer it! D'ye see how it sits?
>
> *Eliza.* Well enough, Cousin, if Dressing be your aversion.
>
> *Olivia.* 'Tis so: and for Variety of rich Cloaths, they are more my aversion.
>
> *Lettice.* Ay, 'tis because your Ladyship wears 'em too long; for indeed a Gown, like a Gallant, grows one's aversion, by having too much of it.
>
> *Olivia.* Insatiable Creature. I'll be sworn I have had this not above three dayes, Cousin, and within this month have made some six more.
>
> *Eliza.* Then your aversion to'em is not altogether so great.
>
> *Olivia.* Alas! 'tis for my Woman only I wear 'em, Cousin.
>
> *Lettice.* If it be for me only, Madam, pray do not wear 'em.

36

The first journal containing reports on current fashions was published in Paris from 1673 onwards. In England in the early eighteenth century, a group of writers, of whom the most famous were Joseph Addison and Sir Richard Steele, published in the *Tatler* and the *Spectator* under the collective name of Isaac Bickerstaff, Censor of Great Britain, and both male and female dress came under "his" censorship. From 3 to 6 December 1709, in the *Tatler*, he judged what Pope called "the nice Conduct of a Clouded Cane": a licence was granted to a man to wear a cane "provided that he does not walk with it under his Arm, brandish it in the Air, or hang it on a Button: in which case it shall be forfeited" and a "Prig" whose cane was "very curiously clouded, with a transparent Amber Head, and a blue Ribbon to hang upon his Wrist" was ordered to replace it with "a plain Joint headed with Walnut" three days a week. I cannot help sympathising with a certain "lively fresh-coloured young Man . . . an *Oxford* scholar, who was just entered at the *Temple*" who "immediately told me, He had a Property in it, and a Right to hang it where he pleas'd, and to make use of it as he thought fit, provided that he did not break the Peace with it". The Censor agreed, insisting only that he should wear it round his neck instead of on a button. He also allowed men to wear scents such as orange-flower water on the grounds that "some of their Persons would not be altogether inoffensive without them".

On 20–22 December of the same year, he announced a judgment on petticoats: "Going out of the Court, I received a Letter, informing me, That in Pursuance of the Edict of Justice in one of my late Visions, all those of the Fair Sex began to appear pregnant who had ran any Hazard of it, as was manifest by a particular Swelling in the Petticoats of several Ladies in and about this great City. I must confess, I do not attribute the Rising of this Part of the Dress to this Occasion, yet must own, that I am very much disposed to be offended with such a new and unaccountable Fashion." He asked ladies to refrain from having petticoats made until his judgment was passed; Addison, in 1711, remarked that "Ladies deffended hoops on grounds that 'They are Airy, and very proper for the Season'".

Bickerstaff's opinions on female finery echo La Bruyère. Steele's essay "On Ladies' Dress", which appeared in the *Tatler* on 25–28 March 1710, begins:

> When Artists would expose their Diamonds to an Advantage, they usually set them to Show in little Cases of black Velvet . . . The present Fashion obliges every body to be dressed with Propriety, and makes the Ladies' Faces

the principal Objects of Sight. Every beautiful Person shines out in all the Excellence with which Nature has adorned her. Gawdy Ribbons and glaring Colours being now out of Use, the Sex has no Opportunity given 'em to disfigure themselves; which they seldom fail to do whenever it lies in their Power. When a Woman comes to her Glass, she does not employ her Time in making herself look more advantagiously what she really is, but endeavours to be as much another Creature as she possibly can.

This, he conceded, was beneficial to ugly women: "Let *Thalestris* change herself into a Motly Party-coloured Animal: the Pearl Necklace, the Flowered Stomacher, the Artificial Nosegay, and Shaded Furbelow, may be of Use to attract the Eye of the Beholder, and turn it from the imperfections of her Features and Shape. But if Ladies will take my Word for it, (and as they dress to please Men, they ought to consult our Fancy rather than their own in this Particular), I can assure them, there is nothing touches our Imagination so much as a beautiful Woman in a plain Dress . . . This I know is a very harsh Doctrine to Womankind, who are carried away with every Thing that is showy, and with what delights the Eye, more than any other Species of living Creatures whatsoever." This applied to men's clothes as well: "Many a Lady has fetched a Sigh at the Toss of a Wig, and been ruin'd by the Tapping of a Snuff-box. It is impossible to describe all the Execution that was done by the Shoulder-Knot while that Fashion prevailed, or to reckon up all the Virgins that have fallen a Sacrifice to a Pair of Fringed Gloves. A sincere Heart has not made half so many Conquests as an open Wastcoat; and I should be glad to see an able Head make so good a Figure in a Woman's Company as a Pair of Red Heels." He tells a story of a great-aunt, Margery Bickerstaff, whose family wanted to prevent her marriage so as to keep her thousand pounds from going elsewhere. This they did by giving her new clothes, which made her so conceited she felt no man was good enough for her. He was lucky that the cost of the clothes did not exceed her fortune.

Addison expressed similar sentiments (*Spectator*, 17 March 1711) on "the numberless Evils that befall the Sex, from this light, fantastical Disposition . . . this Natural Weakness of being taken with Outside and Appearance" but admitted two days later that "Foppish and fantastick Ornaments are only Indications of Vice, not criminal in themselves. Extinguish Vanity in the Mind, and you naturally retrench the little Superfluities of Garniture and Equipage . . . To speak truly the young People of both Sexes are so wonderfully apt to shoot out into long Swords or sweeping Trains, bushy

Head-dresses or full-bottom'd Perriwigs, with several other Incumbrances of Dress, that they stand in Need of being pruned very frequently, lest they should be oppressed with Ornaments, and over-run with the Luxuriency of their Habits. I am much in doubt, whether I should give the Preference to a Quaker, that is trimmed close and almost cut to the Quick, or to a Beau that is loaden with such a Redundance of Excrescences." Even the least fashionable men trimmed their own hair close, however, in order to wear wigs.

Addison disapproved of slovenly dress in both sexes. Any kind of androgynous dress, however, was frowned on, and not only by the Censor. Samuel Richardson wrote of the wearer of a riding-habit: "She looked neither like a modest girl nor an agreeable boy",[34] and Steele expressed similar sentiments: "I am not certain whether she, who in Appearance was a very handsome Youth, may not be in reality a very indifferent Woman." Foreshadowing John Berger, he said that she "appear'd to me to have been educated only as an Object of Sight".

In what would now be called mainstream fashion, riding clothes were the only form of androgynous dressing, but there was one woman who tried to bring about another: Lady Mary Wortley Montagu, active feminist and advocate of women's education. During her travels in Turkey she adopted Turkish dress, and a a portrait was made of her wearing it; that picture alone is enough to show, even if her writings did not, that she was by no means indifferent to how her clothes looked. She also appreciated the freedom with which a woman who was disguised by a veil over her face could contravene accepted rules of behaviour without being found out; as Wendy Frith's essay on her notes, this was why Addison and others condemned masquerades.[35]

A far less well-known writer, Sarah Scott, suggested in her novel *Millenium Hall* (1762) how the inhabitants of a female Utopia might dress. The male narrator describes a household of women living in what would now be called a commune: "The dress of the ladies was thus far uniform, the same neatness, the same simplicity and cleanliness appeared in each, and they were all in lutestring night-gowns, though of different colours, nor was there anything unfashionable in their appearance, except that they were free from trumpery ornaments."[36] ("Night-gowns" must mean something which could be worn during the day; I have seen other instances of this usage.) They too were far from indifferent to beauty in people or clothes, nature or art, as the text makes clear. It is a male writer, Marivaux, who gives an example of what Lewis Carroll called uglification. In his play *La Colonie* (1729), women living on an island league themselves against men in protest at not being allowed to participate in government. To punish men they dress as badly as possible: "vous saurez que les femmes se sont mises tout en un tas pour être laides, elles vont quitter les pantoufles, on parle même de changer de robes, de se vêtir d'un sac, et de porter les cornettes de côté pour vous déplaire", says a male character. He did not believe that women themselves liked to dress badly. In *L'Ecole des Mères* (1732), whose plot harks back to the similarly titled plays by Molière, the daughter of a mother who keeps her in subjection and ignorance complains to her maid: "Ma mère appelle cela un habit modeste: il n'y a donc de la modestie nulle part qu'ici? car je ne vois que moi d'enveloppée comme cela; aussi suis-je d'une enfance, d'une curiosité! Je ne porte point de rubans; mais qu'est-ce que ma mère y gagne? que j'ai des émotions quand j'en aperçois."[37]

He does not mention paint or patches, but both sexes used them. A London clockmaker, James Upjohn, writing a diary of his travels in France and Germany in 1768, notes that "the French Ladies paint themselves more than the English . . . some of them are like the Dolls with round red spots up to their Eyes, and these I find are the Quality, for the fashion, or general maxim is, the more they are painted, the higher they are in Rank and Fortune." He frequently mentions dress as one of the most usual reasons for young men spending too much; this happened to one of his sons. He himself was mistaken at a German inn for the King of Prussia's brother: "I had on a Pompadour colour'd Coat, with a Green Waistcoat, embroidered with a running sprig of Gold, Bag Wig, and Sword."[38]

Another source of information is the diary of William Hickey, born in 1749, who thought himself "as ugly a fellow as need be" but cared passionately about dress. When taking up his first post as an attorney's clerk, he was "gratified by having my hair tied, turned over my forehead, powdered, pomatumed, and three curls on each side, with a thick false tail" and when he joined the army, "not knowing to what corps I should be appointed, I conceived the best thing I could do would be to have a suit of each description . . . some of my brother Joseph's acquaintances enquired what the devil regiment I had got into, for that they met me in half a dozen different uniforms in as many days . . . My father made no complaint of my having such a variety of clothes, but much as to the cut of them." As well as his own clothes, he describes those of his friend Robert Pott, "pronounced by the women to be the handsomest young man in London" who walked with him in St James's Park wearing "a white coat, cut in the extremity of *ton*, lined with a garter-blue satin, edged with ermine, and ornamented with rich silver frogs; waistcoat and breeches of the same blue satin, trimmed with silver twist à la hussar, and ermine edges." Later Hickey practised law in India: "At the time I arrived in Bengal, everybody dressed splendidly, being covered with lace, spangles and foil. I, who always had a tendency to be a beau, gave into the fashion with much goodwill, no person appearing in richer suits of velvet and lace than myself." When he returned to London he went to a party in one of them, "being of scarlet with a rich spangled and foil lace . . . my dress was greatly admired, my brother only remarking he thought it a little too gaudy." Someone else pretended to mistake him for the Lord Mayor's trumpeter: "I was not a little disconcerted. It, however, put me so much out of conceit with my finery that I determined not only to get rid of it immediately, but also of upwards of twenty coats, equally ornamented and rich, that I had brought from Bengal."[39]

It was not only men with no other creative gifts who liked dressing up; even Dr Johnson, who normally did nothing of the sort, wore "a scarlet waistcoat with rich gold lace, and a gold-laced hat" for the opening of his play *Irene*.[40]

The artist Richard Cosway was also criticised for overdressing, and according to Thackeray Oliver Goldsmith, though pock-marked, "liked to deck out his little person in splendour and fine colours. He presented himself to be examined for ordination in a pair of scarlet breeches, and said honestly that he did not like to go into the Church, because he was fond of coloured clothes. When he tried to practise as a doctor, he got by hook or by crook a black velvet suit, and looked as big and grand as he could, and kept his hat over a patch on the old coat: in better days he bloomed out in plum-colour, in blue silk, and in new velvet."[41] He expresses more ambiguous views in his writings. The protagonist of *The Vicar of Wakefield* (1766), "chose my wife as she did her wedding-gown, not for a fine glossy surface, but such qualities as would wear well" and his daughters "were certainly very handsome. Mere outside is so very trifling a circumstance with me, that I should scarce have remembered to mention it, had it not been a general topic of conversation". When he loses his money, he says they should abandon "laces, ribbons, bugles, and catgut . . . their hair plastered up with pomatum, their faces patched to taste" not only because their neighbours would think they were showing off but because "the nakedness of the indigent world may be clothed from the trimmings of the vain."

Goldsmith puts almost exactly the same words (substituting "rich" for "vain") into the mouth of the heroine's father in *She Stoops to Conquer* (1773) but here he sympathises with her: she wears a plain "housewife's dress" in the evening to please him, and in the morning a fashionable one to please herself, and makes a conquest of the young man she wishes to attract in spite, not because, of being seen in the former. He and his friend dress fashionably: the latter intends "opening the campaign with the white and gold" while the former plans "to reserve the embroidery to secure a retreat . . . Don't you think the *ventre d'or* waistcoat will do with the plain brown?"

The heroine of Fanny Burney's *Evelina* (1778) says of her first shopping trip in London: "we were more frequently served by men than by women; and such men! so finical, so affected! they seemed to understand every part of a woman's dress better than we do ourselves; and they recommended caps and ribands with an air of so much importance, that I wished to ask them how long they had left off wearing them." As to her hair, the result of their recommendations was: "You can't think how oddly my head feels; full of powder and black pins, and a great cushion on the top of it . . . When I shall be able to make use of a comb for myself, I cannot tell; for my hair is so much entangled, *frizzled* they call it, that I fear it will be very difficult." She says of one man that "his dress was so foppish, that I really believe he even wished to be stared at; and yet he was very ugly" whereas the hero is "gayly but not foppishly dressed, and indeed extremly handsome". In Burney's play *A Busy Day, or, an Arrival from India*, written in the 1790s, a male character says that "you cannot wear a coat for two years, but what it is out of the mode." The hero of Sheridan's *St Patrick's Day, or the Scheming Lieutenant* (1775) complains that "the London ladies . . . are so defended, such a circumvallation of hoop, with a breastwork of whale-bone that would turn a pistol-bullet, much less Cupid's arrows, – then turret on turret on top, with stores of concealed weapons, under pretence of black pins, – and above all, a standard of feathers that would do honour to a knight of the Bath. Upon my conscience, I could as soon embrace an Amazon, armed at all points." He adds: "bashfulness is a very pretty thing; but, in my mind, there is nothing on earth so impudent as an everlasting blush."

Opposition on moral grounds, as opposed to the Lieutenant's, was expressed by both religious and rationalist authors. Among the former was the hymnodist Dr Watts, who wrote that there was no clothing until after the expulsion from Eden; some women writers agreed with him, such as the children's author Mrs Sarah Trimmer, who condemned the story of Cinderella for encouraging vanity and love of dress, and Mrs Hannah More. She warned women against fashionable men in her poem *The Bas Bleu; or, Conversation*:

> The frigid Beau! Ah! luckless fair,
> 'Tis not for you that studied air,

Ah! not for you that sidelong glance,
And all that charming nonchalance;
Ah! not for you the three long hours
He worshipped the 'Cosmetic powers';
That finished head which breathes perfume,
And kills the nerves of half the room,
And all the murders meant to lie
In that large, languishing grey eye.
Desist – less wild the attempt would be
To warm the snows of Rhodope.
Too cold to feel, too proud to feign,
For him you're wise and fair in vain;
In vain to charm him you intend,
Self is his object, aim, and end.

The most famous of the rationalists who preached simplicity in dress is Rousseau, the "Man of Feeling" and nature-lover. An essay by Linda Walsh[42] refers to the *homme sensible* as "the eighteenth century equivalent of the 'new man'", but this is misleading. The new man is theoretically non-sexist; the Man of Feeling did not think in those terms. Rousseau's books, such as *Emile ou de l'Education*, make it clear: woman's duty is to please man, look after man, defer to man, and bear children for whose sake he will stay with her when he tires of her as he inevitably will. This ideal woman should hate the idea that any artifice or elaboration of dress could add to her charms, so that if anyone compliments her on her appearance when she is more dressed up than usual, she should blush with mortification.

Mary Wollstonecraft, who admired Rousseau in many ways but totally opposed his view of women, devoted a whole chapter of her first book *Thoughts on the Education of Daughters* (1787) to the subject of dress. It reads:

Many able pens have dwelt on the peculiar foibles of our sex. We have been equally desired to avoid the two extremes in dress, and the necessity of cleanliness has been insisted on. 'As from the body's purity the mind receives a sympathetic aid.'

By far too much of a girl's time is taken up in dress. This is an exterior accomplishment, but I chose to consider it by itself. The body hides the mind, and it is, in its turn, obscured by the drapery. I hate to see the frame of a picture so glaring, as to catch the eye and divide the attention. Dress ought to adorn the person, and not rival it. It may be simple, elegant, and becoming, without being expensive; and ridiculous fashions disregarded, while singularity is avoided. The beauty of dress (I shall raise astonishment by saying so) is its not being conspicuous one way or the other; when it neither distorts, or hides the human form by unnatural protuberances. If ornaments are much studied, a consciousness of being well dressed will appear in the face – and surely this mean pride does not give much sublimity to it.

'Out of the abundance of the heart the mouth speaketh.' And how much conversation does dress furnish, which surely cannot be very improving or entertaining.

It gives rise to envy, and contests for trifling superiority, which do not render a woman very respectable to the other sex.

Arts are used to obtain money; and much is squandered away, which if saved for charitable purposes, might alleviate the distress of many poor families, and soften the heart of the girl who entered into such scenes of woe.

In the article of dress may be included the whole tribe of beauty – washes, cosmetics, Olympian dew, oriental herbs, liquid bloom, and the paint which enlivened Ninon [de Lenclos]'s face, and bid defiance to time. These numerous and essential articles are advertised in so ridiculous a style, that the rapid sale of them is a very severe reflection on the understanding of those females who encourage it. The dew and herbs, I imagine, are very harmless, but I do not know whether the same may be said of the paint. White is certainly very prejudicial to the health, and never can be made to resemble nature. The red, too, takes off from the expression of the countenance, and the beautiful glow which modesty, affection, or any other emotion of the mind, gives, can never be seen. It is not 'a mind-illumined face.' 'The body does not charm, because the mind is seen,' but just the contrary: and if caught by it a man marries a woman thus disguised, he may chance not to be satisfied with her real person. A made-up face may strike visitors, but will certainly disgust domestic friends. And one obvious inference is drawn, truth is not expected to govern the inhabitant of so artificial a form. The false life with which rouge animates the eyes, is not of the most delicate kind; nor does a woman's dressing herself in a way to attract languishing glances, give us the most advantageous opinion of the purity of her mind.

I forgot to mention powder among the deceptions. It is a pity that it should be so generally worn. The most beautiful ornament of the features is disguised, and the shade it would give to the countenance entirely lost. The color of every person's hair generally suits the complexion, and is calculated to set it off. What absurdity then do they run into, who use red, blue, and yellow powder! – And what a false taste does it exhibit!

The quantity of pomatum is often disgusting. We laugh at the Hottentots, and in some things adopt their customs.

Simplicity of Dress, and unaffected manners, should go together. They demand respect, and will be admired by people of taste, even when love is out of the question.

("White" means white lead, often used in cosmetics and a source of lead poisoning.) When Wollstonecraft worked as a governess, she wrote to one of her sisters that ladies normally took five hours to dress, "without including preparations for bed". One of her biographers, Ralph M. Wardle, opines that "the gentlemen may have been a bit afraid of women and their subtle powers. So at least one would gather from the statute which Parliament passed in the year 1770, declaring that 'all women of whatever age, rank, profession, or degree, whether virgin maid or widow, that shall from and after such Act impose upon, seduce, and betray into matrimony any of His Majesty's subjects by means of scent, paints, cosmetics, washes, artificial teeth, false hair, Spanish wool, iron stays, hoops, high-heeled shoes, or bolstered hips, shall incur the penalty of the law now in force against witchcraft and like misdemeanours, and that the marriage upon conviction shall stand null and void." Wardle adds that in youth Wollstonecraft deliberately wore coarse clothes and unbrushed hair, but as she grew older she arranged her hair becomingly and embraced the new fashions in dress, which harked back to Greek and Roman styles.[43]

This was not the only manifestation of the desire for a return to simplicity. In 1778 King Gustav III of Sweden passed a law intended to discourage luxury and establishing a national Swedish form of dress, to be worn by everyone except peasants and the clergy. It revived the costume of the reign of Gustav II Adolf (1611–32), and ruled that men should wear blue and white on festive occasions, black and gold on others.

In general, however, the "new simplicity" expressed itself in neo-classicism. When women began to wear Grecian draperies, men might have worn tunics or togas. Instead they turned to sports clothes, and we are still living with the consequences.

3

WHAT HAPPENED TO MEN?

DON'T wear apparel with decided colours or pronounced patterns. DON'T – we address here the male reader – wear anything that is *pretty*. What have men to do with pretty things?

"Censor" (Oliver Bell Bunce)   Don't (1883)

Men became drab. Their clothes were practical instead of decorative. That is the obvious answer to the question, and like all obvious answers is over-simplified. The "masculine renunciation" happened only by degrees: of the changes to men's clothing which began at the turn of the nineteenth century, dark colours were not the first and the straight-up-and-down shape of the modern business suit was almost the last. Equating this process with utilitarianism is tempting, but in some ways it would be more accurate to speak of pseudo-utilitarianism. Many of the changes had as much to do with looking solemn as with practicality. This solemnity became the badge of the supposedly stronger and more rational sex, and any feminist who endorses it should know why.

There is some truth (just enough to mislead) in the common-sense view that the French revolution and the industrial revolution caused the change. They produced a shift of power from the aristocracy to the manufacturers, from the leisured class to those engaged in work (though not manual work). In revolutionary France, being taken for an aristocrat could have meant death. Professional men had always dressed more quietly than their social superiors; doctors, lawyers and teachers had traditionally worn black at a time when a nobleman only did so if he was in holy orders or in mourning. The serious-looking class, therefore, was in the ascendant. Its members found sports clothes, whose appearance was dictated by the need for freedom of movement and fairly hard wear, eminently suitable. These clothes had evolved in England, where unlike France, the traditional epicentre of new fashions, many of the aristocracy lived in the country and where class distinctions had never been as rigid as in the rest of Europe. (Voltaire, in his *Lettres Philosophiques* of 1734, noted with approval that an English lord's brother could be a merchant.) In the United States, according to the historian Lois W. Banner, "Puritan asceticism and revolutionary and republican idealism had made virtues of simplicity of style and demeanor in the postrevolutionary period. American periodicals in the 1790s were filled with attacks on fashion, and prominent public leaders often wore homespun on ceremonial occasions", but this did not last: "The vogues of fashion flew in the face of republicanism, but the growth of fashion consciousness was in keeping with the rampant individualism, materialism, and search for status and success that were as much a part of basic American values as . . . egalitarianism."[1] America came to be seen as the land of opportunity for everyone who could afford it to dress fashionably, without being accused of "aping your betters".

Male rather than female dress was affected because there were fewer women's sports than men's, which meant fewer forms of suitable clothing to imitate, and middle-class women, like aristocratic ones, seldom went out to work. A few did so in the early days of industrialism, but this grew increasingly rare. As men dropped decorative dress, the pressure on women to wear it increased: men made them wear what they had renounced, hence Thorstein Veblen's theory of women's clothes as symbols of "conspicuous consumption" and "pecuniary canons of taste".[2] This is how decorative dress became a symbol both of the upper class and the lower sex.

Neither social snobbery nor aesthetics disappeared from men's clothes, but they took a different form, some aspects of which were paralleled in the dress of women. The source of the new fashion was the clothing worn by country squires, but it was not they who set it, nor was it middle-class business or professional men; it was urban dandies, who were no more concerned with strict practicality than the fops and macaronis of the previous generation. What they did can be seen as the latest form of playing at shepherds and shepherdesses, which had been popular ever since the classical revival of the Renaissance, and whose roots go back to the pastoral poetry of Theocritus and Vergil. The personal contribution of the most famous dandy, George "Beau" Brummell, may have been exaggerated, but it certainly existed. Modern men's "no-nonsense" dress derives at least in part from a man who allegedly reduced the Prince Regent to tears by telling him his breeches didn't fit.

Fit was crucial to the new look: the dandy's clothes were tight. "Splendour has given way to fit, line and cut"[3] writes Germaine Greer of twentieth-century women's dress, and both Emmanuel Ungaro and Vivienne Westwood have described their ambition to dress a woman so that people will admire her appearance but not be able to remember what she wore. Just what Brummell wanted: he said that if anyone noticed what a man was wearing, he was not well-dressed.

Diana de Marly explains: "The new interest in statuary had an impact on menswear, for it meant that bodies were back in fashion. Consequently clothes were made more revealing . . . The vests or waistcoats . . . were now shortened and rose at a rapid rate until they only reached the hips or lower waist. The breeches and the flies were revealed, and given the admiration for classical limbs, breeches became tighter and ever tighter . . . Masculinity at its most blatant was making a comeback. And what style of clothes could best dress this natural man if not the British country look? . . . skin colour became the tone for waistcoats and breeches. This did give an impression of nakedness at a distance."[4] It was nude, not clothed, figures in classical art that men copied, though Jacques-Louis David designed a uniform based on Roman clothing for the members of the French Directoire (Gillray caricatured it in 1798). Men also wore less jewellery, abandoned paint (except on stage) and began to care more about hygiene, also as a result of Brummell's influence. As Elizabeth Wilson puts it: "The skin-tight breeches of the dandy were highly erotic; so was his new, unpainted masculinity. The dandy was a narcissist. He did not abandon the pursuit of beauty; he changed the kind of beauty that was admired."[5] As an example of how this can be misunderstood, one might quote Juliet Ash, who, writing on modern menswear, sees Brummell's concern with his appearance as an act of individual rebellion and makes the astonishing statement that Brummell was not a dandy.[6] Rebellion against what? In his time, for a man to show such concern was normal.

The dandy's female equivalent also imitated classical art. She wore a slender, high-waisted tunic, which clung to the body as much as possible, and in France (though not England) was sometimes transparent. In 1809 a little-known writer, John Scott-Waring, published a book under the pseudonym "B. C." giving his ideas on what women should wear. Its full title is *The Ladies' Monitor, being a series of letters, first published in Bengal, on the subject of female apparel, tending to favour a regulated adoption of Indian costume; and a rejection of superfluous vesture, by the ladies of this country: with incidental remarks on Hindoo beauty, whale-bone stays, iron busks, Indian corsets, man-*

milliners, idle bachelors, hair powder, side-saddles, waiting-maids and footmen. He approved of short waists and condemned

> those vile steel BUSKS, sometimes half a yard in length, which so rudely press against their stomachs, and cannot fail of being ultimately injurious to their health . . . the horrid STAYS, still unhappily in use, that must necessarily, perhaps, somewhat swell out the lower region of the waist, to the great injury of personal grace . . . iron busks must necessarily be dangerous in stormy weather, during the prevalence of thunder and lightning . . . those little triple-headed ivory monsters, styled DIVORCES . . . Not an old dowdy in the country who is not strongly cased with ribs of whale, and monstrous wooden busks; and whose cumbrous stays, right up and down, mocking all shape, terminate in huge bluff points, that hideously puff out her five-fold nether covering . . . let her dress as may best become her: neither totally rejecting fashion, nor yet following servile in its ample train . . . To be always following the track of the fashion dictators of Europe, argues a mental dependence, inconsistent with the dignity of improved understanding.

As neo-classicism in art gave way to romanticism, there was a certain attempt to copy mediæval dress and to revert to bright colours, red waistcoats being especially popular. As might be expected, professional artists were in the forefront of this trend, and they also grew beards and whiskers, the latter framing the face in the same way as fashionable women's ringlets. Mediæval styles did not last, however, and bright colours gave way to black. Both men and women tried to look slim and delicate. James Laver explains: "Schoolgirls in convents drank it [vinegar] in order to have a look of illness, to keep thin; they sat up all night reading to give themselves heavy eyes with black rings underneath them. Among fashionable ladies there was an enormous consumption of belladonna, a drug which dilated the pupils of the eyes and gave them a wild, fixed appearance. There was a rage for the Spanish type, black-haired and green as a lemon. So sallow was the prevailing complexion in 1835 that a memoirist of the period compares the contemporary beauties with the Chinese and Japanese. Some, both men and women, even made up with yellow pigment. Men strove to look pale and distinguished, as if ravaged by some secret sorrow; women to look frail and afflicted with a settled melancholy."[7] In America, writes Lois Banner (who calls this female type the "steel-engraving lady"), a man who looked ill might be thought of as virtuously concentrating on business. She also points out that men adopted the wasp-waisted look, though to a lesser degree than women; French and German soldiers wore corsets, and "Censor" later told men to "adopt no style of cutting that belittles the figure".

Black went well with this look, making figures appear slimmer and complexions paler, and suggesting perpetual mourning. The writer Edward Bulwer Lytton, Baron Lytton, who liked to call himself a "blighted being", was highly influential. Black became the fashion and, for men's formal dress, has remained so ever since.

Why did the darker rather than the more colourful side of romanticism persist, even after looking ill was no longer popular? According to Laver, it "was partly due to the growing ideal of good form . . . It may be defined, in one of its aspects, as a conspiracy of the minor gentry, in alliance with the upper middle classes, against the ostentation natural to the *grand seigneur* . . . In the eighteenth century a duke went about the London streets with his orders glittering on the outside of his coat . . . but the mid-nineteenth century succeeded in making it bad form to distinguish yourself from other gentlemen. No one any longer wore any outside mark of his rank, except on very formal occasions. In the eighteenth century a wealthy peer bought himself a coat more richly embroidered than those of his neighbours . . . This too became bad form, and a gentleman was allowed no more distinction in dress than any good tailor could give him". It is easy to see how this made the transition to what Juliet Ash calls "the male supporting-cast role" in dress less noticeable.

Laver adds: "It was the French Romantics of the eighteen-thirties who succeeded in making the word *bourgeois* a term of abuse" so it is hardly surprising that "In resisting the fashions which the rise of the *bourgeoisie* imposed they were less successful . . . All that remained were the beards"[8] (I suspect because, until electric razors were invented, it was painful to shave a beard once grown). Artists began to be seen as natural rebels, aspiring not to lead society's taste but to distance themselves from it. Society in turn distanced itself from them. Art became remote from ordinary life, something people might go to look at in buildings specially designed for the purpose; this "high art" was the province of men. Artistic values in everyday life were left to those with nothing more important to think about: women.

Dark colours had obvious advantages in a world of coal fires and gas fumes, especially at a period less tolerant of dirt than the preceding one. Light clothes are unsuitable for work, even managerial work, in dirty factories. These considerations combined with the values of the growing moral and religious revival. This, unlike the early church, was not hostile to the material world or to cleanliness, which was now "next to godliness", probably because of growing awareness of the link between dirt and disease. It was widely believed that prosperity was a direct consequence of Christian virtue. Romantic sorrow turned into the kind of seriousness which came to be seen as typically Victorian, or its equivalent in other countries. Deliberately doing something for enjoyment came under suspicion as a form of frivolity, and this affected attitudes to art: whereas the "blighted beings" had an obvious motive for preferring tragedy to comedy, the former was now seen as "deeper" and therefore more conducive to moral virtue. Children were discouraged from reading for pleasure rather than "instruction" or "improvement". Happiness and beauty were both to be regarded as by-products of virtue; if they could not be achieved by this means, they must be ignored. There was even a cult of physical discomfort, with consequences which were anything but practical: Wordsworth among others condemned umbrellas as unmanly, perhaps because of ladies' parasols (I am told this idea still persists in some quarters) and according to Lord Balfour's autobiography, short-sighted schoolboys were not allowed to wear glasses.

This is what I mean by pseudo-utilitarianism and it still remains part of male dress to a greater extent than is sometimes realised. For example, ties became simpler and looser, but why were they retained at all? Why were gentlemen's dark suits invariably contrasted with white shirts, if not to show how well the wearer conformed to the gentlemanly ideal of cleanliness? The first men's fashion article I ever saw, in the 1950s, plaintively asked why, when most men expected to wear a shirt two days, they clung to a colour that "only stays spotless for half a day". The most interesting example, however, is the silk top hat.

James Laver's book *Style in Costume* shows the connection between styles in clothes and in architecture, and the mid-nineteenth century examples are crinolines (compared to such feats of engineering as the Crystal Palace) and top hats. These were known as "stove-pipes" and "chimney-pots" and resembled factory chimneys. Unlike pipes and chimneys, however, their form did not follow their function. They were part of a style derived from nostalgia for a country life which was less and less relevant to the age of industry, and Laver himself notes that they were originally devised as a kind of crash-helmet for horsemen; so why wear them for walking or riding in a carriage? Moreover, if blackness was practical, silk was not. Jerome K. Jerome, who hated top hats, wrote in 1889 that their wearer could no more go out without the previously despised umbrella than a baby without its nurse, and about a dozen years earlier the comic paper *Fun* suggested that silk hats, like wax fruit, should be protected by glass covers.

If men's dress has been thought of as more practical than it was, women's has been thought less so. It would be insane to argue that a lady's clothes didn't hamper her, but the guilt of at least one culprit has been exaggerated. This is the most famous female garment of the century: the crinoline. Ann Oakley writes that its wearers were turned into "caged birds surrounded by hoops of steel" which, according to Evans and Thornton, is typical of modern feminist views.[9] But no skirt forms the wearer's whole environment as a bird's cage does, and hoops were first invented in order to alleviate the weight of petticoats, hence the eighteenth-century ladies who defended them to Mr Bickerstaff as "airy". Laver remarked of children's versions, "A little girl in a crinoline could at least run about inside her swaying cage",[10] which was impossible in the tight skirts that replaced it. Gwen Raverat, who was no slave of fashion, confirms this: "Clothes were a major cause of rows, naughtiness, misery and all unpleasantness, right through my whole youth . . . all the fashions from 1890 till 1914 seemed to me then, and seem to me still, preposterous, hideous and uncomfortable . . . Once I asked Aunt Etty what it had been like to wear a crinoline. 'Oh, it was delightful,' she said. 'I've never been so comfortable since they went out. It kept your petticoats away from your legs, and made walking so light and easy.'"[11] Amelia Bloomer also approved of hoops, and wore one when forced by pressure of opinion to abandon the costume named after her.

Something equally comfortable and less cumbersome could have been devised, but looking decorative was a woman's duty. Ladies were expected to dress quietly but, at least in summer, they wore pale colours, although the problems caused by coal and gas applied to both sexes. They had separate occupations, but not separate air.

Dress was also one of women's few means of self-expression. Bonnie G. Smith has analysed the implications of this in *Ladies of the Leisure Class: The Bourgeoises of Northern France in the Nineteenth Century*, which begins: "What is a bourgeois woman? . . . And if she were rational, why the many depictions of the bourgeois woman as preoccupied with furniture and fashion?" Academics have tended to regard these preoccupations "as signs of mental inferiority" and Smith quotes Veblen's theory that they made a woman "a puppet of her husband's needs" but what, the book asks, did they mean to her? "It was fashion . . . that served as the most insistent and increasingly popular way of drawing attention to a woman's presence and of speaking about that presence . . . simplicity of taste and utilitarian considerations had succumbed to a fondness for a series of ornate garments. Although the bourgeois woman might limit herself to five or six dresses, those five or six were sometimes refurbished daily to fit the latest style or a sudden whim." Some women writers had moral objections, but even convent girls wore discreet ornaments:

> Full skirts, bodices, huge sleeves gave substance to female claims to impor-
> tance by increasing their physical size to at least double that of men . . . Yet
> objects so thoroughly reflected women that they had to tell of weakness as
> well as strength. Pictures of the Northern bourgeoise show her dressed in
> voluminous clothing, but her dress at mid-century has embroidery and tiny
> tucks in the bodice that give a delicate air to the bulk. She has an abundance
> of miniscule [sic] false curls escaping from her bonnet. In 1870 her semi-
> bustled overskirt is ringed with small bows; the sleeves of her dress are
> tightly fitted to make the arms show, and they end in a row of intricate pleats
> at the wrist. She wears, too, a small half-hat with a wisp of veil, a tiny feather,
> a narrow ribbing. At the end of the century her massive upper torso is weak-
> ened with shirred fabric, her skirt banded with slender ribbon, and the
> imposing hat undermined by fluttering ostrich feathers, a cluster of grapes,
> more veil and ribbon, and a final fragile encasement in the sheerest of tulle.
> The emphasis on fragility terminated in the hobble skirt, but throughout
> the century layers of clothing reduced the importance of the body itself while
> simultaneously creating mass. The corset also made a woman tiny and
> insignificant. And the sum of all garments testified to female imprisonment,
> to an unliberated ego, and was voluntarily worn by all women to testify to
> this aspect of their lives.[12]

Smith considers the crinoline was meant to make women look pregnant, but pregnant women don't have tiny waists. Fashion was seen by the most conservative and "Victorian" thinkers as a moral danger, but no man wanted his wife to be ugly or (though he would not have put it like that) sexually unattractive. The spinster who was too ugly to "catch" a husband was a standing joke, as seen in comic papers and most of W. S. Gilbert's operatic libretti (he had written for *Fun*); the new greetings-card industry had a special line in ugly valentines for ugly people, which were apparently sent to men as well as women.

There was one exception to the "great renunciation": ceremonial dress. This applied up to a point to evening dress, for which knee breeches remained compulsory long after trousers had taken over during the day, but even more to uniforms. The protagonist of Stendhal's novel *Le Rouge et le Noir* (1830), who is training for the priesthood and obliged to wear black, is overjoyed to take part in the parade of a guard of honour with sky-blue and silver uniforms, and also when his employer permits him to wear blue in the evenings. Charles Lamb was censured for wearing a black coat to a wedding, and according to one popular historical work "forty years later, in 1861, the high priests of *Minister's Gazette of Fashion* felt obliged to issue a public rebuke to all gentlemen who persisted in the same offence. 'Unfortunately', they sighed, 'invisible green or even black frock coats are occasionally seen at weddings but both are inconsistent with the occasion except in the case of the marriage of a clergyman.' Instead, they advised blue, claret or mulberry frock coats, pale drab or lavender doeskin trousers, and waistcoats of white quilting."[13]

Uniforms, both in and out of the armed services, proliferated. Opponents of royal pageantry, like opponents of what are known as traditional Christmas and wedding celebrations, like to point out that many of the traditions only date from the early nineteenth century, and it is hard not to see their establishment as an attempt to keep colourful dress alive. Holidays, being frivolous occasions, were also excuses for colour. It is ironic that drabness for men should have begun with sports clothes, because some sports, notably boating, became the last refuges for its absence. Jerome K. Jerome wrote in *Three Men in a Boat* (1889), perhaps with some exaggeration for comic effect: "For once in a way, we men are able to show *our* taste in colours . . . I always like a little red in my things – red and black . . . and then I always think a light-blue necktie goes so well with it, and a pair of those Russian-leather shoes and a red silk handkerchief round the waist – a handkerchief looks so much better than a belt."

The influence of Scott's novels made Highland dress, outlawed in the previous century, almost mandatory for holidays in Scotland, especially for children, even when the wearers (Prince Albert, for instance) had no Scottish connections. Wordsworth, in the poem condemning umbrellas, mentioned:

The Roman kilt, degraded to a toy
Of quaint apparel for a half-spoilt boy.

The rules of men's dress did not apply to small boys, who continued to wear dresses until the age of about five. (Kilts may have been a way of prolonging this, and a French fashion plate of 1863 shows one with a visible petticoat underneath.)

Boys too old for dresses wore velvet suits, lace collars and long curling hair, and even adult men had their hair curled on special occasions. My grandfather, born on 31 December 1855, was painted by Abraham Solomon in 1860 wearing black velvet with a white lace collar, a matching feathered hat and a blue cravat. In 1886 this fashion was boosted by Frances Hodgson Burnett's *Little Lord Fauntleroy*; Laver calls the costume "the despair of every decent-minded boy".[14] Alexander Woollcott was not decent-minded: "all the little boys in America had to be rigged out by their mothers in Fauntleroy get-up. All except me, who had to importune my parents for a Fauntleroy costume. At the first sight of my huge bullet head with its five cowlicks rising out of that lace collar, the whole family went into gales of inconsiderate mirth and promptly ordered the entire regalia given [away] . . . Birch did a water-colour sketch of Fauntleroy at Dorincourt Castle, golden curls, velvet pantaloons, huge mastiff and all, with only one variation – my face in the place of Cedric Errol's. The effect was singularly sickening."[15] A French author whose name I forget also longed for a Fauntleroy or sailor suit rather than what he had to wear: pseudo-English tweeds with a bowler hat and starched shirt.

Decorative uniforms had some detractors, including Thackeray, who guyed military ones in *Some Passages in the Life of Major Gahagan* (1838–9). The major serves in the Indian Army: "I, for the first time, put on the beautiful uniform of the Invincibles; a light blue swallow-tailed jacket with silver lace and wings, ornamented with about 3000 sugar-loaf buttons, rhubarb-coloured leather inexpressibles (tights), and red morocco boots with silver spurs and tassels, set off to admiration the handsome persons of the officers of our corps. We wore powder in those days, and a regulation pig-tail of seventeen inches, a brass helmet surrounded by leopardskin, with a bear-skin top and a horse-tail feather, gave the head a fierce and chivalrous appearance". He acquires the command of a regiment, and is

allowed to settle the uniform . . . I . . . gave a carte-blanche to my taste, and invented the most splendid costume that ever perhaps decorated a soldier. I am . . . six feet four inches in height, and of matchless symmetry and proportion. My hair and beard are of the most brilliant auburn, so bright as scarcely to be distinguished at a glance from scarlet. My eyes are bright blue, over-shadowed by bushy eyebrows of the colour of my hair, and a terrific gash of the deepest purple, which goes over the forehead, the eyelid, and the cheek, and finishes at the ear, gives my face a more strictly military appearance than can be conceived. When I have been drinking (which is pretty often the case) this gash becomes ruby bright, and . . . I have another which took off a piece of my under-lip, and shows five of my front teeth . . . I . . . allowed my hair to grow very long, as did my beard, which reached to my waist. It took me two hours daily to curl my hair in ten thousand little corkscrew ringlets, which waved over my shoulders, and to get my mustachios well round to the corners of my eyelids. I dressed in loose scarlet trousers and red morocco boots, a scarlet jacket, and a shawl of the same colour round my waist; a scarlet turban three feet high, and decorated with a tuft of the scarlet feathers of the flamingo, formed my head-dress, and I did not allow myself a single ornament, except a small silver skull and cross-bones in front of my turban. Two brace of pistols, a Malay creese, sharp on both sides, and very nearly six feet in length, completed this elegant costume . . . I rode my black horse, and looked . . . like Mars . . .

You may fancy what a figure the Irregulars cut on a field-day – a line of five hundred black-faced, black-dressed, black-horsed, black-bearded men . . . the . . . officers in yellow, galloping about the field like flashes of lightning: myself enlightening them, red, solitary, and majestic, like yon glorious orb in Heaven.

Jos Sedley, the dandy in *Vanity Fair* (1847–8), "never was well-dressed; but he took the hugest pains to adorn his big person, and passed many hours daily in that occupation. His valet made a fortune out of his wardrobe: his toilet-table was covered with as many pomatums and essences as ever were employed by an old beauty: he had tried, in order to give himself a waist, every girth, stay, and waistband then invented. Like most fat men, he *would* have his clothes made too tight, and took care they should be of the most brilliant colours and youthful cut." A "swell" in *Pendennis* (1849–50) "had a bull-dog between his legs, and in his scarlet shawl neck-cloth was a pin representing another bull-dog in gold. He wore a fur waistcoat laced over with gold chains; a green cut-away coat with basket buttons, and a white upper-coat ornamented with cheese-plate buttons, on each of which was engraved some stirring incident of the road or the chase; . . . you would hesitate to say . . . whether he was a boxer *en goguette*, or a coachman in his gala suit."

In *The Book of Snobs, by One of Themselves* (1848) Thackeray parodies the *Court Circular*'s descriptions of presentation dresses:

MISS SNOBKY.

Habit de Cour, composed of a yellow nankeen illusion dress over a slip of rich pea-green corduroy, trimmed en tablier, with bouquets of Brussels sprouts: the body and sleeves handsomely trimmed with calimanco, and festooned with a pink train and white radishes. Head-dress, carrots and lappets.

LADY SNOBKY.

Costume de Cour, composed of a train of the most superb Pekin bandannas, elegantly trimmed with spangles, tinfoil, and red-tape. Bodice and under-dress of sky-blue velveteen, trimmed with bouffants and nœuds of bell-pulls. Stomacher, a muffin. Head-dress, a bird's nest, with a bird of paradise, over a rich brass knocker en ferronière. This splendid costume, by Madame Crinoline, of Regent Street, was the object of universal admiration.

. . . How can you help being the mothers, daughters, &c. of Snobs, so long as this balderdash is set before you?

The words "one of themselves" show why he was so angry. He argued that people could do their jobs just as well without fancy dress as with it, and drew attention to the cost of outfitting an officer in a smart regiment, which could virtually bankrupt a family of moderate means, but he could not help being affected by what he despised. In *Sketches and Travels in London* (1847) an uncle advises his nephew: "let your dress be perfectly neat, polite, and cleanly, without any attempts at splendour . . . Be it yours decently to conform to the fashion, and leave your buttons in the hands of a good tailor, who will place them wherever fashion ordains" (like La Bruyère). He believed women were less interested in men's appearance: "brutes that we are . . . we sidle up naturally towards the prettiest woman".

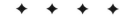

Victorian Heroines and Modern Misreadings

Some misconceptions need clearing up, the first being that fictional heroines were always blonde. Fashion did slowly shift from the slim brunette to the voluptuous blonde, but the older type did not disappear. Kimberley Reynolds and Nicola Humble, in *Victorian Heroines*,[16] give Laura in Wilkie Collins's *The Woman in White* (1860) as an example of the blonde archetype, but in his equally famous *The Moonstone* (1868) the heroine's butler states: "If you happen to like dark women (who, I am informed, have gone out of fashion latterly in the gay world) and if you have no particular prejudice in favour of size, I answer for Miss Rachel as one of the prettiest girls your eyes ever looked on. She was small and slim, but all in fine proportion from top to toe . . . Her hair was the blackest I ever saw. Her eyes matched her hair." Robin Tolmach Lakoff and Raquel L. Scherr, in *Face Value: The Politics of Beauty*,[17] print what I can only call a howler. Rightly pointing out that dark women in Victorian literature tend to have strong characters, whether good or evil, they describe Becky Sharp in *Vanity Fair* as a brunette. Thackeray repeatedly says her hair is sandy (innocent-looking blonde crossed with red). She and the blonde Blanche in *Pendennis* are both hypocrites, and both books have brown-haired heroines.

Dickens's heroines vary in hair colour, if little else, the only golden-haired ones being in *Bleak House* and *A Tale of Two Cities*. In *Hard Times* (1854), two children appear: "whereas the girl was so dark-eyed and dark-haired, that she seemed to receive a deeper and more lustrous colour from the sun, when it shone upon her, the boy was so light-eyed and light-haired that the self-same rays appeared to draw out of him what little colour he ever possessed. His cold eyes would hardly have been eyes, but for the short ends of lashes which, by bringing them into immediate contrast with some-thing paler than themselves, expressed their form. His short-cropped hair might have been a mere continuation of the sandy freckles on his face. His skin was so unwholesomely deficient in the natural tinge, that he looked as though, if he were cut, he would bleed white."

He draws a surprising number of attractive older people. Mrs Skewton in *Dombey and Son* (1848) is repulsive, with her "wrinkled face . . . with that patched colour on it which the sun made infinitely more dismal than any want of colour could have been"; so is Mr Turveydrop in *Bleak House* (1853): "a fat old gentleman with a false complexion, false teeth, false whiskers, and a wig . . . He was pinched in, and swelled out, and got up, and strapped down, as much as he could possibly bear. He had such a neckcloth on (puffing his very eyes out of their natural shape), and his chin and even his ears so sunk into it, that it seemed as though he must inevitably double up, if it were cast loose."

In *David Copperfield* (1850), however, Peggotty is "handsome" in his "ruddy, hearty, strong old age" and Mrs Lupin in *Martin Chuzzlewit* (1844), though "not exactly what the world calls young" has "roses in her cheeks, – ay, and roses, worth the gathering too, on her lips . . . She had still a bright black eye, and jet black hair; was comely, dimpled, plump". Mrs Varden in *Barnaby Rudge* (1840–1), who has a marriageable daughter, is "symmetrical in figure, buxom in bodice, ruddy in cheek and lip, faultless in ankle . . . delicious to behold". Older still is Mrs Crisparkle in *Edwin Drood* (1870), whose seventh son is thirty-five: "What is prettier than an old lady – except a young lady – when her eyes are bright, when her figure is trim and compact, when her face is cheerful and calm, when her dress is as the dress of a china shepherdess: so dainty in its colors, so individually assorted to herself, so neatly moulded on her?"

He also throws light on contemporary attitudes to cosmetics, which were not so uniformly condemned as is usually thought. A character in *Bleak*

House describes a doctor's wife of about fifty: "If I add, to the little list of her accomplishments, that she rouged a little, I do not mean that there was any harm in it" and when the author says that "a young lady (of sixty) . . . is a little dreaded . . . in consequence of an indiscreet profusion in the article of rouge" he suggests that she is not immoral but embarrassingly old-fashioned. Rouge had become semi-secret. Miss Mowcher, the beauty specialist in *David Copperfield*, based on a real person, says that dowagers called it lip-salve, gloves, tucker-edging and fans: "*I* call it whatever *they* call it. I supply it for 'em, but we keep up the trick so, to one another, and make believe with such a face, that they'd as soon think of laying it on, before a whole drawing-room, as before me. And when I wait upon 'em, they'll say to me sometimes – *with it on* – thick, and no mistake – 'How am I looking, Mowcher? Am I pale?'"

In Thackeray's *The Newcomes* (1854–5) a young lady has "her full lips slightly shaded, – how shall I mention the word? – slightly pencilled after the manner of the lips of the French governess". Trollope in *The Eustace Diamonds* (1876) refers, with regret, to the use of rouge by older women and Lady Eustace (a dark-haired hypocrite) "had begun to use a little colouring . . . there was the faintest possible tinge of pink colour shining through the translucent pearl powder. Any one who knew Lizzie would be sure that, when she did paint, she would paint well."

More familiar to us is Gwen Raverat's description of middle-class circles in the nineties: "less favoured ladies did use powder, with discretion; but never young girls. And never, never rouge or lipstick. That was definitely only for actresses, or 'certain kinds of women', or the wickedest sort of 'fashionable lady'."[18] Mrs Beeton, when a magazine editor, snubbed readers who wrote for advice on cosmetics: "painting the face, dyeing the hair, or any other artifice, spoils the real beauty of a handsome woman, and makes an ugly woman ridiculous". In the United States, again, Lois Banner gives a different picture; after a short period when make-up was rejected as a symbol of the ancien régime, it was openly used until the seventies, when moral objections arose, and it did not return until the end of the century. Consuelo Vanderbilt, the American wife of an English duke, regretted it: "it seemed to me then unfair that *ces dames du demi-monde* should be permitted to enhance their beauty with cosmetics which were forbidden to *la femme du monde*. For the respectable woman, as she was called, had to observe a neutral role; her clothes as well as her 'make-up' had to be discreet".[19]

The most important misunderstanding of all, however, is the most relevant to this book. So far we have been studying male writers' attitudes, but were women's different? Thackeray wrote in *Vanity Fair*:

> What is there in a pair of pink cheeks and blue eyes forsooth? these dear Moralists ask, and hint wisely that the gifts of genius . . . are far more valuable endowments for a female, than those fugitive charms which a few years will inevitably tarnish. It is quite edifying to hear women speculate upon the worthlessness and the duration of beauty.
>
> But though virtue is a much finer thing, and those hapless creatures who suffer under the misfortune of good looks ought to be continually put in mind of the fate which awaits them; and though, very likely, the heroic female character which ladies admire is a more glorious and beautiful object than the kind, fresh, smiling, artless, tender little domestic goddess, whom men are inclined to worship – yet the latter and inferior sort of women must have this consolation – that the men do admire them after all . . . so I am tempted to think that to be despised by her sex is a very great compliment to a woman.

Feminist readers might feel it a compliment to be despised by Thackeray. But did women writers' heroines lack those "fugitive charms"? When we examine what they wrote as opposed to what some later feminists would like to think they did, we find unmistakable signs of a theory being pushed too hard, and even some more howlers.

Frankie Finn, for instance, writes of "conventionally unattractive" heroines: "Dorothea, Emma, Lucy Snowe are not pretty women."[20] A reader who assumes that they were plain would be wrong about two of them. Jane Austen begins *Emma* with the words: "Emma Woodhouse, handsome, clever, and rich . . . " and none of her heroines is plain, even Catherine in *Northanger Abbey* (1816): "To look *almost* pretty is an acquisition of higher delight to a girl who has been looking plain the first fifteen years of her life, than a beauty from the cradle can ever receive." At seventeen she is "pleasing, and, when in good looks, pretty". As to Marianne in *Sense and Sensibility* (1811): "her face was so lovely, that when, in the common cant of praise, she was called a beautiful girl, truth was less violently outraged than usually happens. Her skin was very brown, but, from its transparency, her complexion was uncommonly brilliant; her features were all good; her smile was sweet and attractive; and in her eyes, which were very dark, there was a life, a spirit, an eagerness, which could hardly be seen without delight." Those of her male characters who turn out to be worthless are all handsome, but so are some of her heroes, notably Mr Darcy. It would be hard to imagine a more prosaic introduction than that of Mr Knightley in *Emma*, "a sensible man about seven or eight and thirty", but when Emma sees him at a party, "so young as he looked! He could not have appeared to greater advantage perhaps anywhere, than where he had placed himself. His tall, firm, upright figure, among the bulky forms and stooping shoulders of the elderly men, was such as Emma felt must draw everybody's eyes; and, excepting her own partner, there was not one among the whole row of young men who could be compared with him." This is before Emma falls in love with him. Austen explores the influence of feelings on judgments of appearance in *Pride and Prejudice*, *Sense and Sensibility* and *Persuasion* (1816), which contains her vainest character, Sir Walter Elliott. He believes "every face in the neighbourhood worsting" except his own and his eldest daughter's: "'there certainly were a dreadful multitude of ugly women in Bath; and as for the men! They were infinitely worse. Such scarecrows as the streets were full of! It was evident how little the women were used to the sight of anything tolerable, by the effect which a man of decent appearance produced. He had never walked anywhere arm-in-arm with Colonel Wallis (who was a fine military figure, though sandy-haired), without observing that every woman's eye was sure to be upon Colonel Wallis.' Modest Sir Walter! He was not allowed to escape, however. His daughter and Mrs Clay united in hinting that Colonel Wallis's companion might have as good a figure as Colonel Wallis, and certainly was not sandy haired."

Charlotte Brontë, who disliked her own looks, is well known for plain heroines (and heroes) but this is not the whole truth. In Jane Eyre's words: "I ever wished to look as well as I could, and to please as much as my want of beauty would permit. I sometimes regretted that I was not handsomer; I sometimes wished to have rosy cheeks, a straight nose, and small cherry mouth; I desired to be tall, stately, and finely developed in figure; I felt it a misfortune that I was so little, so pale, with features so irregular and so marked . . . I had a reason, and a logical, natural one too." Though she tells her pupil Adèle that she thinks too much of her clothes ("there was something ludicrous as well as painful in the little Parisienne's earnest and innate devotion to matters of dress"), she expects the reader to recoil from the "brown stuff frocks of quaint fashion" of the girls at her charity school, where the treasurer's wife and daughters "ought to have come a little sooner to have heard his lecture on dress, for they were splendidly attired in velvet, silk, and furs. The two younger of the trio . . . had grey beaver hats . . . shaded with ostrich plumes, and from under the brim of this graceful headdress fell a profusion of light tresses, elaborately curled; the elder lady . . .

wore a false front of French curls." This is based on the Clergy Daughters' School which the Brontës attended, and whose director, the Rev. Carus Wilson, put his pupils into "a very simple and uniform attire . . . to nip in the bud any growing symptom of vanity".[21]

Saintly Miss Temple, the headmistress, is "tall, fair and shapely" and dressed "in the mode" and the Misses Rivers, Jane's cousins, have "faces full of distinction". Their brother St John is "a handsome man: tall, fair, with blue eyes, and a Grecian profile." This indicates neither intellectual nor moral weakness: he is a "profound scholar" and a ruthlessly dedicated missionary. The woman he loves has "a face of perfect beauty . . . a strong expression; but I do not retrace or qualify it: . . . sweet features . . . pure hues of rose and lily . . . justified . . . the term. No charm was wanting, no defect was perceptible; the young girl had regular and delicate lineaments; eyes shaped and coloured as we see them in lovely pictures, large, and dark, and full; the long and shadowy eyelash which encircles a fine eye with so soft a fascination; the pencilled brow which gives such clearness; the white smooth forehead, which adds such repose to the livelier beauties of tint and ray; the cheek oval, fresh, and smooth; the lips, fresh too, ruddy, healthy, sweetly formed; the even and gleaming teeth without flaw; the small dimpled chin; the ornament of rich, plenteous tresses – all . . . were fully hers." St John, when moved, "looked nearly as beautiful for a man as she for a woman."

Jane regards handsome men as not for her. When she first meets Mr Rochester, "I had hardly ever seen a handsome youth; never in my life spoken to one. I had a theoretical reverence and homage for beauty, elegance, gallantry, fascination; but had I met those qualities incarnate in masculine shape, I should have known instinctively that they neither had nor could have sympathy with anything in me, and should have shunned them as one would fire, lightning, or anything else that is bright but antipathetic." Even when she is in love with him, she says: "I don't call you handsome, sir, though I love you most dearly: far too dearly to flatter you. Don't flatter me."

This doesn't mean Charlotte thought beauty was only for women, as St John proves. The "showy, but not genuine" Blanche Ingram, talking to impress Mr Rochester, condemns "Creatures so absorbed in care about their pretty faces, and their white hands, and their small feet; as if a man had anything to do with beauty! As if loveliness were not the special prerogative of woman – her legitimate appanage and heritage! I grant an ugly *woman* is a blot on the fair face of creation; but as to the *gentlemen*, let them be solicitous to possess only strength and valour". Would she have said it if Mr Rochester had looked like St John?

In the author's first and last novels, *The Professor* (not published until 1856) and *Villette* (1853), both the heroes and heroines are schoolteachers. "I am not handsome, and no dressing can make me so" says the "Professor" and, like Jane, he scorns flattery. When his employer's mother laughs at her daughter for saying he looks like Apollo, he agrees: "her sensible, truthful words seemed so wholesome, contrasted with the morbid illusions of her daughter."

Yet he disapproves "of the high-flounced, slovenly, and tumbled dresses in costly silk and satin; of the large, unbecoming collars in expensive lace; of the ill-cut coats and strangely fashioned pantaloons" of the English in Brussels, and finds himself more influenced by the heroine's appearance than he thought: "I began to suspect that it was only my tastes which were unique, not my power of discovering and appreciating the superiority of moral worth over physical charms. For me Frances had physical charms: in her there was no deformity to get over; none of those prominent defects . . . which hold at bay the admiration of the boldest male champions of intellect (for women can love a downright ugly man if he be but talented) . . . Frances' mental points had been the first to interest me . . . but I liked the graces of her person too . . . and that pleasure I could ill have dispensed with. It appeared, then, that I too was a sensualist, in my temperate and fastidious way."

Such conceit might seem typically masculine, but it is paralleled in *Villette*. Lucy, certain she is plain, insists on wearing dun-colour when every other woman of her generation is in white, and, when given a pink evening dress, "I thought no human force should avail to put me into it. A pink dress! I knew it not. It knew not me." She passes a mirror while wearing it: "No need to dwell on the result. It brought a jar of discord, a pang of regret; it was not flattering, yet, after all, I ought to be thankful; it might have been worse." Her colleague Paul Emmanuel expresses moral doubts about the dress, although his own "taste in colours decidedly leaned to the brilliant", leaving Lucy rather pleased that someone exists by whose standards even she looks "too airy and cheery". When he is dressed for a picnic, "his figure (such as it was, I don't boast of it) was well set off by a civilised coat and a silken vest quite pretty to behold . . . The little man looked well, very well; there was a clearness of amity in his blue eye, and a glow of good feeling on his dark complexion, which passed perfectly in the place of beauty: one really did not care to observe that his nose, though far from small, was of no particular shape, his cheek thin, his brow marked and square, his mouth no rose-bud; one accepted him as he was", evidently in the same spirit as the Professor accepted Frances.

Lucy reveals her attitude to herself when Paul worries about her pallor:

'Ah! I am not pleasant to look at ——?'

I could not help saying this; the words came unbidden: I never remember the time when I had not a haunting dread of what might be the degree of my outward deficiency; this dread pressed me at the moment with special force . . .

'Do I displease your eyes much?' I took courage to urge: the point had its vital import for me.

He stopped, and gave me a short, strong answer; an answer which silenced, subdued, and profoundly satisfied. Ever after that I knew what I was for him; and what I might be for the rest of the world, I ceased painfully to care. Was it weak to lay so much stress on an opinion about appearance? I fear it might be; I fear it was; but in that case I must avow no light share of weakness.

In this book, there is another example of male beauty: "his face and fine brow were most handsome and manly. *His* features were not delicate, not slight like those of a woman, nor were they cold, frivolous and feeble; though well cut, they were not so chiselled, so frittered away, as to lose in power and significance what they gained in unmeaning symmetry." He loves a woman who like Jane Eyre is "small, slight, white" but whom Lucy calls beautiful.

The heroines of *Shirley* (1849) are the least closely based on the author, and by far the best looking. It is the only complete work by any of the Brontës to be narrated in the third person, meaning that we see the characters through Charlotte's eyes instead of their own. When Mr Rochester calls Jane's eyes hazel and she calls them green, who is right? With Shirley we know: "she was gracefully made, and her face, too, possessed a charm as well described by the word grace as any other . . . Her features were distinguished" and when dressed for a special occasion "there was style in every fold of her dress and every line of her figure; the rich silk suited her better than a simpler costume . . . the attention to fashion, the tasteful appliance of ornament in each portion of her dress, were quite in place with her". She also shocks her governess by whistling and being interested in politics. Her friend Caroline, champion of single women's rights, inherits her looks, though nothing else, from her dissolute father: "Each lineament was turned with grace; the whole aspect was pleasing. At the present moment – animated, interested, touched – she might be called beautiful."

Shirley also contains the only exception to Charlotte's rule that characters may marry out of their social sphere but not their level of physical attractiveness. The character most like the author had to be plain. Socially, Shirley and Louis Moore are the mirror-image of Jane and Mr Rochester: he is a tutor, she an heiress. "He had the shorter nose and longer upper-lip of his sister, rather than the fine traits of his brother" and as Shirley says: "You have a habit of calling yourself plain. You are sensitive about the cut of your features, because they are not quite of an Apollo-pattern. You abuse them more than is needful, in the faint hope that others may say a word in their behalf – which won't happen. Your face is nothing to boast of, certainly: not a pretty line, nor a pretty tint, to be found therein."

Roszika Parker's essay *Images of Men*[22] quotes the description of Louis' brother Robert when ill, with "beauty in his pale, wasted features" in support of her theory that: "In order for men to appear desirable they have to resemble *the* objects of beauty and desire in our society – women." But even when Robert first appears, "his features are fine, . . . they have a Southern symmetry, clearness, regularity in their chiseling" though the anxious expression and "haggard outline of face" caused by business worries "disturb the idea of beauty with one of care".

We have little information on what Emily Brontë's Cathy looked like, but she was certainly not plain; her daughter has "the most exquisite little face . . . small features, very fair; flaxen ringlets, or rather golden" (her mother was darker). Heathcliff as a boy has misgivings about his appearance, wishing for Edgar Linton's "great blue eyes and even forehead", to which Nelly Dean answers: "tell me whether you don't think yourself rather handsome? I'll tell you, I do. You're fit for a prince in disguise."

Anne Brontë's work shows the same pattern as Charlotte's: the heroine of her autobiographical novel is plain. Helen in *The Tenant of Wildfell Hall* (1848) is not: "Her hair was raven black . . . the features in general, unexceptionable" says the hero. She does, however, have quiet tastes: "to please him [her husband] I had to violate my cherished predilections – my almost rooted principles in favour of a plain, dark, sober style of dress; I must sparkle in costly jewels and deck myself out like a painted butterfly, just as I had, long since, determined I would never do – and this was no trifling sacrifice".

The heroine and narrator of Anne's first novel, *Agnes Grey* (1847), is a governess, like its author. Like Helen she is pale and dark-haired, but there the resemblance ends. When she begins to fall in love (with a not particularly handsome man) she reflects:

hitherto I had been a little neglectful . . . but now, also, it was no uncommon thing to spend as much as two minutes in the contemplation of my own image in the glass; though I never could derive any consolation from such a study. I could discover no beauty in those marked features, that pale, hollow cheek, and ordinary dark brown hair; there might be intellect in the fore-head, there might be expression in the dark grey eyes, but what of that? – a low Grecian brow, and large black eyes devoid of sentiment would be esteemed far preferable. It is foolish to wish for beauty. Sensible people never either desire it for themselves or care about it in others. If the mind be but well cultivated, and the heart well disposed, no one ever cares for the exte-rior. So said the teachers of our childhood; and so say we to the children of the present day. All very judicious and proper, no doubt; but are such asser-tions supported by actual experience?

We are naturally disposed to love what gives us pleasure, and what more pleasing than a beautiful face – when we know no harm of the possessor at least? . . . They that have beauty, let them be thankful for it, and make a good use of it, like any other talent; they that have it not, let them console themselves, and do the best they can without it; certainly, though liable to be over-estimated, it is a gift of God, and not to be despised . . . I might dive much deeper, and disclose other thoughts, propose questions the reader might be puzzled to answer, and deduce arguments that might startle his prejudices, or, perhaps, provoke his ridicule, because he could not compre-hend them; but I forbear.

Mrs Gaskell is also quoted as rejecting the current ideal. Some of her short stories have heroines like the "very plain" one in *The Three Eras of Libbie Marsh*, and her best-known book, *Cranford*, is mostly about elderly women. In one passage, the narrator finds some letters written in the late eighteenth century by the mother of one of them: "six or seven letters were principally occupied in asking her lover to use his influence with her parents (who evidently kept her in good order) to obtain this or that article of dress, more especially the white 'Paduasoy.' He cared nothing how she was dressed; she was always lovely enough for him, as he took pains to assure her, when she begged him to express in his answers a predilection for particular pieces of finery, in order that she might show what he said to her parents. But at length he seemed to find out that she would not be married till she had a 'trousseau' to her mind". When she became a mother, "It was pretty to see . . . how the girlish vanity was being weeded out of her heart by love for her baby. The white 'Paduasoy' figured again in the letters, with almost as much vigour as before. In one, it was being made into a christening cloak for the baby . . . It added to its charms when it was 'the prettiest little baby that ever was seen . . . I do think she will grow up a regular bewty!'"

For Mrs Gaskell, as Reynolds and Humble point out, love of clothes could represent a moral danger. They cite *Mary Barton* (1848), in which a factory worker is driven to prostitution by her desire for upper-class habits, especially fine clothes, which she buys out of her pay: "as I had no more sensible wants, I spent it on dress and on eating." Mary nearly makes the same mistake: "trust a girl of sixteen for knowing it well if she is pretty; concerning her plainness she may be ignorant. So with this consciousness she had early determined that her beauty should make her a lady . . . the rank to which she firmly believed her lost aunt Esther had arrived." Esther, in "faded finery" and "glaring paint", is walking the streets. The heroine of *Ruth* (1853) is a dressmaker's apprentice who knows she is pretty, and she too is seduced.

Again, this is only half the picture. According to Reynolds and Humble "There is notably very little sense in Victorian literature of dress as explicitly pleasurable for women. It is rarely . . . represented . . . as an aesthetic phenomenon." They make an exception for a scene near the beginning of *North and South* (1855) in which the heroine tries on her cousin's Indian shawls. Her "tall, finely made figure . . . set off the long beautiful folds of the gorgeous shawls . . . She . . . took a pleasure in their soft feel and their brilliant colours, and rather liked to be dressed in such splendour, enjoying it much as a child would do, with a quiet pleased smile on her lips." When the gentlemen appeared, however, "the ladies started back, as if half ashamed of their feminine interest in dress".

Cranford apart, all Gaskell's full-length novels have good-looking heroines. Molly, in her last, unfinished work, *Wives and Daughters* (1866), has a stepsister, Cynthia ("a glowing beauty") mistakenly described by one writer as the heroine.[23] She suffers a far less drastic version of Ruth and Esther's fate: she borrows money to buy clothes from a man who later blackmails her. Michèle Roberts has drawn attention to Cynthia's French education, which for both Mrs Gaskell and Charlotte Brontë was morally suspect. Molly, though anxious not to be vain, likes dress and profits from lessons in grooming given by Cynthia and her mother: "Mrs Gibson had tried to put her through a course of rosemary washes and creams to improve her tanned complexion; but about that Molly was either forgetful or rebellious, and Mrs Gibson could not well come up to the girl's bedroom every night and see that she daubed her face and neck over with the cosmetics so carefully provided for her. Still her appearance was extremely improved" and when she goes to a ball she says: "I should like to be pretty!" Cynthia answers: "The French girls would tell you, to believe that you were pretty would make you so." Something does; by the end of the book "she scarcely knew the elegant reflection to be that of herself . . . a very pretty, lady-like, and graceful girl." The hero is "a tall powerfully-made young man" with a large mouth and small eyes, of whom Molly's first impression is: "'I would rather never be married at all,' thought she, 'than marry an ugly man – and dear good Mr Roger is really ugly; I don't think one could even call him plain.' Yet the Miss Brownings, who did not look upon young men as if their natural costume was a helmet and a suit of armour, thought Mr Roger Hamley a very personable young fellow, as he came into the room, his face flushed with exercise, his white teeth showing pleasantly in the courteous bow and smile he gave to all around."

George Eliot's position is more complex, because of contradictions in her own views. As a young and fervently Evangelical woman, she repudiated not only dancing but church music and even imaginative literature, and when she lost her faith she still faced a struggle between her need for these things and her suspicion of anything self-indulgent (though Edmund Gosse reported seeing her in a fashionable bonnet in later life). She also disliked her own appearance, as others did. All this was reflected in her fiction: while some of her heroines frankly enjoy dress and dancing, like "bewitching" Nancy in *Silas Marner* (1861), with her silvery twilled silk and coral necklace, and Hepzibah in the same book with her decided views on the ideal fabric for a wedding dress, others share the attitudes of the Puritans (all are immaculately clean). In *Adam Bede* (1859) the heroine Dinah is a Methodist preacher, and first appears in a cap like a Quaker's, looking "as unselfconscious of her appearance as a little boy. It was one of those faces that make one think of white flowers with light touches of colour on their pure petals. The eyes had no peculiar beauty, beyond that of expression" and she has a musical voice. Vain Hetty could hardly be more different: "Hetty's cheek was like a rose-petal, . . . dimples played about her pouting lips, . . . her large dark eyes hid a soft roguishness under their long lashes, and . . . her curly hair, though all pushed back . . . stole back in dark delicate rings on her forehead, and about her white shell-like ears." Her "dreams were all of luxuries" and this indicates moral weakness, as it does in *Felix Holt* (1866).

Maggie in *The Mill on the Floss* (1860) is a tomboy as a child, and during her family's troubles renounces worldly pleasures on religious grounds: "Maggie, in spite of her own ascetic wish to have no personal adornment, was obliged to give way to her mother about her hair, and submit to have the abundant black locks plaited into a coronet on the summit of her head . . . So Maggie, glad of anything that would soothe her mother . . . consented to the vain decoration, and showed a queenly head above her old frocks – steadily refusing, however, to look at herself in the glass." At sixteen she is told:

> 'You are very much more beautiful than I thought you would be.'
> 'Am I?' said Maggie, the pleasure returning in a deeper flush. She turned her face away from him and took some steps, looking straight before her in silence, as if she were adjusting her consciousness to this new idea. Girls are so accustomed to think of dress as the main ground of vanity, that, in abstaining from the looking-glass, Maggie had thought more of abandoning all care for adornment than of renouncing the contemplation of her face.

A year or two later, "The culmination of Maggie's career as an admired member of society in St Ogg's was certainly the day of the bazaar, when her simple noble beauty, clad in a white muslin of some soft-floating kind . . . appeared with marked distinction among the more adorned and conventional women around her." When "taken before Lucy's cheval-glass, and made to look . . . Maggie had smiled at herself then, and for the moment had forgotten everything in the sense of her own beauty."

Middlemarch (1871) opens with these words: "Miss Brooke had that kind of beauty which seems to be thrown into relief by poor dress. Her hand and wrist were so finely formed that she could wear sleeves not less bare of style than those in which the Blessed Virgin appeared to Italian painters; and her profile as well as her stature and bearing seemed to gain the more dignity from her plain garments, which by the side of provincial fashion gave her the impressiveness of a fine quotation from the Bible, – or from one of our elder poets, – in a paragraph of to-day's newspaper." She is descended from "a Puritan gentleman who served under Cromwell" and we are told that the minor gentry's code of behaviour "in those days made show in dress the first item to be deducted from, when any margin was required for expenses more distinctive of rank . . . but in Miss Brooke's case, religion alone would have determined it . . . to her the destinies of mankind, seen by the light of Christianity, made the solicitudes of feminine fashion appear an occupation for Bedlam. She could not reconcile the anxieties of a spiritual life involving eternal consequences, with a keen interest in guimp and artificial protrusions of drapery."

This contrasts with her attitude to other pleasures: "Riding was an indulgence which she allowed herself in spite of conscientious qualms; she felt that she enjoyed it in a pagan sensuous way, and always looked forward to renouncing it." She cannot help responding to the beauty of her family jewels but: "All the while her thought was trying to justify her delight in the colours by merging them in her mystic religious joy." She would never consider wearing them, and has difficulty in justifying art (though, unlike some of Cromwell's followers, she would like to). She pays a social call wearing some "thin white woollen stuff soft to the touch and soft to the eye . . . always in the shape of a pelisse with sleeves hanging all out of the fashion" in contrast to her hostess Rosamond's "infantine blondness and wondrous crown of hair-plaits, with her pale-blue dress of a fit and fashion so perfect that no dressmaker could look at it without emotion, a large embroidered collar which it was to be hoped all beholders would know the price of, her small hands duly set off with rings, and that controlled self-consciousness of manner which is the expensive substitute for simplicity."

One of Eliot's biographers, Jennifer Uglow, calls Dorothea Brooke "plain"![24] (Uglow is right that Rosamond's husband finds her unattractive, but this is "notwithstanding her undeniable beauty".) *Middlemarch* contains a sympathetically drawn plain woman who is loved: "Rembrandt would have painted her with pleasure, and would have made her broad features look out of the canvas with intelligent honesty."

Finally, *Daniel Deronda* (1876) begins: "Was she beautiful or not beautiful?" The first part of the book, which introduces Gwendolen, the subject of Daniel's question, is called "The Spoiled Child". The real heroine of the story is small though beautifully made, unlike Maggie and Dorothea whose tall stature contrasts with the merely pretty "little ladies", Dorothea's sister Celia and Maggie's cousin Lucy. Gwendolen behaves in a way which Joanna Russ, writing of Bella in Dickens's *Our Mutual Friend* (1864–5) declares that no woman does: she "flirts (impossibly) with her mirror. Women speaking of mirrors and prettiness make it all too clear that even for pretty women, mirrors are the foci of anxious, not gratified, narcissism. The woman who knows beyond a doubt that she is beautiful exists aplenty in male novelists' imaginations; I have yet to find her in women's books or women's memoirs or in life."[25] In fact Bella, though she talks to her reflection and asks its advice, does not flirt with it, but we have already seen Maggie's reaction to hers and here is Gwendolen's: "Her beautiful lips curled into a more and more decided smile, till at last she took off her hat, leaned forward and kissed the cold glass which had looked so warm." Later, Margaret Mitchell made Scarlett in *Gone With the Wind* kiss her reflection.

What of children's books? A poem by Jane and Ann Taylor runs:

Sophia was a little child
Obliging, good, and very mild,
Yet, lest of dress she should be vain,
Mamma still dress'd her well, but plain;
Her parents, sensible yet kind,
Wish'd only to adorn her mind.
No other dress, when good, had she,
But useful, neat simplicity.

Though seldom, yet, when she was rude,
Or ever in a naughty mood,
Her punishment was this disgrace,
A large fine cap, adorn'd with lace,
And feathers and with ribbons too,
The work was good, the fashion new,
Yet, as a fool's cap was its name,
She dreaded much to wear the same.

A lady, fashionably gay,
Did to Mamma a visit pay;
Sophia stared, then whispering said,
'Why, dear Mamma, look at her head!
To be so tall, and wicked too,
The strangest thing I ever knew!
What naughty tricks, pray, has she done,
That they have put that fool's cap on?'[26]

(The illustrator, Kate Greenaway, had almost as much effect on girls' clothes as Frances Hodgson Burnett on boys', with her drawings of simple, high-waisted dresses, influenced by the Regency and the Pre-Raphaelites.) In Louisa M. Alcott's *Little Women* (1868) Meg is sometimes vain, Amy almost always. When Meg's rich hosts dress her up for a party ("they powdered and squeezed and frizzled, and made me look like a fashion-plate", she says) we are meant to disapprove; but when in the sequel, *Good Wives* (1869), Amy, who has artistic ambitions, "covered poverty with flowers" by contriving a ball-dress out of cast-offs, we are not. In *Jo's Boys* (1886) Amy is married and no longer has any poverty to cover, and embraces the principles of Brummell, Ungaro and Westwood: "a stately, graceful woman, who showed how elegant simplicity could be made by the taste with which she chose her dress and the grace with which she wore it. As someone said: 'I never know what Mrs Laurence has on, but I always receive the impression that she is the best-dressed lady in the room.'" The same author's *An Old-Fashioned Girl* (1870) takes a strong line on women's right to work and vote, and deplores the clandestine use of cosmetics by society women, but shows sympathy for the desire to dress well; and *Eight Cousins: or, The Aunt-Hill* (1875) stresses that girls should not only take exercise, including football, but wear pretty as well as practical clothes for it.

In Susan Coolidge's *What Katy Did* (1872) Katy is "comfortably indifferent to what became of her clothes", but looks forward to growing up: "Her eyes, which were black, were to turn blue; her nose was to lengthen and straighten, and her mouth, quite too large at present to suit the part of a heroine, was to be made over into a sort of rosy button. Meantime . . . Katy forgot her features as much as she could"; her younger sisters quarrel because Clover wants to be "the most beautiful lady in the world" and Elsie "*more* beautiful than the most beautiful". Katy, seeing the bracelets and lace-trimmed nightgown of their "saintly invalid" Cousin Helen, asks: "Is it worldly to have pretty things when you're sick?" Helen answers: "Pretty things are no more 'worldly' than ugly ones, except when they spoil us by making us vain, or careless of the comfort of other people." In *What Katy Did Next* (1866), however, we are told: "Pretty dresses are very pretty on pretty people – they certainly play an important part in this queer little world of ours – but depend upon it, dear girls, no woman ever has established so distinct and clear a claim on the regard of her lover as when he has ceased to notice or analyse what she wears, and just accepts it unquestioningly, whatever it is, as a bit of the dear human life which has grown, or is growing, to be the best and most delightful thing in the world to him."

Among lesser-known English writers for girls and young women, Charlotte M. Yonge, certainly no feminist, criticises both excessively fashionable dress and eccentric-looking intellectuals, whom she also blames for neglecting domestic duties. Theodora, heroine of *A Life for a Life* (1859) by Dinah Maria Mulock (Mrs Craik) describes herself at twenty-five': "'Tis a good thing to be good-looking. And next best, perhaps, is downright ugliness, – nice, interesting, attractive ugliness – such as I have seen in some women; nay, I have somewhere read that ugly women have often been loved best . . . But to be just ordinary; of ordinary height, ordinary figure, and, oh me! let me lift up my head from the desk to the looking-glass and take a good stare at an undeniably ordinary face. 'Tis not pleasant." This is based on the author's experience, as she told friends: "I was always a plain girl and no one came near me to ask me to dance. I could have cried."[27] The hero, himself not "either particularly handsome or particularly young", says: "In repose her features are ordinary; nor did they for one moment recall to me the flashing, youthful face, full of action and energy, which amused me that night at the Cedars. Some faces catch the reflection of the moment so vividly that you never see them twice alike. Others, solidly and composedly handsome, scarcely vary at all, and I think it is of these last that one would soonest weary. Irregular features have generally most character. The Venus de' Medici would have made a very stupid fireside companion, nor would I venture to enter for Oxford honours a son who had the profile of the Apollo Belvidere."

Theodora has a "statuesque" sister with "a pure Greek profile", as does plain (Mrs Craik's own word) Edna in *The Woman's Kingdom* (1869): "Letty actually suffered, mentally and morally, from a worn-out shawl or an old-fashioned bonnet; while as to herself, so long as she was neat and clean, and had colors matching — no blues and greens, pinks and scarlets, which poverty compelled to be worn together — it did not materially affect her happiness, whether she had on a silk dress or a cotton one." Edna has more character in all respects.

Young girls were not allowed to read some of the most famous popular novelists, such as "Ouida" (Marie Louise de la Ramée). She leaves no doubt about the hero's beauty in *Under Two Flags* (1867): "a face of as much delicacy and brilliancy as a woman's, handsome, thoro'bred, languid, nonchalant, with a certain latent recklessness under the impassive calm of habit, and a singular softness given to the large, dark hazel eyes by the unusual length of the lashes over them. His features were exceedingly fair, fair as the fairest girl's; his hair was of the softest, silkiest, brightest chestnut; his mouth very beautifully shaped; on the whole, with a certain gentle, mournful love-me look that his eyes had with them, it was no wonder great ladies and gay lionnes alike gave him the palm as the handsomest man in all the Household Regiments."

Girls were also unlikely to be allowed Ellen (Mrs Henry) Wood's *East Lynne* (1861). When erring Lady Isabel first meets her future husband, "the extraordinary loveliness of the young girl before him almost took away his senses and his self-possession. It was not so much the perfect contour of the exquisite features that struck him, of the rich damask of the delicate cheek, or the luxuriant falling hair; no, it was the sweet expression of the soft dark eyes . . . there was in its character a sad, sorrowful look . . . a sure index of . . . suffering". Virtuous Barbara is merely "a pretty girl, very fair" though she does look "very lovely" at her wedding.

(Wood also gives a pretty girl a happier fate than a great beauty in her *St Martin's Eve* of 1866.)

Isabel sometimes dresses down when her neighbours, including Barbara, dress up, and sometimes the reverse. This shows that her heart is better than her judgment, which is why she is seduced by a man whose attributes are the opposite of her "pleasing and distinguished" husband's: "He was considered handsome, with his clearly-cut features, his dark eyes, his raven hair, and his white teeth; but, to a keen observer, those features had not an attractive expression." In *Verner's Pride* (1863) Wood says of the hero in mourning, "A handsome man never looks so well in any other attire" and the villain always wears a "large clear blue sapphire ring". She sums up her views in *The Channings* (1862), the story of a family moral enough for any Victorian parent:

> For one thing, she [the mother] had never allowed them to put on new clothes upon the Sunday. The very best of us are but human; and one, to whom God gave great wisdom, has told us that childhood and youth are vanity. When our hair grows gray and our body drooping, then we may be wise enough to begin to put vanity away from us; but, in earlier life, we no doubt possess our share. 'This new suit of broadcloth, home last night from the tailor's, how does it fit me? – how does it look, I wonder? Are you, who are staring at me, admiring the taste I have displayed in the selection? – are you thinking how tall and well my figure appears in it? But the coat is tight under the arms. Bother the fellow! he must alter it to-morrow. I feel like one in a vice.'
>
> 'Oh this charming bonnet! I am sure I never had on so becoming a one before! I am so glad I chose it white! – it contrasts so well with this lovely new lilac dress. Let me glance round! there's nobody looking *half* so well as I, I declare! I don't see a single new bonnet or dress out to-day, except mine. What a set of dowdies! Goodness me, though! she has dreadfully pinched my waist in, that dressmaker! I can't breathe. I shall be miserable all day.'
>
> Now all this – this self-complacency, self-absorption, self-torture – are very legitimate at times and seasons, for there's no help for it; and all the preaching of all the world could not put such feelings away from the young. In a greater or less degree, they do and must prevail; new things must be donned for the first time, and we must grow accustomed to their fresh aspect – to their misfit. Very good. But Mrs Channing did not choose that Sunday should be wasted in these idle thoughts; any day in the week, from Monday to Saturday, they might put on their new clothes to get seasoned to them; but not on Sunday. I think the rule was a good one.

Women writers were more realistic than men about what dressing well involves. Harriet Beecher Stowe's book of sketches *The Chimney-Corner*

(1868) includes one on "Woman's Sphere" (women should vote and be able to have careers, but: "The talents and tastes of the majority of women are naturally domestic") and two on dress. The narrator says: "Your nice young girl, of good family and good breeding, is always a pretty object . . . All their mysterious rattle-traps and whirligigs – their curls and networks and crimples and rimples and crisping-pins, – their little absurdities, if you will, – have to me a sort of charm, like the tricks and stammerings of a curly-headed child." His daughter and her friends say the work of keeping up with fashion interferes with other pursuits, but one asks, "*Is* it necessary to go without hoops, and look like a dipped candle, in order to be unworldly?" The daughter answers that the woman who does "injures the cause of goodness by making it outwardly repulsive . . . Her *outré* and repulsive exterior arrays our natural and innocent feelings against goodness; for surely it is natural and innocent to wish to look well." Her father agrees: "the love of dress and outside show has always been such an exacting and absorbing tendency, that it seems to have furnished work for religionists and economists, in all ages, to keep it within bounds." He quotes, and disagrees with, a poem by Thomas Moore (rather out of keeping with most of Moore's work), "suggested" by St Jerome:

> I chose not her, my heart's elect,
> From those who seek their Maker's shrine
> In gems and garlands proudly decked,
> As if themselves were things divine.
> No: Heaven but faintly warms the breast
> That beats beneath a broidered veil;
> And she who comes in glittering vest
> To mourn her frailty still is frail . . .

He continues:

But . . . all these modes of warfare on the elegancies and refinements of the toilet . . . were too indiscriminate. They were in reality founded on a false principle. They took for granted that there was something radically corrupt and wicked in the body and in the physical system . . . the body was a loathsome and pestilent prison, in which the soul was locked up and enslaved, and the eyes, the ears, the taste, the smell, were all so many corrupt traitors in conspiracy to poison her. Physical beauty of every sort was a snare . . . to be valiantly contended with and straitly eschewed. Hence they preached, not moderation, but total abstinence from all pursuit of physical grace and beauty.

75

Now, a resistance founded on an over-statement is constantly tending to reaction. People always have a tendency to begin thinking for themselves; and when they so think, they perceive that a good and wise God would not have framed our bodies with such exquisite care only to corrupt our souls, – that physical beauty, being created in such profuse abundance around us, and we being possessed with such a longing for it, must have its uses, its legitimate sphere of exercise . . . It is, therefore, neither wicked nor silly nor weak-minded to like beautiful dress, and all that goes to make it up. Jewelry, diamonds, pearls, emeralds, rubies, and all sorts of pretty things that are made of them, are as lawful and innocent objects of admiration and desire as flowers, or birds, or butterflies, or the tints of evening skies.

He mentions a Quaker lady who loved looking at jewels, concluding that a Christian woman loves dress too much only if it takes up "*All* her time. *All* her strength. *All* her money." But "the state of morals in France is apparently at the very lowest ebb . . . Women who can never have the name of wife, – who know none of the ties of family, – these are the dictators whose dress . . . and appointments give the law, first to France, and through France to the civilised world." The "sources of beauty in dress" are appropriateness "to our climate, to our habits of life and thought, and to the whole structure of ideas on which our life is built", which in the United States meant simplicity ("our public men wear no robes, no stars, garters, collars, &c."); unity of effect ("the same effect which is produced in mourning or the Quaker costume may be preserved in a style of dress admitting colour and ornamentation"), and truthfulness: "false jewelry and cheap fineries of every kind are in bad taste; so also is powder instead of natural complexion, false hair instead of real, and flesh-painting of every description."[28] Compare "Censor", Mrs Stowe's compatriot (though this passage, so far as I know, only appears in the British edition): "DON'T supplement the charms of nature by the use of the colour-box. Fresh air, exercise, the morning bath, and proper food, will give to the cheek nature's own tints, and no others have any true beauty."

"That we should all as far as our means allows [*sic*] us be beautifully and gracefully apparelled is proved by the fact that God never made a wave but He gilded it with golden sunbeams," agrees the Rev. T. DeWitt Talmage, Pastor of Brooklyn Tabernacle, in *Marriage and Home Life* (1892):

I have no prim, precise, prudish, or cast-iron theories on the subject of human apparel; but the goddess of fashion has set up her throne in this country . . . Her altars smoke with the sacrifice of the bodies and souls of ten thousand victims . . . Men are as much the idolaters [sic] of fashion as women, but they sacrifice on a different part of the altar . . . men do not abstain from millinery and elaboration of skirt through any superiority of simplicity. It is only because such appendages would be a blockade to business. What would sashes and trains three and a-half yards long do in a stock market? . . . Some of them wear boots so tight that they can hardly walk . . . and there are men . . . who go through the streets in great stripes of colour.

The results are Indelicate Apparel ("the womanly costume of our time is the cause of the temporal and eternal damnation of a multitude of men"), Drawing-Room Rivalry ("The parlour and drawing-room are now running a race with the theatre and opera bouffe . . . Immodest apparel always means a contaminated and depraved society"), Extravagance, An Incentive to Dishonesty which Curtails Benevolence, Distracts Attention (from religion), Mental Impoverishment ("Extravagant costume belittles the intellect . . . Can you imagine anything more dwarfing to the human intellect than the study of dress? I see men . . . who . . . must have taken two hours to arrange their apparel"), Bars Heaven ("Give up this idolatry of fashion or give up heaven") and produces Perpetual Envy ("The rivalries and the competitions of such a life are a stupendous wretchedness . . . *The two most ghastly death-beds* on earth are the one where a man dies of *delirium tremens*, and the other where a woman dies after having sacrificed all her faculties of body, mind and soul in the worship of costume.")[29]

How did the emerging feminists react? Another American historian, William Leach, devotes a chapter of *True Love and Perfect Union: The Feminist Reform of Sex and Society* to this. It begins: "Fashion was a powerful adversary to feminism . . . In the 1850s [American] middle-class dress, male and female, struck the eye with its variety and color, but by the 1870s men had relinquished color and style for unrelieved drabness, while women had become subject to every wave and flutter of fashionable style."[30] It was part of the "femininity" from which feminists were struggling to break away, just as, if men wanted to vary their dress, they had no-one to imitate but women. "For the early reformers especially", says Leach, "fashion was a poison, a 'pestilential excrescence' of a new society, 'a vile breath of pollution' that spread slowly until it struck and disabled the very heart of a woman's identity . . . Influenced by the model of Quaker costume . . . by a general Protestant dislike for all gewgaws and artificiality, and by a utilitarian naturalism, they also demanded an overdress free of all superfluous ornament." Mrs Bloomer's long trousers, reminiscent of Lady Mary Wortley Montagu, and the pressure on her to give them up, are well known, but it was not always for such reasons that feminists dressed in a "feminine" way. Some, including Susan B. Anthony, Elizabeth Cady Stanton and Lucy Stone, actually enjoyed it. The writer Sarah Grand, of whom her biographer says: "All her life she cared inordinately about clothes, her first involvement with the suffrage movement stemming from her interest in the Rational Dress Society", believed a "New Woman" should be "careful of her appearance", wore elaborate hats and kept notes of the details of her outfits.[31] Silk, satin, lace and bright colours reappeared (I am tempted to say by the back door) as feminist fiction shows.

Annie Denton Cridge's *Man's Rights; or, How Would You Like It?* (1870) depicts a world of reversed *rôles*, with "gentlemen-housekeepers" in

> calico suits, trimmed with little ruffles . . . red, green, yellow, drab, and black suits, trimmed in such fanciful styles! Some of these suits were parti-colored . . . Some . . . were trimmed with lace . . . almost covered with elaborate embroidery, or satin folds, or piping, or ribbon, while bows and streamers of the same or contrasting colors, according to taste, were placed on the backs of the coats' shoulders; or here and there, on the vest and pants . . . Their head-dresses, too, were most fantastic; flowers, bits of lace, tulle or blonde, feathers, and even birds, were mixed in endless profusion with ribbon, tinsel, glitter, and . . . grease . . . Many of these gentlemen carried little portemonnaies . . . Others carried fans . . . Each of these gentlemen seemed particularly interested in every other gentleman's costume.

The champion of men's rights, however, wears "a suit of black silk . . . bordered with broad black lace . . . no ornaments, except ear-rings, a plain breast-pin, and one or two rings on the fingers. Very good taste, I thought".[32]

This love of simplicity is practically a constant in feminist fiction. The parthenogenetic inhabitants of Charlotte Perkins Gilman's *Herland* (1915) have "short hair, hatless, loose, and shining; a suit of some light firm stuff, the closest of tunics and kneebreeches, met by trim gaiters. As bright and smooth as parrots". Like several other feminists, she admired the flowing uncorseted dress pioneered by the Aesthetic Movement. In Gilbert and Sullivan's *Princess Ida; or, Castle Adamant* (1884), based on Tennyson's poem *The Princess*, the educated women, like those in Marivaux, are good-looking but dress badly to punish male intruders:

> Let no-one care a penny how she looks –
> Let red be worn with yellow – blue with green –
> Crimson with scarlet – violet with blue!

Let all your things misfit, and you yourselves
At inconvenient moments come undone!

Feminists' opponents depicted them as dowdy – for instance Sir George du Maurier in the *Punch* cartoons and Mrs Humphry Ward in her novels. Suffragette posters deliberately suggest the opposite. An eye-witness report from 1909 notes that "The suffragette campaign [in Preston] opened in earnest with a meeting . . . addressed by Margaret Hewitt. Daringly modern, she wore a jaunty hat and a trace of lipstick."[33]

Modern writers have taken up the *rôle* reversal theme. In Gerd Brantenberg's *The Daughters of Egalia* (1977) the "menwim" (as opposed to "wim") have to wear skirts and constricting "pehos" (penis holders) and remove body hair; they long to be fat with small penises, trying to look not only female but pregnant. The narrator of Esmé Dodderidge's *The New Gulliver* (1979) finds himself in a world where women wear "an unbecoming tubular garment" and men "gaudy breeches . . . All that area where a decent man keeps his private parts in a kind of modest seclusion is here encased in a highly coloured, tightly fitting three-pronged bag . . . Not even to please my dear wife, however, will I wear the very latest fashion, which is to encase the middle member in a bag of a separate and most distinctive colour, which is also designed to keep the member in an upright position at all times".[34] In contrast, Margaret Atwood's *The Handmaid's Tale* (1987) shows a world of triumphant religious fundamentalism, with cosmetics and adornment outlawed except for prostitutes.

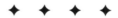

In the male sex, beauty is a defect.
> *Rev. Horace Bushnell*   Woman Suffrage: The Revolt Against Nature (1869)

No man can expect his children to respect what he degrades.
> *Charles Dickens*   Martin Chuzzlewit

So where are we now? Confused. In this field, at least, the conflation of anti-sexism with being like men is almost as complete as anti-feminists say it is. Caroline Bird prophesied in 1979, "Women will become more like men than men will become like women. Unisex clothing is a good example. Women have borrowed pants, utilitarian suits, and hair styles that require only cutting and combing from men, while men have borrowed only bright colours and jewelry from the sartorial repertoire of women . . . 'Femininity', it appears, is not an inborn female sex characteristic, but an artifact of powerlessness that will never be missed."[35] Masculine egalitarianism with a vengeance.

If she is right, how does one explain the historical evidence? Letty Cottin Pogrebin writes: "skirts have always been worn by men: the loin cloth, Egyptian apron, Turkish caftan, Greek chiton, Roman toga, Japanese kimono, Polynesian sarong, medieval tunic, and today's Arab jalaba, Scottish kilt, and priestly robes come immediately to mind . . . little boys continued wearing dresses into the early twentieth century – and to this day men sometimes wear a vestigial male skirt: formal tails."[36] She might have added countrymen's smocks, worn even after the First World War, and the long robes of Chinese mandarins, outlawed by Mao in 1927; the modern cheongsam derives originally from male, not female, Chinese dress. (I have heard the writer Jung Chang, lecturing at the Royal Society for Asian Affairs in London, say that on arriving in the West she was confused by the skirted and trousered figures on lavatory doors; to her they did not represent a sex difference.) If there is nothing innate about the current form of male dress, why, as Aileen Ribeiro has asked in *Dress and Morality*,[37] do women imitate it?

Montaigne's theory has been proved right: men made decoration compulsory for the inferior sex while spurning it themselves, so women who wanted equality rejected it. While men monopolised the sphere they thought of as theirs, women, in a kind of sexual trade unionism, retaliated by guarding their own; hence such beliefs as "only a woman can make a home". Decorative dress was taken over by "feminine" women who carried it to extremes, having nothing to lose by doing so. The "superior" sex treated their looks with indifference to show they could afford to, and women rebels copied them as a way of saying "I'm as good as you." Since boys outgrew dresses and girls didn't, both sexes may have felt the latter remained children for life (there are proverbs to that effect) and seeing the plainly dressed sex taken seriously, girls probably hoped that if they dressed plainly they would be taken seriously too. `Nineteenth-century writers on evolution, write Joanne B. Eicher and Mary Ellen Roach-Higgins, sometimes attributed differences in the dress of females and males to differences in the sexes' respective levels of social evolution, with males being at a higher level.[38] Modern feminists would not agree, but they dress as if they did.

Men's business clothes have become even more aesthetically and sexually neutral than they were at the end of the nineteenth century. The frock coat has become the sack suit. Only the most casual or the most formal men's clothes show the distinctive shape of their bodies, while "feminine" women's clothes continue to show theirs, which does not merely reinforce but exaggerate sexual differences by suggesting not that male and female torsos are differently shaped, but that only women's have any shape at all.

Do men like dressing that way? Not all of them. Some men have tried to reject the "great renunciation" ever since it happened. In Disraeli's novel *Coningsby* (1844) a gallery of family portraits contains "courtiers of the Tudors, and cavaliers of the Stuarts, terminating in red-coated squires fresh from the field, and gentlemen buttoned up in black coats, and sitting in library chairs, with their backs to a crimson curtain. Woman, however, is always charming", and in his last novel *Endymion* (1880) a tailor advises a young man: "In youth a little fancy is rather expected, but if political life be your object, it should be avoided – at least after one-and-twenty . . . No man gives me the trouble which Lord Eglantine does; he has not made up his mind whether he will be a great poet or a Prime Minister." Disraeli was Prime Minister twice and a successful novelist, and wore lace, gold chains and ringlets all his life; but in his youth decorative male dress was not quite dead, and by the time it was, he was well-known enough to please himself. Other flamboyant dressers were Balzac, Dickens, Offenbach, Turgenev and Wagner, who liked pink silk dressing-gowns with long sashes, and his patron "Mad" Ludwig II, King of Bavaria: a king could do as he pleased and eccentricity is tolerated in artists.

The Aesthetic Movement of the late nineteenth century sought to make beauty a reality in everyday life by extending the artist's care for it to the design of all objects, including both men's and women's clothes. It was ridiculed, and such influence as it had on mainstream fashion applied much more to women than men. One historian wrote of its decline: "The experimentation with boundaries and gender through aesthetic fashion that existed in the 1870s and 1880s for both men and women was over" when women moved "into the 'male' sphere of sports, higher education, and the professions."[39]

In 1881 Jerome K. Jerome's *Idle Thoughts of an Idle Fellow* drew an analogy between modern dress and old age: "We have been through the infant period of humanity when we used to run about with nothing on but a long, loose robe, and liked to have our feet bare . . . after that, the world grew into a young man, and became foppish . . . we are more sensible in this age . . . I wish, though, it were not so, and that one could be good, and respectable, and sensible without making oneself a guy . . . Why should we all try to look like ants crawling over a dust-heap? . . . Very young men think a good deal about clothes, but they don't talk about them to each other. They would not find much encouragement. A fop is not a favourite with his own sex." He still isn't, as one can see from agony columns: one teenage boy wrote that his parents kept telling him his spots didn't matter because he was male. Anna Ford notes in her book of interviews, *Men*: "Some men denied the importance of their looks and clothes entirely, although I fear they were not without a certain vanity. That is not a criticism, but it made me wonder why men, particularly those of the old school, are rather ashamed to admit that they have thought about their appearance . . . I use the word 'vanity' because these particular men so often chose their clothes with an attention to colour, arrangement and material that could not have been achieved without some thought."[40] Some men hate their natural looks as much as any woman. One was Edward Lear, whose light verse so often mentions noses and who always drew himself with a small one although, or rather because, his was large; another was the eighteenth-century painter Richard Wilson, known as Red-Nosed Dick, who used to pull his hat so far over his eyes that he had to pay small boys to see him across the road.

Various attempts to loosen male dress codes have been made since the Second World War, but they were almost entirely confined to youth culture, having little influence beyond it, and they were even less unisex than the Aesthetic Movement. The Teds, Mods and Rockers all stressed masculinity, and though the hippies (whose dress was most like that of the Pre-Raphaelites) nominally rejected it, they did not abandon sexism, as autobiographies of feminist ex-hippies show. From the sixties onwards, men's casual clothing has become slightly more colourful, and some kinds of jewellery (hair clips and bands, for instance) and cosmetics more acceptable, but on the whole Quentin Bell's summing-up of the nineteenth century's influence in *On Human Finery* (1976) still holds:

> Look at those sober hard-working men in their sober hard-working clothes, with never a hint of prettiness or provocation, colour, carnality or caprice; the body sufficiently liberated for the pursuit of business but in no way displayed, the hair, as the century progressed, shortened to almost penal brevity above, trimmed to luxuriant but masculine ferocity below . . . It was felt to be right and proper that men should form a sober black and white background to the various, lustrous and many-coloured ladies, that woman should submit to the bondage of her stay maker, display her neck, her arms

and an appetising portion of her bosoms to the public, spend in one year on dress that which her husband would spend in twenty, and embark on twenty changes of fashion while he had barely completed one . . . And while the first brave effort at emancipation, the 'divided skirt', was greeted with unkind derision, the merest hint of femininity in a man's wardrobe was regarded with deep visceral aversion. Even today, after twenty years of permissive innovation, older people, at all events, are still shocked by long curls, cosmetics, bracelets or necklaces on a man, so thoroughly have we been indoctrinated with the belief that it is only women who should, in a direct sense, be consumers.[41]

Nearly thirty years later, "masculinity" is almost incompatible with skirts (celebrities like David Beckham occasionally wear them), or anything which suggests its maker put aesthetics first. Designers and wearers of fashionable clothes for men try to combine visual appeal with pretending they don't care about it, which cancels itself out. Scent for men is called "aftershave", though putting it on freshly shaved skin must hurt, with tough-sounding "manly" names (one had a cardboard padlock on every bottle and the slogan "Tame it's not!"). Men have started using skin care products, but many are allegedly so embarrassed that they send women to buy them; I only once saw a man at a make-up counter, and he felt it necessary to tell the saleswoman, "I'm NOT gay!" "So why not put boys in pretty dresses for parties, with ribbons in their hair?" asks Polly Toynbee. "The fact that to subject a boy to such ridicule would be a bizarre cruelty shows how deeply and fundamentally differently we still view boys."[42] It is cruel to make boys imitate girls, but not the other way round, because conventional wisdom still says, in Letty Cottin Pogrebin's phrase, "Boys Are Better."[43] Some boys know what they are missing, however. Angela Phillips in *The Trouble with Boys* quotes a mother who "told me rather sadly: 'He loves pretty things but knows they are not for him. He sublimates his own desire to dress up and takes a great interest in what I wear . . . for a boy, pretty is what you look at, not what you are.'"[44]

So women are still under pressure to be aesthetic for two, as well as domestic for two, while men are under even greater pressure to pretend they don't care even when they do (a man who paints his face is condemned far more than a woman who doesn't paint hers) and wear clothes which look practical even when they are not. Laver wrote of the late-Victorian "New Woman"'s stiff collar: "She adopted . . . the one element of male attire which did not help her in the least."[45] Pseudo-utilitarianism isn't dead; the tie, still "throttling you all your life for no reason"[46] as Santayana wrote in 1936, proves this, though unlike Brummell's cravat it no longer takes a whole morning to arrange. Its colour and pattern, being among conventionally dressed men's few signs of individuality, are highly important to some of them: Minna Thornton told me floral ties in the sixties were considered revolutionary.

Elizabeth Hawes, an American designer, published a book in 1939 advocating reforms which would free men from collars, ties and excessively heavy clothes.[47] Every hot summer brings letters to the press from men forced to wear jackets when women's arms are bare. Safari suits exist but men hesitate to wear them, so, as one writer to *The Times* pointed out, air-conditioning in hot climates is boosted, wasting energy and making the air outside even hotter, so that men can wear hot clothes. One African High Commissioner wore an open-necked shirt at the Travellers' Club in London, which allowed the removal of jackets for the first time in 1995; he said he had worn it when presenting his credentials to the Queen because it was his national dress, and she commented on its practicality.

Businesswomen are expected to wear similar suits to men, but with skirts; trousers are frowned on, but so is the "femininity" of bright colours, decoration or obvious cosmetics.[48] Both sexes in conservative circles must keep their hair tidy, men must cut it short. (Some extreme Protestant sects still insist on long hair in women, and in 1988 a Missouri woman was refused custody of her children because of her "un-Christian" bob.) The Rev. Jerry Falwell, former head of the American Moral Majority, banned long hair on men at Liberty College, Massachusetts, of which he was President, though he must know the story of Samson; Bob Jones University, South Carolina, which awarded Falwell a doctorate, also bans beards and moustaches (though Jesus Christ is bearded in most pictures), short skirts and inter-racial dating, but not nail varnish.[49] An American Mormon recalls that in Brigham Young University in the sixties, a "strict dress code still forbade miniskirts anywhere on campus and mandated that young women could not wear slacks of any kind to classes . . . young men . . . were brutally barbered and clean-shaven . . . And in an era when much of the university-aged world had embraced a concept of beauty that relied on the mixed blessings of nature, my new sisters and I were swabbed with a quantity of makeup that would have camouflaged burn victims."[50] In Afghanistan, the Taliban, who made beards and short hair on men compulsory, punished users of cosmetics with beatings, and those who wore nail varnish risked having the tops of their thumbs cut off.

What can a boy who cares about dress do, except pretend not to? He may be able to find some excuse for historic costume; uniforms make an excellent one. He can always say he only wears the clothes because he belongs to the group, even if he joined the group to wear the clothes. It is someone else's responsibility, and he doesn't lose masculine status. Sir Philip Gibbs wrote of his youth at the end of the nineteenth century that "there was an epidemic of pageants . . . It was, I believe, due to a national craving for colour and pageantry after the drabness of the Victorian era. It was also an extension of the childish instinct for 'dressing up', and young men, limited in their wardrobes to black and grey and tubular trousers and felt hats or top hats, enjoyed themselves in the costumes of the Elizabethan days, or in the splendid foppery of the Plantagenets, or the white wigs and knee-breeches of Dick Sheridan's time."[51] Marie Corelli wrote in *Ziska* (1897), before trouser creases came in, that men had legs like elephants.

It is said that when the American feminist lawyer Florynce Kennedy was rebuked by a judge for her trousers, she pointed to his robes and said that if he would overlook what she was wearing, she would overlook what he was wearing. No modern reform has abolished ecclesiastical robes, though they have been simplified; the Italian word *sottana* means both a priest's robe and a petticoat. Virginia Woolf wrote of men in *Three Guineas*: "After the comparative simplicity of your dress at home, the splendour of your public attire is dazzling . . . Not only are whole bodies of men dressed alike summer and winter – a strange characteristic to a sex which changes its clothes according to the season, and for reasons of private taste and comfort – but every button, rosette and stripe seems to have some symbolic meaning . . . the wearer is not to us a pleasing or an impressive spectacle. He is on the contrary a ridiculous, a barbarous, a displeasing spectacle."[52] (It can have serious consequences; when the First World War began, graduates from the French military academy at St Cyr allegedly went into battle wearing gloves.)

The American radical feminist Robin Morgan adds: "The costumes, uniforms, disguises, worn by men of the church and the military . . . *and* by men of the corporation, *and* by the hip-radical or the Yuppie, the biker or the chieftain"[53] are all forms of concealment, and has written in an earlier book: "Women . . . are fit to be the objects of gently patronizing ridicule or even direct scorn when, for instance, we wear the very cosmetics we are assured men demand – and which are relentlessly advertised and sold to us by men . . . When the Pict warriors painted their bodies blue . . . when the leftist student sported his blue denim shirt as a sign of solidarity with 'the working class,' . . . this is Serious Business . . . such a double standard . . . reflects – in fact it doubles – objective power."[54]

What should people wear? Saying "anything" isn't good enough: someone must decide how clothes are designed and made. Morgan's tone in these passages, unlike almost everything else in her books, would appear to endorse practicality at any price. She even seems to assume trousers are intrinsically better than skirts: in *The Anatomy of Freedom* she refers to the "religious transvestism" of male priests' and rabbis' "dresses". Letty Cottin Pogrebin's list of skirt-wearing men throughout history answers this. Elsewhere in these and other books, Morgan shows passionate enthusiasm for aesthetics; besides, she includes business and casual clothes in her indictment. Elizabeth Hawes suggested both robes and flared skirts, as well as "slack suits" and breeches, for men, and encouraged them to wear any colour they chose. Virginia Woolf didn't think the dress of a liberated future would be purely practical, as *Three Guineas* shows: "the outsiders [women] will dispense with pageantry not from any puritanical dislike of beauty. On the contrary, it will be one of their aims to increase private beauty . . . the beauty of flowers, silks, clothes".

In the meantime, men still have to shelter behind a set of rules and "symbolic meaning" to have an excuse to dress up, or they must persuade women to. As Jerome K. Jerome says in the essay quoted, "Women, at all events, ought to dress prettily. It is their duty . . . the world would be dull enough without their pretty dresses and fair faces." Is it surprising that when boys like the one mentioned by Angela Phillips grow up, they try to enforce this, if necessary by taking over the job of designing women's clothes? Uniforms don't offer the same opportunities, since by definition they are designed once and for all. The first male couturier, Charles Frederick Worth, was born in 1825, beginning his career just at the time of the "great renunciation." A final quotation from Carol Lee: "For the enemies of beauty in its many forms – whether physical, artistic, or emotional – are those who have given away beauty."[55]

So much for the stereotypes of the elegant, useless woman and the sternly practical man. In the strict as well as the slang sense of the word, they are myths. Here are some older ones: Narcissus was male, and so were the Ugly Duckling and the Beast who married Beauty.

4

TWO KINDS OF FREEDOM

Servility creates despotism.

Charlotte Brontë   The Professor

He who goes against the fashion is himself its slave.

Logan Pearsall Smith   All Trivia

I've no desire to be ill-dressed; but I hate the feeling that I daren't be ill-dressed if I want to.

John Braine   Room at the Top

Freedom is indivisible, and either we are working for freedom or you are working for the sake of your self-interest and I am working for mine.

June Jordan

Throughout history freedom fighters have replaced one tyranny with another. Robin Morgan noted in *The Demon Lover* that the literal meaning of the word "revolution", which it still has when used as a technological term, is going round in circles. Feminists have tried to escape this trap; did they succeed?

If the same word were used for both love and hate, it would hardly be more ambiguous than the word "freedom". It has two mutually exclusive meanings: freedom of choice and freedom from it.

In terms of clothes, the perfect example of freedom from choice is uniform. Even an elaborate and uncomfortable one saves its wearers from worry about what to put on. Its principal drawback was pointed out by Juvenal in the phrase *Quis custodiet ipsos custodes?*, usually translated as "Who watches the watchdogs?" If uniform is to be worn, someone has to decide what it will be, and all wearers may not like it.

This applies to any task: delegate it to others and you put yourself in their power, do it yourself and you have all the responsibility and all the work. Birth control is a well-known example: every time the possibility of a pill for men arises, somebody says "Can you trust them to take it?"

For nearly two hundred years men have been enjoying the freedom conferred by delegating the task of dressing decoratively to women, and the lack of power doesn't seem to worry them much. Why? Because fashion is a luxury. It saves them trouble to ignore it, and if we do likewise, they won't lose anything they need for survival. They can always withdraw from us or grumble about our lack of personal attractions. At the same time, they have been protected by a rigid convention making it impossible for us to say, "All right, let's see you do better!"

These are real advantages, but negative ones. They appeal principally to people with no interest in the subject, which is exactly what men are supposed to be. What is more, to such people the possibility of having to wear something you dislike isn't serious, since what you wear doesn't matter. Only for those to whom it does matter is lack of choice potentially important.

One of the arguments levelled against fashion, and not only by feminists, is that it restricts women's choice. "Tyranny" is a word frequently used, by "Censor" for instance. Feminist books for teenagers are full of denunciations like those of Joyce Nicholson: "make-up . . . makes all girls look alike, all painted to the fashionable pattern",[1] and Carol Adams and Rae Lauriekitis: "Girls often say that one good thing about being female is being able to dress how they like and to wear nice clothes. But is it really? What it means is that . . . you have to follow the latest fashion craze . . . it must be the look of the moment, with all the right accessories to go with it."[2] All this sounds like an argument for more choice, not less. That would certainly be consistent with feminist attitudes to other aspects of life, from sex to work. But what was their solution? Susan Bassnett's analogy is telling: "for a time in the 1970s, dungarees, laced boots and short-cropped hair were every bit as emblematic of a group identity as the old serviceman's tie and blazer".[3] This she found truer of Britain than of the other countries she examined (the former East Germany, Italy and the United States). Is this "uniform" so superior to any other form of dress that no-one, given freedom of choice, would ever choose anything else?

Some feminists would argue that it is, but there is another explanation: in Elizabeth Janeway's words, "It is easier for each side to do the opposite of what was done before than to create something new."[4] Easier because it is always tempting to defy orders, easier because it proves one's identity as a rebel, easier because it saves thinking and in this instance, easier physically. Any uniform saves trouble and this one was simple, cutting out jewellery, cosmetics, all grooming not essential for hygiene, seasonal changes and dressing differently for different occasions. What would feminists have done if, instead of being the adorned sex, theirs had traditionally been the unadorned one? Adornment had become associated exclusively with women, so it was bound to be attacked when women rebelled not just against the current definition of women's *rôle*, but the whole idea of any such definition; no wonder, to quote the opening words of Evans and Thornton's *Women & Fashion*, "In the early years of the Women's Liberation Movement, the entire package of fashion was condemned by feminists. Liberation meant breaking out of the straitjacket of a controlled femininity. Dress, fashion and cosmetics were considered to be trivialities which functioned ideologically to construct a false femininity. Femininity was something that women had been forced to apply, to dress up in; liberation and the search for an authentic self meant taking it off, getting out of it."[5] And into what? Another straitjacket.

Pressure to adopt the old one took the form not so much of ordering women to dress fashionably (as Monica Dickens wrote in her *Woman's Own* column in about 1957, "The dress shops do not stand over us with a gun") as trying to prevent them realising that it was possible not to. This is how "brainwashing" really works. Gloria Steinem explains why *Ms.*, the magazine she and later Robin Morgan edited, stopped carrying advertisements: the advertisers wanted to dictate the editorial policy. Maidenform would not allow their bras to be advertised next to anything relating to "illness, disillusionment, large size fashion, etc."; Procter & Gamble's products "were not to be placed in *any* issue that included *any* material on gun control, abortion, the occult, cults, or the disparagement of religion. Caution was also demanded in any issue that included articles on sex or drugs, even for educational purposes . . . There had to be an overall 'look' compatible with beauty and fashion ads." This excludes

> women who are not young, not thin, not conventionally pretty, well-to-do, able-bodied, or heterosexual . . .We hear that women in the (then) Soviet Union have been producing feminist samizdat (underground, self-published books) and circulating them throughout the country . . . four of the main organizers have been exiled . . . and so are free to talk for the first time. Though *Ms.* is operating on its usual shoestring, we solicit contributions for plane fare and send Robin Morgan to interview them in Vienna.

The result is an exclusive cover story; a rare grassroots, bottom-up view of Russian life in general and the lives of Russian women in particular. The interview also includes the first news of a populist peace movement against the Soviet occupation of Afghanistan, and prediction of *glasnost* to come . . . The story wins a Front Page award.

Nonetheless, this journalistic coup undermines years of hard work trying to get an ad schedule from Revlon. Why? Because the Soviet women on our cover *are not wearing makeup*.[6]

They might have been only too glad to. Sir Reader Bullard, a former British Ambassador to Moscow, wrote: "In the early days after the revolution many highly placed communists were deliberately careless about their clothes, and even went about looking dirty. This had its good side: university dons, who were miserably paid and had few privileges, could wear without loss of dignity clothes that were worn, ill-fitting and patched . . . The bad side was the hostility sometimes shown to the better dressed. It was almost dangerous to be smart in appearance, and a woman wearing a hat ran the risk of being called a lady to her face."[7] In Nikolai Ostrovsky's novel of the revolution, *How the Steel Was Tempered*, the hero's girlfriend reveals the "cheap individualism" which leads to their break-up by dressing up for a Komsomol meeting.[8] In 1990, Francine du Plessix Gray wrote of asking a floor attendant in a Georgian hotel why Soviet women showed such enthusiasm for fashion: "To heighten their self-esteem? To be more seductive to men? . . . 'For *men*! Do you think they ever get out of their selfish little brains to *notice* what we wear? . . . life is black, and this is one of the few inner joys I can buy. And the girls at work – *they* will be so impressed." The author was "amazed and appalled, at first, that highly educated women should dedicate so many hours of the day to what many of us look on as frivolous trifles; awed, after the first few weeks, when it becomes clear that their obsession with an impeccable, attractive appearance has little or nothing to do with narcissism but is more akin to the compulsive grooming instinct of a healthy cat or bird, and may be the only way of brightening the uniform drabness of Soviet life." A Siberian designer told her that "for decades . . . a person wearing a bright-green skirt to the office, or say, an imaginative homemade hat, was singled out for reprimand, could even be sent to prison for unorthodox dress."[9]

In China during the Cultural Revolution all adults wore uniform; cosmetics were outlawed (this is not too strong a word[10]) but even then, Paul Theroux was told, "the women workers showed up at their factories with bright sweaters and frilly blouses under their blue baggy suits; it was customary to meet in the women's washroom and compare the hidden sweaters before they started work."[11] When I visited China in 1975, my female guide asked me about Western fashions; women have tried hard to follow them in post-Ceausescu Romania and, according to Slavenka Drakulić, Croatia:

> the communist ideal was a robust woman who didn't look much different from a man. A nicely dressed woman was subject to suspicion, sometimes even investigation . . .
>
> But aesthetics turned out to be a complex question that couldn't be answered by a simple state decree. By abolishing one kind of so called 'bourgeois' aesthetic, not with a plan . . . but more as the natural result of ideology, the state created another aesthetic, a totalitarian one. Without a choice of cosmetics and clothes, with bad food and hard work and no spare time, it wasn't at all hard to create the special kind of uniformity that comes out of an equal distribution of poverty and neglect of people's real needs. There was no chance for individualism – for women or men . . . To avoid uniformity, you have to work very hard . . . [Women] are over-dressed, they put on too much make-up, they match colours and textures badly . . . But where could they learn anything about a self-image, a style? In the party-controlled magazines for women, where they are instructed to be good workers and party members first, then mothers, housewives, and sex objects next, – never themselves? To be yourself, to cultivate individualism, to perceive yourself as an individual in a mass society is dangerous. You might become living proof that the system is failing. Make-up and fashion are crucial because they are political.[12]

Just what feminists in capitalist countries were saying, with the opposite result.

The "uniform" Susan Bassnett describes seems suspiciously like a hangover from a male ideology which only pays lip-service to feminism, and even its practicality is more apparent than real. Elizabeth Wilson writes of dungarees: "the contortions necessary in the lavatory, and the discomfort in cold weather of having to undress completely in order to relieve oneself, should prove conclusively that this form of dress is worn not to promote rational apparel, but to announce the wearer's feminism in public."[13] Boots can also be uncomfortable in hot weather; and I can't help being reminded of the "New Woman's" starched collar.

There was also what Nicci Gerrard called "the shaved-leg debate, worrying about wearing clothes that give out the 'right' message".[14] What debate? Why shouldn't women shave if they wish and not if they don't? Apparently it's not so simple. Robin Morgan, after she "rediscovered" the coolness of skirts, notes that "I, who stopped shaving my legs and armpits in my mid-twenties (Feminist Enlightenment, remember?) recently began to shave them again. I'm not even that certain *why*: part of the generalized celebration in being slender and feeling limber? the resurrection of the ultra-Right flesh-loathing fundamentalists in my own pores? the Domino Theory (aha! heels lead to skirts lead to shaving . . .) a cranky affirmation of what *I* and *not* some Central Feminist Committee wanted to do for a change? or an exhausted capitulation to the internalized standard of Woman implanted in me so long ago when I first was born into the patriarchy and which has been reinforced daily ever since?"[15] When I told Minna Thornton I found skirts comfortable, she mentioned the same problem, which she and Caroline Evans describe: "the question of depilation raged . . . What could be more of a capitulation to arbitrary male tastes? Bodily hair of any sort is associated with sexual power in Western iconography; its removal then amounted to submission. Somehow the problem had not been solved if you did not shave your legs but always wore trousers."[16]

Why not? First, there is nothing liberated about wearing trousers when, for whatever reason, you would rather wear a skirt. Secondly, if the link between hair and power is false, so is the link between shaving and submission and it need not concern us. Thirdly, if male tastes are arbitrary, going out of our way not to submit to them is letting ourselves be ruled by them just as much as "capitulating" by shaving hair or dyeing it (a compromise some feminists adopted including, allegedly, Susan Brownmiller). In Sara Maitland's novel *Daughter of Jerusalem*, the heroine's doctor blames her feminism for her infertility. His other female patients show their admiration for him by dressing up to go to his surgery; she insists on wearing jeans, a donkey jacket and a T-shirt with the slogan "I Am a Humourless Feminist", and is not pleased when her husband points out that this is just another way of dressing up for him.[17] Finally, what is liberated about worrying about whether you are "giving out the 'right' message?" An advertisement for a cosmetic surgery clinic asks, "Do you reflect the right image?" and "image" is the right word for the difference between the two. The new fear reflects the old one like a mirror.

Kathy Davis treats this particular aspect of beauty culture in *Reshaping the Female Body: The Dilemma of Cosmetic Surgery*.[18] She began by assuming that no-one would ever undergo it except as the result of social pressure, and it is easy to see why: for example, breast augmentation has a forty percent failure rate, and one woman she interviewed had permanently damaged health as a result of eighteen unsuccessful operations. A large majority of applicants for surgery were women, many of whom complained that they had not been given the full facts about side-effects (and also that the surgeons ignored their wishes as to the precise changes they wanted made) and were indignant about this, but many said they would have gone ahead even if they had known. Davis's field of research was The Netherlands, where cosmetic surgery is available at public expense, but moves have recently been made to restrict it because of increased demand. Doctors were therefore obliged to assess which applicants really needed it, and found it all but impossible to establish criteria. "Here," says Davis, "it is the patient who knows what's wrong and the surgeon who often has a hard time seeing it", and she considered all the applicants she saw looked normal or even attractive except for one "man with a cauliflower nose". Women, she insists, don't have surgery to look more beautiful but just to look normal. A woman who already does so may think she doesn't: "The fact that our evaluations did not match did not make her suffering any less tangible."

She deduces that the cliché that beauty is in the eye of the beholder is true; one can, however, take issue with this. It may not be so much the idea of what beauty is that varies, as the importance which a given person attaches to it, just as two people may agree that a certain house is ugly, but one may regard having to remain in it as a real misfortune, while the other says "So what, provided it's comfortable and weatherproof?" Also, a woman who says she wants to look "normal" rather than "beautiful" isn't saying she's uninterested in beauty, but that she only feels the need for an average, rather than ideal, amount of it. There may be another reason which Davis herself suggests: "that their disclaimers merely reflect the discourses of Dutch Calvinism – discourses which make excessive vanity reprehensible, at best, and sinful, at worst. In The Netherlands, it is difficult to admit to having cosmetic surgery at all. How, then, could a woman possibly justify going to such lengths for something as trivial and ignoble as beauty?" (Their country produced the Concertgebouw Orchestra and many of the world's most famous painters.) It seems to me at least possible that these women were exaggerating the abnormality of their looks because it was the only way to get their problems taken seriously, and that in doing so they had convinced themselves. It takes courage to admit that the standard of beauty which is supposed to be adequate, and appears to be so for most of the people you know, is not so for you, because you run the risk of being accused of thinking yourself too good for them. Small wonder if some seekers after beauty disguise their feelings even from themselves.

She reports that many patients had faced opposition from their friends and families, and quotes comments such as: "You're married, you have a husband, children, why do you want something like that now? You don't have to look good any more." (This seems to me exactly like saying, "You've passed your exams so you no longer need to be well-read.") They felt they were acting in accordance with feminist principles: making their own decisions, standing up for their rights. Her own opinion is that women are under such pressure to conform that it may not be possible to take this at face value: "Choice presupposes that the individual has viable options to choose from." She quotes another writer, Kathryn Morgan, who concludes that these women must have been "coerced" into having surgery and who, unlike Davis, has based her research not on patients' own accounts but on the reports in women's magazines, which have been rewritten according to editorial policy. When both writers spoke at a conference on the subject, however, Davis was met with "rows and rows of faces with blank expressions and . . . the low rumble of whispered comments . . . I watched my plea for a feminist approach which took the needs of the recipients into consideration disappear unheeded and unheralded and there I stood . . . a feminist scholar of tarnished alloy" whereas Morgan was met with "a palpable sense of *this-is-more-like-it* in the air". The speaker whose research was based on first-hand testimonials was ignored in favour of the one whose research was not, because she told the conference what the participants wanted to hear. We shall not discover the truth like that.

Davis concludes: "we simply cannot afford the comfort of the correct line", which brings us to political correctness. Nobody seems sure how the term originated, but the most likely explanation is that it was invented as a parody of a certain rigidity of attitude in the political left. It has since become a political football. Opponents of sexual and racial equality use it as an insult, and many people wish us to believe it is only an insult. Gloria Steinem quotes Robin Morgan's suggestion that the initials ought to stand for "Plain Courtesy".[19] Unfortunately, it isn't quite so simple, because others have produced evidence that they might stand for "Philistine Coercion."

They claim that it is now mandatory to reject the traditional scale of cultural values, that it is now "incorrect" to have traditional or even any ideas of artistic merit or beauty, including dress. Allegedly this is in the name of opposing élitism, a word which according to Milan Kundera was coined in 1967. The idea behind it is that the notion of an élite, tradition-ally regarded as desirable and even essential, is an evil to be eradicated. Kundera pointed out that nobody wanted to abolish an administrative élite, but in art and culture the idea became suspect.

Confusingly, there are two ways of challenging traditional values, and "anti-élitism" is used for both. They are less diametrically opposed than the two definitions of freedom, but still incompatible. One is relativism, the idea that no form of culture can be seen as "better" than another, and the other is actual hostility to what is loosely described as "high art", not only denying it a higher status but giving it a lower one. I shall call them PC Mark 1 and PC Mark 2; and according to the process we have already observed, as soon as the first becomes current there is a temptation to adopt the second, because it's the line of least resistance: popular culture is more accessible physically (because it surrounds us), intellectually and sometimes financially, so, other things being equal (and the PC Mark 1 principle is that they are) it will inevitably take over. Levelling down is easier than level-ling up. This appeals to people, of whatever political complexion, who have always disliked anything they think of as "highbrow" and are delighted to have an intellectually respectable reason for being anti-intellectual. Freedom not to prefer the high becomes an obligation to prefer the low, then to reject the high altogether, which logically leads to its abolition: not just a new hierarchy, but a new monopoly.

We already saw in chapter 1 that this attitude exists; the question is how far it has become identified, not just with left-wing politics, but with oppo-sition to racial and sexual prejudice. Traditional opinion was not only that some aesthetic experiences were better than others, but that women's art was generally inferior to men's art, and women to men. Similar beliefs were held about race. There is therefore a tendency for reaction against the second and third of these beliefs, which is implicit in the idea of sex and race equality, to lead to automatic reaction against the first, which is not. It is perfectly possible to deny that "only a white man could have written Shakespeare" without denying that Shakespeare was a better writer than most others. Political correctness, however, is supposed to mean that one must deny it, either by saying that the word "better" is meaningless, or that the fact of Shakespeare being a DWEM (dead white European male) makes him a worse one.

If cultural hierarchies are meaningless, how can one writer be worse than another? To speak in these terms is creating a new hierarchy, with a new élite at its head. The supporters of PC Mark 2 say the type of art represented by Shakespeare, Michelangelo, Beethoven and their kind is by its very nature acceptable only to a privileged class of the sort which ought not to exist, and thus incompatible with equality and democracy. (Just to make confusion worse confounded, there is some doubt as to whether this vaguely-defined group is bourgeois, aristocratic or what; hence the label "bourgeois art" given to the work of artists who, ever since the Romantic Movement, have regarded "bourgeois" as an insult , and the habit of using "middle class" to mean both "middle" and "upper". I have seen it used of the women who buy *haute couture* in Paris, of whom only a few hundred exist; if they are in the middle, who, at least in economic terms, is above them?) As Slavenka Drakulić said of the Communists, "aesthetics were considered a superficial, 'bourgeois' invention." This is the anti-intellectuals' line, as can be seen from two accounts taken from *The Independent* on the same day. Nicholas Kenyon, Controller of BBC Radio 3, defends himself against accusations of "dumbing down" with the words: "Radio 3 is élitist, and so it should continue to be; it would not have survived nearly 50 years as the envy of the world if it were not . . . Elitist must never mean exclusive." A few pages earlier, Kenan Malik writes of criticism (from both Labour and Conservative politicans) of lottery money being awarded to the Royal Opera House and Sadler's Wells: "Opera and ballet, apparently, are élitist arts that are of interest only to toffs who can afford to pay for their own entertainment. Lottery money should go to things that are of genuine interest to ordinary punters – such as bingo halls, according to [Terry] Dicks. But what could be more élitist than the argument that high art and ordinary people don't mix, and that working-class people would prefer bingo halls to opera houses? . . . a performance at Covent Garden or Sadler's Wells need cost no more than a ticket to a premiership football match. Try telling a supporter outside Anfield or Old Trafford on a Saturday afternoon that they are being extravagant."[20]

Fashion too, at least at "high" as opposed to "street" level, can be described as élitist; it certainly imposes a hierarchy of taste, if only a temporary one. Therefore, though fashion-lovers would not necessarily have anything to fear from PC Mark 1, and logically should not (if anything is acceptable, smart clothes must be) they have everything to fear from PC Mark 2. So is it true that it has become compulsory?

According to many of the left, certainly not. *The War of the Words*, a book of "for and against PC" essays edited by Sarah Dunant, contains statements from the pro-PC contributors such as: "Public opinion was swayed by stories like those about 'loony' councils banning black bin-liners (because they

were offensive to Blacks) . . . most of which were later proved to be false"
(Yasmin Alibhai-Brown) and "Forget about the tabloid scare-headline
fantasies about policing the language and erasing tradition from the canon.
I travel a lot, and teach in a lot of universities here and in the United States,
and I have yet to encounter one real life example of such bowdlerising or
crass strait-jacketing" (Lisa Jardine).[21]

I have unfortunately lost the reference, but I read in about 1998 that an
American university sacked a theatre teacher for refusing to "reinterpret"
several Shakespeare plays by changing their endings. A school official said
they were "works from a sexist European canon" and the theatre department
substituted *Betty the Yeti: An Eco-Fable*, about a logger becoming an envi-
ronmentalist after having sex with a sasquatch.[22] My father received this
letter from a friend on 18 March 1997:

> About two years ago, a good friend living in Vermont and having been a
> member of the state Library Board was forced to resign. He explained that
> it was because the public library of that state wanted to go 'modern', 'demo-
> cratic' and 'politically correct', which meant that they wanted to only keep
> on their shelves those books that have something 'relevant' to the lives of
> library users, and/or those books that have been taken out with certain
> frequency ('top ten best sellers', many of them about that ever popular
> American preoccupation: 'self-improvement').
>
> 'That meant, my dear,' my friend said to me shaking his head, 'they lit-
> erally threw out Shakespeare, Gibbon, Dickens, James . . . even the recently
> 'popular' writers such as Saki and Hemingway . . . and in their place went
> . . . Oh I don't even know the silly titles of some more recent and very pop-
> ular books . . . but you know, 'How to feel Okay about yourself' or
> 'Robocop' or 'My diary as an anorexic . . .'
>
> And I have put up a good fight on behalf of some great writers, fiction or
> otherwise, and I was so effective on my corner that even the old ladies (nowa-
> days all 'women's libbers') threw rotten tomatoes at me because Shakespeare,
> of course, was an anti-semite (Merchant of Venice) according to those silly
> people, and Hemingway was not sympathetic to women's causes . . . all polit-
> ically incorrect!

If this happens in public libraries it is almost more serious than if it
happens in universities, as they are the only source of literature for people
who can't afford higher education or even bookshops. Peter Vansittart
writes that, in America, "Lionel Trilling was perplexed when students told
him that, by teaching Jane Austen, he was assisting the Americans in
Vietnam", that British school editions of classics cut out not only words

judged to be sexist or racist but those that were simply unusual, and that "teachers were complaining of the tyranny of syntax . . . When an educational secretary demanded stricter attention to language, its precision, subtleties and literature, he was abused as *reactionary*."[23]

In 1984 the *New Statesman* printed an article by Alison Hennegan of the Women's Press, saying she had been told at a feminist conference that it was élitist to know classical Greek: not to refuse to translate it, just to know it (Victorian feminists were told it was unfeminine). British publishing, for economic reasons, is heavily influenced by America, and writers for children in particular report that books have been rejected for including references to ballet or riding lessons, and even to children going to the seaside or washing their hands before meals, on grounds of élitism; one article claims that children "must be clothed in a quasi-uniform of trainers, jeans and patterned jumpers".[24] (Sir Reader Bullard's parents, at the turn of the last century, managed to take their family to the seaside every year on an income of 35s. (£1.75) per week.[25]) The columnist Janet Daley reported that a school had stopped violin lessons because it was a "bourgeois instrument", and Simon Jenkins wrote of modern buildings in *The Sunday Times* on 15 November 1987: "Invisible access – real entrances were elitist – left people lost and confused." Who is supposed to benefit from not making it clear how to enter a building? I hope nobody applied the same theory to fire exits.

Vansittart's remarks on language suggest they might. People have been deprived of skills that are not just desirable but necessary. Lack of linguistic precision means not knowing which sounds or visual symbols mean what, which makes it difficult, and in the last resort impossible, to convey meaning. That is language's job. Carried to its logical conclusion, this reduces people to the level of babies screaming with frustration because nobody knows what they want. Jonathan Kozol, a black American teacher writing about "free" schools in places like Harlem, has attacked the "bad jargon and unexamined slogans" of teachers who belittle the importance of reading, resulting in "kids who just can't do a damn thing in the kinds of cities that we live in",[26] which simply widens the gap between poor and rich children. Even environmentalists, concerned with whether the earth is becoming incapable of supporting life, have had to defend themselves from attacks on class grounds. Anne Phillips writes: "I once heard a working-class woman complain at a Labour Party meeting about the way that concern for the environment was thought to be a middle-class fad. 'Don't *we* care whether our children see trees?'"[27]

Art is less vital than the environment, but the question I asked in chapter 2 remains: should the élite's culture be made available to all or scrapped? The latter would seem illiberal even to people with no interest in it, but calling it "irrelevant" does what banning couldn't: it makes the narrowing of options look democratic. This destroys democracy's essence, defined by Michael Foot as giving people a choice: of course violins and ballet will be "bourgeois" if only the privately educated know about them. An education which ignores them is as limiting as textbooks where all the girls are gentle and all the boys tough; just another stereotype and a self-fulfilling prophecy, because it produces people to whom it won't occur to use subsidised access to the arts, leading to calls to cut the subsidy, which makes them truly inaccessible or even extinct. Similarly, clothes other than jeans and jumpers will become uneconomic to make in large quantities if they don't sell, thus forcing up the price until ordinary, perhaps all, people are unable to buy them. Jonathan Kozol, in *Free Schools*, asked the same question as Elizabeth Wilson in *Adorned in Dreams*: why, among people supposedly "doing their own thing", did everybody do the same kind of thing? He answered: "Children can only 'choose' what they see *as* choices; people can only 'opt' for what they see *as* options. Children will never ask spontaneously to learn of things which they have never heard of."

Naomi Wolf describes a "senior seminar of women's studies majors . . . One woman charged that I was too elitist – I had used compound sentences [in her book *The Beauty Myth*] . . . Isn't the act of writing a book, asked a young woman accusingly, exclusionary to women who cannot read?"

When she met "some of the same undergraduates" informally, they were able

> to talk about their real concerns . . . safe from the arbitration of peer pressure . . . Tutored into an arid rhetoric of political self-righteousness, and shaken by the pedagogical mood that turned intellectual inquiry into a grim battle over who would get to make the rules for everyone else under the flimsy banner of 'consensus', they seemed to me to have formed a carapace as uncomfortable and unproductive as the intellectual machismo that had been fashionable when I was in college . . . The only difference was that the boxed-in decision about what women should do and think was under *their* control, rather than under the control of men. The undergraduates seemed to have little understanding that true radicalism in education is a woman who is thinking under nobody's control, and reaching no one's conclusions but her own . . . A collective mentality can be just as authoritarian as the 'authority' of Western and Masculine Truth that deconstructionist inquiry has attempted to unseat.[28]

This doesn't only apply to aesthetics. In the sixties, the Oxford branch of the Revolutionary Socialist Students' Federation had a slogan: "Absolute Control By All." In practice, an ex-member wrote to the undergraduate magazine *Isis*, this meant absolute control by seven unelected people who shouted down everyone who disagreed with them. Maybe they were men, but feminist collectives, wrote *Everywoman* in May 1993 about the closure of another feminist magazine, *Spare Rib*, "are easily hijacked by powerful personalities, allow their members to evade personal responsibility and lack structures to deal with disputes." Unresolved conflicts caused the end of national feminist conferences in the seventies. Barbara Grizzuti Harrison describes a consciousness-raising group whose rules against criticism led to something very like old-fashioned "feminine" spitefulness: "Direct confrontations were not allowed; but nothing prevented us from rehashing offenses with our intimates . . . One woman wanted to gag me . . . The rules didn't allow her verbally to tell me . . . so she rolled her eyes, cracked her knuckles, flung herself around in her chair . . . I felt as if I were being punished."[29] This could be straight out of Steele's play *The Lying Lover: or, the Ladies' Friendship* (1704) in which "friends" try to make each other look ugly. A feminist architect I met said: "A collective is a place where it takes you two years to find out who the boss is."

Rosie Boycott, one of *Spare Rib*'s founders, wrote that when it was launched in 1972 she argued with her colleague Marsha Rowe:

> "I wear make-up, so do you, and I buy clothes, and I like them, and I like parties and I like men, and you like all these things too . . . you can't pretend that they don't exist."
>
> "Oh, go and work for *Vogue* then."

When it became a collective "the items of lighter interest . . . were usually dropped for the more serious stuff, which stood up to the feminist critique. The cookery, fashion, beauty were phased out . . .. [The first issue had a feature on jeans and one on skin care.] . . . Though politically more correct the magazine was undeniably duller . . .There was a leaden feel to the pages."[30] One contributor, Eileen Fairweather, said decisions were made according to a "hierarchy of oppression" but according to another, it was the least privileged who had the lighter interests: "'we were . . . trying to transform a white middle-class readership into broad-based internationalist revolutionaries. So they recruited people like me, to broaden their appeal to black women, then watched in horror as I trotted around in full make-

up and cute little clothes' . . . Inevitably, it was those cute little clothes –
and what they were deemed to represent – that became a central focus for
all this aggro."[31] Leah Fritz mentions groups in which "every written piece
was put together collectively – sentence by sentence. This tedious method
led inevitably to tedious results, but many of the participants insisted they
were setting new 'collective' standards of beauty!"[32]

Marcia Cohen's book *The Sisterhood* describes a Congress to Unite
Women held in 1970, including an event at which women had their hair
publicly cut and "there seemed to be pressure for everyone to submit to the
ritual. Rumblings could be heard, a few shaky objections were percolating.
The beautiful actress Anselma dell'Olio [also a feminist writer] stood up
with tears in her eyes, her long chestnut hair flowing like velvet over her
shoulders. Her hair, she explained tremulously, was essential to her career,
her means of surviving." Not long after this, *No More Fun and Games*
exhorted women "to chop their hair short because it was long only for male
pleasure, not their own." In the same year Susan Brownmiller was asked to
review a play by a feminist writer, Myrna Lamb:

> Once before . . . Susan had reviewed – unfavorably – one of Lamb's plays, and
> the flak ('How can you do this to a sister?') had been more than she bargained
> for . . . The new play was, in her opinion, no better than the last.
>
> 'It was just,' Susan would remember, 'god-awful theater.'
>
> Which is what, according to the most basic standards of journalistic
> integrity, she should have and normally *would have* – written.
>
> But for the first time . . . a higher priority loomed. Susan fudged . . . forcing
> herself to hammer out a critique of a sister's work that was far kinder than
> she believed it deserved.

Much good it did her. She was publicly condemned at a feminist meeting
for having dared to speak for feminism as a whole by writing an article about
it: this was "élitism." Her boyfriend

> 'understood . . . He gave me a Vonnegut short story to read. It was a sort of
> Orwellian piece about a society after the revolution where everyone was being
> equalized. The dancers who were too graceful were forced to wear weights
> on their legs and the smart people had to wear a headset that scrambled their
> brains . . .'
>
> Yet crazy as it was – nutty, bizarre – she would endure, Susan concluded.
> This movement was that important.
>
> In the months to come, in fact, she even capitulated to that 'elitist'
> notion.[33]

More important than the difference between truth, if only a personal truth, and falsehood? We shall only be freed for telling lies, and lies won't liberate us. (In Elizabeth Wilson's novel *Prisons of Glass*, it was "a secret never to be admitted: that you could envy another woman's beauty, or even admit that some were more beautiful than others".)[34] Many people believe there are no objective standards in aesthetics, but that is no reason for denying subjective ones. I have seen rubber stamps on sale saying "Passed for political correctness" and others saying "I am a feminist because I object to people telling me what's right"; the two are incompatible. "One may discover integrity in the companionship of others," writes Andrea Dworkin, "but one does not ever discover integrity by bowing to the demands of peer pressure".[35] Ask yourself how happy you would have been to go to that Congress to Unite Women with long hair, make-up and the sort of clothes to which *No More Fun and Games* objected. Wouldn't it feel like trying to enjoy a glass of wine in a room full of disapproving teetotallers, and if so, wasn't it more of a Congress to Divide Women?

It was the fear of being divided that made people cave in, as Susan Brownmiller did. Being condemned by one's allies, or having to condemn them, is far more painful than even the worst insults from one's opponents. All they need do is create a hostile atmosphere. George Eliot wrote of Dorothea Brooke's younger sister, who did not share her disapproval of jewels: "There was a strong assumption of superiority in this Puritanic toleration, hardly less trying to the blond flesh of an unenthusiastic sister than a Puritanic persecution."

For a modern example, see Rose Shapiro's essay "Prisoner of Revlon": "The use of cosmetics is supposed to mean feminine vanity, but in fact it means precisely the opposite – the belief that your face is unattractive and even ugly, and money and time has to be spent in compensating for its inherent unpleasantness. Kept in thrall to that belief, women could never be liberated." But "the paint and powder have slowly crept back on to the faces of some of my friends. .. they recognise that the use of it does amount to a basic dissatisfaction with their own faces . . . but say that it helps them to cope in other ways . . . And some now say that make-up can be a creative form of self-expression, exactly the same as the choice of clothes . . . Punks are always given as an example of liberated use of make-up. They don't do it to look 'naturally beautiful', they do it to annoy, as a personal statement. But how many new wave-ettes would be seen with naked faces?"

(Punks and similar groups like crusties and moshers are certainly as conformist in their way as women in, say, tweeds and pearls in theirs; but so are some feminists. Not only is "doing it to annoy" others a form of dependence on them, but isn't it possible that some people join these groups because their friends do?) Shapiro contiues: "I know of no face that is actually improved by make-up . . . Women with make-up don't *look* better — they feel it . . . putting make-up back on our political agenda need not mean a crude rejection of it . . . It's not make-up itself but the ideas about what's underneath it that have got to change."[36] But what room do her ideas leave for wearing it, especially if you prefer "naturally beautiful" to deliberate outrage? "Cosmetics could and should be fun", wrote Kathy Myers in an article immediately following, but could you enjoy them in Shapiro's company? In practice people just give them up, inevitably strengthening the objectors' conviction that their enjoyment wasn't real: a self-fulfilling prophecy.

Breaking rules and incurring clearly defined penalties is much easier than defying intangible unpleasantness. Rules, however unjust, at least let us know where we are with them; in the totalitarian nightmare of Orwell's *Nineteen-Eighty-Four* there were officially no laws, which meant the Ministry of Love could arrest anyone for anything. I hope I have made it clear that PC can produce a state very close to this.

I have said that fashion suffers from lack of artistic status: it is condemned on the same socialist and anti-masculine grounds as high culture, but not seen as part of it or equally worthy of defence. Some feminists agree with Barbara Grizzuti Harrison's review of Adrienne Rich's *On Lies, Secrets and Silence*, which calls Matisse's chapel at Vence a monument to men's culture: "I do not wish to be told that Matisse, Michelangelo, Donne, Yeats, et al, do not belong to me because I am a woman. If what feminism says is that women are fully human, then Vence belongs to me as much as Jane Austen belongs to me and as much as Georgia O'Keeffe belongs to me."[37] Catherine Itzin, looking back on socialist struggles for "popular art forms and arts for the people", admits: "we (on the left) made some serious mistakes . . . wrongly we wanted to get rid of the old (high) art . . . the real problem has always been the hierarchy itself . . . The reality must be that there are different kinds of art and literature (culture), all of value and importance: a continuum or network (rather than a hierarchy) which *includes* (rather than excludes) Shakespeare and stand-up comedy . . . Excellence is not the issue, but who defines it."[38] I am not so sure; it is perfectly possible to admit the "value and importance" of several art forms but still consider that some have more than others, though the implications go far beyond the scope of this book. The question is not, as I have said, whether fashion (which Itzin doesn't even mention) should have the same status as other arts, but whether it should have any. I am even less sure that "excellence is not the issue"; with some feminists, it seems to be. Elaine Hobby writes of neglected women authors, "One final question . . . that has been posed to me repeatedly: were they any good? . . . ideas about 'good writing' help support many of the values of the establishment, of white, heterosexual, middle-class men . . . I am much more interested in what women's writings show us about female struggles . . . than I am in their use of rhyme or complexity of characterisation."[39] I am a woman and when I read, say, a novel, it matters to me whether the characters seem real or not. Is this because I am corrupted by the values of men? A black American academic, Henry Louis Gates, Jr., has said that "some people around on the Left . . . feel that the only way you can teach literature by women, or literature by people of colour, is to say, 'Well, yes, this is bad, but we'll hold our noses and pretend that these standards are some sort of white Western hegemonic strategy to oppress us'."[40] Again, it patronises the people it is supposed to help; by what right does Hobby suggest that writers who are working-class, female, homosexual or all three are less capable of writing books which stand up to criticism, or that readers in those categories can't appreciate them? Professor Gates has been criticised for defending not just literary values but historical accuracy: "because I try to insist on things like standards and rigour . . . I'm some kind of Uncle Tom."

Where fashion is concerned, almost the only people who defend it do so on "anti-élitist" grounds. This leads to the same sort of attitude as it does with other arts: a bias in favour of the "street" as opposed to the "high" variety, and a reluctance to apply critical standards, or to assume that only the reverse of the traditional ones can be valid. Calling punks the only liberated cosmetic users is very like saying pop is the only music anyone really enjoys. Mary Quant, interviewed in the *Guardian* at the height of her career, claimed to have "taken the snobbery and gracious living out of fashion" but was nobody ever snobbish about her clothes? What about the conspicuous labels on jeans and trainers? In the seventies there was a brand of clothes called "Mother Wouldn't Like It" and I read that the Spice Girls were losing popularity with teenagers because younger children liked their songs.[41] How does that differ from a Victorian (or earlier) socialite giving away her new dress because the housemaid had managed to copy it?

Andrea Dworkin, in the preface to the British edition of *Right-Wing Women*, quotes a letter from someone at the Women's Press telling her "that in England right-wing women . . . wore hats and were prudes and fascists and left-wing women . . . didn't and weren't"; her compatriots Esther Newton and Shirley Walton, speaking at the Scholar and Feminist IX Conference, "Towards a Politics of Sexuality" at Barnard College, New York in 1982, described the lesbian feminist look as middle class (as opposed both to the "decadent and elite" upper class and the working class, who, they say, reject it). They define it thus: "The dyke look is supposed to be androgynous, but leans towards masculine gender symbols . . . a modified butch look, we speculate, because femininity is the mark of difference and inferiority which must be eliminated. Paradoxically, the look is downwardly mobile."[42] Evelyn Tension, a British working-class feminist, agrees: "I don't find poverty, dirt and ugliness groovy. I don't like wearing old shirts about ten sizes too big". So does Jonathan Kozol: "It is only the child of the owner of the biggest shoe store in New Jersey who finds it radical to go in bare feet in the streets of Harlem . . . those streets of broken glass and in those canyons of cracked asphalt and concrete."[43] This appears to echo what Rosie Boycott said of the dispute at *Spare Rib.*

Mary Evans, in *A Good School: Life at a Girls' Grammar School in the 1950s*, describes how uniform was imposed as part of an anti-fashion "set of moral attitudes about appearance and vanity. 'Good' girls did not bother about whether their shoes were fashionable . . . To care about one's appearance was therefore part of an unacceptable attitude to the world." It didn't work: "A complete lack of interest in dress was quite uncommon among my contemporaries; what was much more common was a studied and affected apparent lack of interest that masked either a complete or a near complete obsession. Admitting to caring about the matter was about the same as saying that you were in favour of sin."[44] Meanwhile, like women under Communism, they spent a lot of time trying to modify their uniforms.

It happened with the feminist uniform too. Liz Heron recalls that "behind the sartorial rhetoric of intransigent practicality there was abundant compromise. My dungarees were a good deal tighter than some, I wore a touch of mascara, a dash of perfume . . . I was not alone. Gender was only bent so far." But so was the new orthodoxy: "In pretty pastel or brilliant primary colours, in velvet and cords, satin and sheeny cotton, designer jump-suits retained the basic shapes of serviceability, but these were transformed and accessorised to the height of artifice."[45]

She expresses worry about whether this is betraying the cause, and is not alone there either. Amanda Sebestyen describes how male interviewers remarked on her wearing lipstick: "Something I'd hoped was my personal frivolous choice was being used to set me up against other women.

'Normal', 'pretty', or at least trying hard, not one of those *ghastly* combat-booted libber types . . . Well, I've stopped wearing lipstick again. But that's not a solution if I'm just conforming to another hierarchy of correct feminist style."[46] Marie Maguire writes: "many women admit to a terror of being judged not to be, look or sound 'feminist' enough."[47] Anna Coote and Beatrix Campbell call themselves "old lags who have often been beset by fears that others will catch us while we are either literally or metaphorically painting our toenails!" and young feminists have complained of "suspicion . . . if we turn up at a party wearing 'frivolous' clothes", even wondering if they were wrong to mind having spots.[48] Carol Irving, writing in a magazine called *Out* (March 1986) felt "guilty about feeling bad" because she was tired of sludge-coloured clothes. Some freedom!

They may even react like the narrator of June Burnett's novel about the Greenham Common peace camp: "Although I don't wear make-up any more, I still get the occasional impulse to run into the bushes and return wearing the whole damned business, blusher, mascara, everything, just to get up the flared nostrils of the woman . . . who seems to think you measure commitment by appearance."[49] If Greenham really was like this, Caroline Blackwood, who visited it, was wrong to praise it as a place where people could look exactly as they liked.[50] Emma Healey writes that lesbian clubs "often provided an easy and accessible social life where it didn't matter what you wore or what you looked like (as long as you didn't wear lipstick)."[51]

Some feminists have seen what this freedom is worth, like Muriel Dimen ("When the radical becomes correct, it becomes conservative . . . the road to false consciousness is paved with politically correct intentions"), Sheila Rowbotham ("denial of delight in the body and appearance can limit as much as being defined only by one's looks and dress") and Jane O'Reilly: "Trying to be the perfect feminist, with daily examinations of conscience, is not really a big improvement on trying to be a perfect wife, mother, and lady . . . Inflexible guidelines are probably antifeminist by definition."[52] Joanna Russ, who wrote that "the demand for 'attractiveness', like the existence of pornography, is sexual harassment, neither more nor less", added: "Makeup, for example, is a feminist issue *not because using makeup is anti-feminist and scrubbing your face is feminist but because makeup is compulsory*. Those who don't see the distinction are building a religion, not a politics. 'Whatever isn't prohibited is compulsory' is not the banner under which I want to march."[53]

Neither do I. It should go without saying that women shouldn't have to follow fashion if they don't want to, and that there should be no more women sacked from their jobs if they don't wear make-up or bras, or do wear trousers. Women have every right to protest at this (except perhaps at make-up if the job is selling cosmetics, which you shouldn't do if you disapprove of them). Forcing themselves to conform is giving in to what Mao called a paper tiger (literally made of paper when it's the fashion press), like the man in a story attributed to Mark Twain, who stayed in prison for years until it occurred to him to find out whether the door was locked, then opened it and walked out. Feminism has shown the way out of one sartorial prison; we must not let it put us in another. If we want to dress decoratively and use cosmetics, we must say so clearly, or we shall find we have thrown off the burden of having words put into our mouths by men only to have them put there by other women. If anyone accuses us of only saying this because male chauvinists think we should, we can always ask how she knows she isn't saying the opposite because they think she shouldn't, and how she knows a desire to wear jeans all the time is any more authentic than a desire to wear something else.

5

Who Are We Trying
to Please?

Pleasure, after all, is a safer guide than either right or duty.

Samuel Butler   The Way of All Flesh

Spayley had grasped the fact that people will do things from a sense of duty which they would never attempt as a pleasure. There are thousands of respectable middle-class men who, if you found them unexpectedly in a Turkish bath, would explain in all sincerity that a doctor had ordered them to take Turkish baths; if you told them in return that you went there because you liked it, they would stare in pained wonder at the frivolity of your motive.

"Saki" (H. H. Munro)   Filboid Studge

Conventional wisdom answers the question this chapter poses in one word: men. If women care how other women look, it is supposed to be in a spirit of competition, either for men's attention or for its own sake; women dress either to please men or to annoy other women. To dress fashionably, there-fore, is to give the impression that you oppose both women's independence and women's solidarity. It also suggests that you are so stupid that you buy whatever the trade tells you to, which helps to give the subject a bad name among socialists and leads to terms like "slave of fashion" and "fashion victim". To understand why fashion has so many enemies, consider some of its friends.

The clearest description I know of what is now called "being a sex object" is in *Sense and Sensibility*. Elinor and Marianne's half-brother calls on them and, hearing that the latter has been ill, says:

I am sorry for that. At her time of life, anything of an illness destroys the bloom for ever! Hers has been a very short one! She was as handsome a girl last September as any I ever saw, – and as likely to attract the men. There was something in her style of beauty to please them particularly. I remember Fanny used to say that she would marry sooner and better than you did; not but what she is exceedingly fond of *you*, but so it happened to strike her. She will be mistaken, however. I question whether Marianne, *now*, will marry a man worth more than five or six hundred a year at the utmost, and I am very much deceived if *you* do not do better.

John Robert Powers, an American writer on beauty culture, wrote in 1960: "It is a woman's birthright to be attractive and charming. In a sense, it is a *duty* as well. A woman's most important role is *giving*. Others turn to her for guidance, sympathy, love and understanding. She is a source of inspiration. She is the bowl of flowers on the table of life."[1]

A year later, the health food specialist Gayelord Hauser made women responsible not only for their own appearance but also their men's: "Once you are on your way to your own radiant perfection, then I ask you to use your womanpower to help your Adam."[2] Women were also responsible for men's reactions to them: a woman's magazine quiz of about the same time, headed, "Are You Just Like a Woman?" asked "Do you make yourself beautiful and if a wolf says hello, slap him?" But if they stopped beautifying, a popular song of 1963 warned:

Hey, little girl, comb your hair, fix your make-up, soon he will open the door.
    Don't think because there's a ring on your finger you needn't try any more
. . .
    . . . I'm warning you.
    Day after day there are girls at the office and men will always be men.
    Don't send him off with your hair still in curlers, you may not see him again . . .[3]

So do anti-feminist women who make a career out of telling other women to be submissive housewives. Some of the best known belong to the American religious right: Helen B. Andelin, author of *Fascinating Womanhood* (1965, revised 1974 and 1992) and Marabel Morgan, author of *Total Woman* (1973). Both founded organisations in which they gave classes in womanliness, and quote testimonials from former pupils. One of Andelin's writes: "I came into the class thinking it was a women's lib oriented course . . . I was hoping to find ways to get my husband to help with domestic duties . . . Our marriage has improved now that I've . . . been gathered up into the enthusiasm of our teachers and class members who really believe in two sexes . . . I'm also happier with housework." The book, based on some anonymous 1920s booklets, advises: "When expressing your viewpoint use words that indicate insight such as 'I feel'. Avoid the words 'I think', or 'I know.' . . . trying to convince a man so often fails. . . because the woman will appear as an *equal partner* to him." The chapter on "Femininity" begins with appearance, which involves *"accentuating the difference between yourself and men* . . . Men never wear anything fluffy, lacy, gauzy or elaborate. Use such materials, therefore, whenever you can." After over two pages in this vein come more testimonials, including this: "When my husband and I worked in our yard or lemon orchard I used to wear pants, boots and a sweat shirt. My husband expected a man's work from me. After studying Fascinating Womanhood . . . I lowered the neckline of my sweat shirt, added rickrack and try to wear crisper looking clothes when helping him. Now he does not expect as much of me." Women are encouraged to imitate the mannerisms of Victorian characters like David Copperfield's "little blossom child-wife" Dora (though not her chaotic housekeeping) and to "visit a little girls' shop . . . Another source of girlish styles is in the children's section of pattern books, some of which are repeated in women's sizes . . . If you think it a bit ridiculous for grown women to wear these youthful styles, wear them in your own home and let your husband be the judge."[4]

Marabel Morgan has similar ideas without Andelin's "refinement" and distaste for "coarse or vulgar language". Whereas Andelin offers no direct advice on sex (that has to be sent for by mail order) Morgan gives it two chapters ("Eat by candlelight; you'll light his candle!") which, some feminists have observed, shows "the spread of women's sexual revolution into the otherwise closed-minded culture of right-wing Christian fundamentalism".[5] She advises women to dress up for their husbands when they come home: "You may be a smoldering sexpot, or an all-American fresh beauty. Be a pixie or a pirate – a cowgirl or a show girl. Keep him off guard." A Baptist Total Woman "welcomed her husband home in black mesh stockings, high heels, and an apron. That's all. He took one look and shouted 'Praise the Lord!' . . . He could hardly eat his dinner!"[6]

How to Become The Sensuous Woman by "J."(1970), gives the same message without a religious angle: "Playing glamorous roles makes Sue less irritable over the repetitive household chores that she's stuck with everyday."[7] In 1972 Barbara Cartland wrote: "men marry women for their looks . . . Far too many women become unrefined when they have landed their fish".[8]

Does anyone still take this seriously? Yes. Melissa Sadoff's *Woman as Chameleon* ("A real woman would want to dress, not for herself, not for other women, not for the sake of fashion, but for her husband") appeared in 1987 and Ellen Fein and Sherrie Schneider's *The Rules* in 1995 (in a sequel, they claim to be feminists): "Don't aspire to the unisex look . . . Remember that you're dressing for men, not other women, so always strive to look feminine. Don't talk so much. Wear black sheer pantyhose and hike up your skirt to entice the opposite sex! You might feel offended by these suggestions and argue that this will suppress your intelligence or vivacious personality. You may feel that you want to be able to be yourself, but men will love it!"[9]

Do they? If women do this for men, they seem to be making a poor job of it. Ask a man if he is interested in women's fashions, and will he say yes? The closer he comes to that mythical being known as Mr Average, the less likely it is. Any such interest would be regarded in conservative male circles as evidence of homosexuality; it's beneath a "real man's" notice. This idea is so much a part of conventional wisdom that an article in *Cosmopolitan* devoted a whole paragraph to refuting it.[10] Jane Austen wrote in *Northanger Abbey* : "man only can be aware of the insensibility of man towards a new gown. It would be mortifying to the feelings of many ladies could they be made to understand how little the heart of man is affected by what is costly or new in their attire . . . Neatness and fashion are enough"; many men would deny the latter. Dale Carnegie wrote in *How to Win Friends and Influence People*: "Men should express their appreciation of a woman's effort to look well and dress becomingly. All men forget, if they have ever realised it, how profoundly women are interested in clothes."[11] A. S. Neill, founder of Summerhill School, had similar ideas but a wholly different viewpoint:

> A mere man can never understand the enormous importance a woman attaches to dress and appearance. If all men were like me the women would be wasting their time and money, for I can never see what a woman wears . . . This feminine concern with outer appearance is slightly depressing.
>
> Men like to be esteemed for their activities, their success in business or academia or acting, meaning that in the main they are less shallow than women . . . Men lack the frailties that make cosmetics and dress important to a woman; they feel more manly; the exhibitionism of women gives them a status . . . I wonder if the feminine desire for outward show has anything to do with the inferior status of women in a patriarchal society . . . So when the men build bridges and make motor cars and tend most of the sick, the women can stress their importance only by being ornamental. One of the most cheering trends of modern life is the rebellion of many women against this inferior role they have to play . . . All the cosmetics and fancy hats and

dresses mean: I am desirable sexually: feast your eyes on me and take me. And many a woman has said that she dresses for other women and not for men. That cannot be true.

Since he claims not to understand women, how does he know? He adds: "when I see the modern girl . . . her carelessness in dress with her blue jeans and blouse, I sigh and wish that women had been as sincere and honest in my early days."[12]

James Laver, who did know about clothes, shared Neill's opinion of their sexual purpose: "Man's strongest desire in choosing his clothes is *not* to belong to the Present, but to reproduce some ideal from the Past; the Time-Spirit, however, is too strong for him. Women, on the other hand, do their utmost to be contemporary. That is the meaning of Fashion . . . woman advancing wears a hat, woman retreating wears a bonnet."[13] This appears in the same book in which he likens a top hat to a factory chimney, and though we have seen that it was part of a style derived from riding clothes and which was adopted because it revealed the figure in the same way as an antique statue, we have also seen that women wore Grecian dresses at the same time; wasn't that at least as backward-looking? I can only assume Laver was so convinced of the existence of "that competition for the attention of men which is the basis of Fashion", as he calls it in the same passage, and the absence of such a motive in men, that all his knowledge of history couldn't prevent him twisting the facts to fit his theory.

The crudest examples of this attitude are books like Paul Tabori's *Dress and Undress* (1969) whose chapter headings include "Sex and the Bed; Sex and the Corset; Shirt, Shift and Sex; Sex and Trousers; Stockings, Garters, Shoes and Sex". In the chapter on cosmetics he writes: "Both fashion and cosmetics have only one purpose – sexual attraction."[14] It really would be surprising if he thought otherwise.

Such men see women as expressing "the eternal feminine", by definition the antithesis of "manliness", and so proving that they cannot escape it. This implies the absence of such "manly" virtues as strength, independence, even intelligence. Virginia Novarra has asked if "femininity" is "a genteel way of saying 'sex appeal'",[15] and we know that what appeals to male chauvinists is weakness in all the areas in which they pride themselves on being strong. A "feminine" appearance, therefore, becomes a symbol of this weakness. Paul Ableman wrote *The Doomed Rebellion* (1983) to demonstrate this theory: "A woman gazing at her image in a mirror, endlessly attentive to her make-up, tensely trying on clothes, bathing and cosseting her body is not engaged in some perverse and masturbatory enterprise. She is, in fact, exploring her empire, looking deep into her nature and her body and preparing the latter for its destiny."[16] He means motherhood. On the other hand J. C. Flugel, who called fashion "a perpetual blush on the face of civilisation" and looked forward to a future when everyone would dress rationally, saw it as masturbatory. Doris Langley Moore, founder of the Costume Museum in Bath, enjoyed attacking him:

> Professor Flugel of the University of London, more than any other psychoanalyst, has afforded me the perverse pleasure of laughter unintentionally evoked. His Psychology of Clothes (which displays a very much more limited knowledge of fashion than we are entitled to expect in one who is laying down the law about it . . .) is enlivened with the most agreeably startling interpretations of ordinary customs and habits.
>
> We learn, for instance, that a woman who removes her hat at the earliest opportunity is suffering from 'the female form of the castration complex . . .' Equally remarkable is his diagnosis of the feminine practice of making up the face in public as narcissistic and implying 'a preoccupation with self and a relative indifference to other things and persons . . .' It is curious for a psychologist not to observe that, on the contrary, make-up implies a preoccupation with appearances (i.e. outwardness) and women who frequently have recourse to powder and lipstick are clearly concerned with the impression they are making upon others . . . As to the reason why public attention to make-up is annoying to men, the Professor has one of his inimitable footnotes:
>
> . . . Another factor in this irritation may come from the auto-erotic elements involved in the practice, in virtue of which powdering the nose, like any other manipulation of the person's own body, is apt to be unconsciously identified with . . . masturbation (sometimes, of course correctly, for the identification may unconsciously exist for the manipulator also).[17]

Flugel says making up is masturbatory and Ableman says it isn't, but both conclude that it isn't feminist.

Watered-down versions of these ideas are ubiquitous. Dr Clifford Longley, formerly religious correspondent of *The Times*, supported objections to women priests because women were too passive, citing as evidence that "girls still dress prettily, with an instinct to attract by vulnerability";[18] Terence McLaughlin[19] speculated, like Susan Brownmiller, that professional women only wear cosmetics because they are uncertain of their competence. Dr Ainslie Meares, in *The New Woman*, reached these conclusions: *"The Woman of Tradition dresses in a way designed to communicate her*

THE OLD WAIL ABOUT WOMAN'S DRESS!

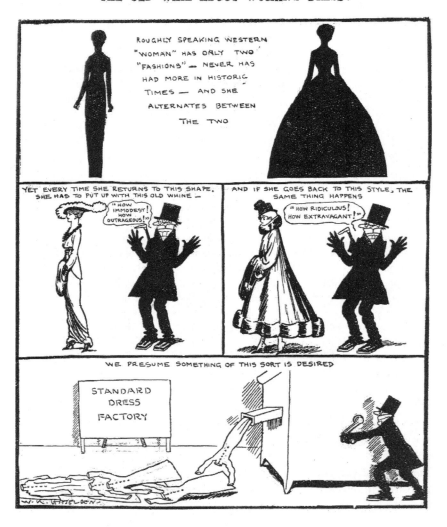

Always the conventional male wants her to "dress sensibly". And always he is amazed when her very ancient fashions refuse to conform to his taste for uniformity.

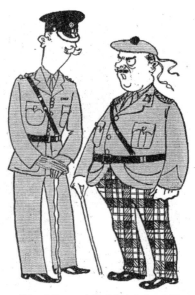

"Fine sights we shall all look in berets!"

'Fine sights we shall all look in berets!'   Osbert Lancaster, 1943

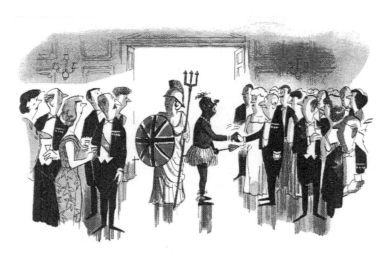

'I fear we must have misread the invitation.'

'I fear we must have misread the invitation'   Alex Graham (*Punch*, 26 January 1963).
Courtesy Punch Cartoon Library, London.

'Don't tell me . . .' Alex
Graham (*Punch*, 7 November
1962). Courtesy Punch Cartoon
Library, London.

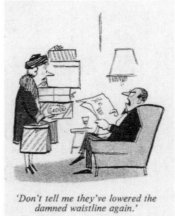

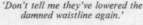

*'Don't tell me they've lowered the
damned waistline again.'*

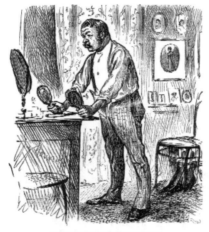

MASCULINE INCONSISTENCY.

Lovelace de la Poer Spinks (his usual soliloquy before his glass). "AFTER ALL—
IT 's NOT A MAN'S PERSONAL APPEARANCE WOMEN CARE FOR. IT 's HIS CHA-
RACTER, IT 's HIS INTELLECT, IT 's——"
*[Proceeds, as usual, to squeeze his neck into a collar which prevents him from
turning his head, his feet into tight boots which prevent him from walking,
and his waist into a belt which prevents him from drawing his breath.]*

Masculine Inconsistency, Sir
George du Maurier (*Punch*, 2
April 1885). Courtesy Punch
Cartoon Library, London. The
caption reads:

Lovelace de la Poer Spinks (his
usual soliloquy before his glass).
'After all, it's not a man's *personal*
appearance women care for. It's
his *character*, it's his *intellect*, it's
—' [Proceeds, as usual, to
squeeze his neck into a collar
which prevents him from
turning his head, his feet into
tight boots which prevent him
from walking, and his waist into
a belt that prevents him from
drawing his breath.]

concept of femininity . . . The woman expresses her femininity to attract a man
. . . But I have the feeling that the woman's expression of her femininity
runs even deeper. For the most part it is certainly not a conscious manoeuvre
to attract men. The evidence for this is that woman's expression of her femininity continues in the absence of male company . . . *In a different way the
New Woman dresses to communicate her new concept of femininity* . . . She wears

clothes much more like those of a man . . .The meaning is clear,'You can see I am just another human being, like a man.' And of course there is a secondary meaning, 'I am really just one of you. Treat me like one of your-selves.'"[20] Meares seems to assume not only that all new women are alike and all traditional women alike (would he treat men like this?) but that there is only one way of being "human": like a man. He believes the Woman of Tradition's behaviour says "I am not very strong. I am not very clever. I am a woman."

Many men say so too: Shulamith Firestone, for instance, quotes the psychoanalyst Theodor Reik (whom she calls "the crackerbarrel layman's Freud") as saying to a patient who swore at him on being accused of wanting to be a man, "I am glad to see a remnant of femininity" when she tidied her hair.[21] You might think no feminist would hold such views, but a woman interviewed in Mette Ejlersen's polemic on women's sexual dissatisfaction, *I Accuse!*, says: "The girl's liking for pretty dresses and make-up is animated by the desire to make herself look feminine and attractive, and perhaps, a little weak and helpless."[22]

This brings us to an enemy of both fashion and feminism, Esther Vilar. The thesis of her book *The Manipulated Man* is: "Men have been trained and conditioned by women, not unlike the way Pavlov conditioned his dogs, into becoming their slaves." One chapter is headed "The Fair Sex": "It is lucky for the adult woman that men do not consider themselves beautiful, since most men are beautiful. Their smooth bodies, kept trim by hard work, their strong shoulders, their muscular legs, their melodic voices, their warm, human laughter, the intelligent expression of their faces, and their calibrated, meaningful movements overshadow those of women com-pletely, even in a purely animal sense . . . after the age of fifty, [women] are nothing but indifferent heaps of human cells . . . she thinks of him as a machine . . . for the production of material goods." (A previous reader of my secondhand copy has written in the margin, "it's a man's world/beauty is culturally defined . . . men look at women as if they're sex machines.") Another chapter, "The Mask of Femininity", describes women's "slavish narcissistic primping" and men's reaction to it: "They [men] will never understand the pleasure a woman takes in housework, and to them the make-up process is just as degrading. Every man knows that he himself could not care less if a woman wears three colors of eye shadow or one."[23] Feminists should be suspicious when they find themselves agreeing with someone who believes that "a movement that fights for yet more of women's rights is reactionary, and, as long as the screaming for female equality does not stop, man will never get the idea that he is actually the victim".

Vilar wasn't the first. I expected an endorsement of "feminine" dress in the notorious expression of post-war anti-feminism, Ferdinand Lundberg and Marynia F. Farnham's *Modern Woman: The Lost Sex* (Simone de Beauvoir allegedly wrote *The Second Sex* in reaction to it) but theirs is highly qualified: "Women dress for other women, according to one theory. They do. But only competitively. Here it is a struggle of female egos. The modern preoccupation with female adornment and embellishment is more positively directed at men, a legitimate female aim, true enough. Here it is libidinal. But this aim, always legitimate in a woman, has attained such fantastic overstress that entire industries, in which are invested millions of dollars, have been erected upon it. Only constant frustration could have resulted in this heavy overemphasis upon one aspect of living . . . If women through this narcissistic overemphasis attained their aim there would be little to say about it. But that they do not attain it is evident from the continued narcissistic overemphasis through all the years of life."[24]

Some of the men quoted above would agree. If one can believe stereotypically masculine men, when they do notice what women wear, they actively dislike it. Hats are almost a standing joke; as the American humourist Art Buchwald put it in 1961, describing a fashion show: "It's hard enough to keep a straight face when your wife comes home with a new hat, but when you see about a hundred at one time I challenge any man who isn't in the business to keep from doubling up with hysterics."[25] (In the same volume he suggests, or pretends to, that women would be happier without the vote, and in another, that no women would buy clothes their husbands liked.)

Twenty-five years earlier, the tone of A. P. Herbert's sketch *Eat Less Lipstick* is anything but humorous: "every man of sense and courage continually tells his favourite lady that he prefers her mouth to look like a mouth and not like a sea-anemone or a piece of raw meat. So I know that women know that nearly all men think that what nearly all young women do is disgusting."[26] John Brophy wrote in 1945: "considering all the adverse criticisms passed by men it must be difficult now to maintain the argument that women adapt their appearance to please masculine taste . . . what it [lipstick] does is to paint another and false mouth on the face: a mouth, moreover, unduly prominent yet makeshift, obtaining a startling effect at twenty yards' distance and a repulsive one at close quarters."[27] Books aimed at women in offices regularly warn that men dislike red nails.

The ultimate in male patronage might seem to be Kenneth C. Barnes's 1958 sex education book, *He and She*: "the overwhelming . . . importance of feminine attire and fripperies is due more to the intense competition of business interests than to the nature of women . . . there must be a large section of the female population open to this sort of persuasion. But my impression is that most girls can laugh at it all, even if they indulge themselves for a while. Perhaps their boy friends can help them with a little laughter too, and an elementary exposition of the working of the capitalist system."[28] But here are the ecologists John Seymour and Herbert Girardet in 1987: "You cannot make yourself truly beautiful by smearing cosmetics on your face, but you can create the illusion of a sort of beauty . . . an appalling waste of time, energy and money . . . Cosmetics are, of course, quite unnecessary, but there is no point in being too puritanical about them . . . self-adornment is not a habit which we humans are likely to give up."[29] On 4 August 1996, Andrew Billen, interviewing the editor of British *Vogue* in the *Observer*, said: "most of the models are . . . thinner than any male ideal of what a woman should look like, and if women are not remodelling themselves to make themselves attractive to men, what the hell are they wasting their time for?" That month's *Harpers & Queen* contained an article on men who hate make-up,[30] and Andrew Marr, then editor of *The Independent*, asked on 19 April 1997: "wouldn't things be far more satisfactory if we all wore standard-issue blue pyjamas?"

So women go to all that trouble and expense to please men by doing something men either don't notice or don't like. No wonder men think women stupid. But how true is it? I can't improve on the description in a guide to dressing well written in 1937 (a year after A. P. Herbert's diatribe) by Alison Settle, a journalist who did believe women dressed for women. The chapter headed "What Men Like in Women" tells the reader "to discount what they actually say" which is that they prefer her old clothes, not in order to save money but because

a remark like that saves him from thinking . . . You can tell that your husband is only saying the things he feels should be said and not the things he urgently wants to say by the difference he accords in opinion to the other women and to you. To you, his wife, he says he hates smartness and all that kind of thing; neatness is all he asks for. Only for goodness' sake don't let's have anything conspicuous or queer, nothing too new. And you buy some little dowd of a dress that wipes out your character only to see him making a beeline for the smartest woman in the place who uses, yes, all the make-up of eyeshadow, brighter lipstick, darkened lashes, that he says he hates, wears one of those slinky dresses you ached to have, and yes, has her nails polished and coloured when he begged you to leave yours alone. Do you remember that time, looking back? The truth was, of course, that he had to make no decision about that other woman; he wasn't asked his opinion, and you know quite well that when his opinion is asked it is always given in a safe negative form. He didn't notice that she used blue-green cream shadows on her eyelids, and would have thought you a cat if you had said she did (you were wise enough to keep silent), and he believed that her eyelashes always were that wonderful hyacinth black

. . . Even the great dressmakers, steeped in the atmosphere of women, have their decidedly masculine prejudices well preserved. I remember Monsieur Patou . . . saying he had always hated red fingernails (although every man has said that, women have gone on wearing them for years, have they not?), disliked any noticeable perfume, and above all exotic ones. A faint flower perfume is all any woman should allow herself [he founded the firm that makes "Joy, the Costliest Perfume in the World"].

Another couturier, Lucien Lelong, "told me he could only bear make-up when it was so carefully . . . done that it did not occur to you that the woman was wearing any".[31]

A character in a story by Abioseh Nicol says: "when I wear African clothes you point to other women who wear modern frocks; when I wear a frock you say I look much nicer in African dress".[32] Men seem about as reliable as people who say they drive better after a double Scotch.

What makes them say one thing and mean another? Settle's explanation is only partially convincing: mindlessly praising new clothes would save thinking just as much as claiming to prefer old ones. I agree, however, that men think they ought to prefer old ones: why?

I think because clothes are supposed to be an unworthy preoccupation, and because of the legacy of moral condemnation of sexuality, especially in women. If a man unconsciously divides women into "bad girls" and Madonna-like mothers and regards looking sexually attractive as an attribute of the former, he will resent any signs of, say, his wife trying to do so. No feminist would blame men for thinking that partners should be chosen for character rather than looks, though her idea of character may not be the same as theirs. Their moral code, wrote Doris Langley Moore, tells them they should not fall in love with someone because she is "pretty, and soft, and scented, and exquisitely attired, and flattering", only with "goodness, and common sense, and domesticity"; though if that's all a woman can offer, "she will not be besieged with suitors".[33] So they convince themselves they are indifferent to appearances; I have heard a man who chooses his wife's clothes, with her full consent, say he doesn't notice what people look like, and I have no doubt he meant it.

But why do men like A. S. Neill, who don't disapprove of sex or other sensuous pleasures, feel obliged to decry this one? To say character is more important than looks is not to say people should care nothing for the latter, or feel guilty if they do. In the last resort character is more important than brains, as schoolteachers used to say, but people don't feel ashamed to say they wouldn't marry someone stupid. The difference is that intelligence has high status and appearance doesn't (I am not suggesting it should be equally high).

Men who admit to being interested in sex but don't care about fashion judge women's dress from one point of view only: whether it is conducive to their favourite activity. Anything which isn't obviously "sexy" doesn't interest them, just as someone who likes dancing but is otherwise unmusical has no interest in music to which one cannot dance. That is why some of the most sexist men dislike the style which Andelin recommends and Settle calls fussy, adding "which is funny when you think how many women choose taffetas and nets and ruches and curls because they think men like that kind of ultra-girlish effect!"[34] I recall a man who told a *Sunday Times* reporter that he hoped mini-skirts would survive because "I'm not interested in women's clothes, I'm interested in women", meaning their bodies.

The other factor which can be identified from Settle's account is sheer ignorance, which the subject's low status reinforces; men are almost encouraged to be proud of it. This explains their hostile reaction to novelty. Women may also find a new style shocking at first, but before actually buying one they "get their eye in", as fashion professionals call it, by looking at different examples in pictures and shops; a man doesn't notice it until one of the women in his household wears it, and he may well think she will be the only person who does. (I have seen the same reaction in unfashionable women.) When he finds other women are wearing it, however, he will be shocked if she doesn't. Jean Rook summed up the "short-haired man" (in 1968, when every man with the slightest pretension to fashion was letting his hair grow at least a little) as one who thinks the whole subject a joke, but will explode if the women in his family are not "suitably dressed" on important occasions, his definition of suitable being just like everyone else.[35]

The most pernicious effect of this ignorance, however, is that men don't realise dress and grooming mean work. They don't believe there is any, just as many of them imagine that running a home, even with young children in it, isn't really doing anything. No-one who had done so would go on believing that women are really passive. Men who are not in the trade also underestimate the money involved. Thackeray wrote in *Vanity Fair*: "how many of you have surreptitious milliners' bills? How many of you have gowns and bracelets, which you daren't show, or which you wear trembling? – trembling, and coaxing with smiles the husband by your side, who does not know the new velvet gown from the old one, or the new bracelet from last year's, or has any notion that the ragged-looking yellow lace scarf cost forty guineas, and that Madame Bobinot is writing dunning letters every week for the money!" In 1991, an article in the women's magazine *best* describes a woman pretending her new coat was old as "far from unusual".[36] This wouldn't work if the man knew the latest fashion when he saw it, which means that men's ignorance makes deceiving them easy; but who wants to live by deceit?

Mrs Humphry's *Manners for Women* hasn't dated either: "A man of mediocrity has his own ideal of a wife . . . She must shine on nothing a-year . . . [She must] Be sympathetic so long as his pocket is not touched . . . Cheerful, though he cuts her to the quick . . . And intellectual, though not to fathom his shallowness."[37]

Just the same complaints that Sally Cline and Dale Spender made ninety years later in *Reflecting Men at Twice Their Natural Size*, which also touches on the cosmetic issue: "Dale pointed out that not only does [body] hair have to be removed but the *signs of removal must be removed*. Dale's own ex-husband had a fit if he saw her razor lying about because it made it clear that she actually did grow hair (just as he did),"[38] exactly like Ruskin, who was so shocked by his wife's body hair that he was unable to consummate the marriage. Alison Settle advises: "Make up your mind what is most successful with men if you value your husband's attention and subconscious (not spoken) opinion; analyse the thing, and then go out and do your darndest. *But do not let him see the works*."[39] No feminist could be happy with that, or with pretending not to know that other women have used cosmetics for fear of being called a "cat".

An American writer, Herb Goldberg, sums up: "*Either way she loses.* If she is casual about her physical appearance, he accuses her of 'letting herself go.' If she is attentive to it, he interprets this as her superficiality and vanity or her interest in attracting other men."[40] Feminists have reason to suspect him as he belongs to the "men's movement" whose members often claim to be just as oppressed as women, but here he agrees exactly with his feminist compatriot, Paula J. Caplan: "Fat is not feminine in North America, and vanity is not compatible with the self-sacrificing, selfless aspect of feminine identity."[41] Goldberg brings us to the question of male jealousy; sexist men want attractive wives but worry about their effect on other men. It isn't even that they want wives who attract them but nobody else, which would be hard enough unless they had most eccentric tastes, because they want other men to envy them. A book by Martine Bourrillon quotes a young woman whose escort walked out on her because of her *lamé* dress, saying "Je ne suis pas le prince consort d'une star" and who had seen other men object to her wearing anything except drably coloured jeans and T-shirts, and then go off with women dressed as she had before she met them. Men who were proud of their anti-feminism, interviewed in *Marie-Claire*, all wanted women to look attractive but condemned them for talking or even thinking about clothes and cosmetics.[42] They are like the parents, all too familiar to teachers, who want their children to learn music and complain about the noise whenever they practise. They want the end without the means.

Thackeray was more honest in *Vanity Fair*: "Nor was Mrs Amelia at all above the pleasure of shopping, and bargaining, and seeing and buying pretty things. (Would any man, the most philosophic, give twopence for a woman who was?)"

Janet Radcliffe Richards, quoting feminist remarks like, "To make yourself attractive is to make yourself a male plaything", refers to the models in fashion magazines as beauty objects (as opposed to sex objects) and asks: "why does everyone presume that the beautification of women is all for men?"[43] Men do, and for most of history, what men said went. The more sexist the man, the more he feels that everything we do is aimed at him. If he likes the result, it must be because we are successfully trying to please him; if not, we must be trying unsuccessfully. If even he can see we haven't tried, we are so conceited we think we can please without trying, or neglecting our duty (for which we deserve to be "taught a lesson"), or have given up in despair. Just think how many times you hear or read, "They're only women's libbers because they're too ugly to get a man." Since sex is supposed to be so important, every human action without clear practical motives (and even actions with them) must be sexual. Alison Lurie's *The Language of Clothes*, for instance, gives examples of supposed sexual meanings in behaviour which common sense could explain: tying laces in a double knot means sexual repression rather than wanting them to stay

tied.[44] One of the easiest ways to misunderstand a language is to overesti-
mate the number of sexual references; I have seen one work of so-called
scholarship which claimed that almost all words (with a few exceptions like
"and", "the" and "but") derived from words for genitals.

Since women are supposed to be inferior to and envious of men, everything they do is regarded as an expression of inferiority and envy. This
applies not only to attempts to behave like men but also to behaviour that
is seen as distinctively feminine: either we are trying to be men or to
compensate for not being men. It also follows that any attempt on men's
part to draw closer to female behaviour is degrading. Naturally Theodor
Reik thought so: "Not only the greater modesty of women, but their never
ceasing striving towards beautifying and adorning their bodies is to be
understood as displacement and extension of their effort to overcompensate
for their original impression that their genitals are ugly."[45] An Indian
novelist has the same idea:

> A nice face and a gown of gold brocade
> A haw of rose, aloes, paint and scent
> All these a woman's beauty aid
> But man, his testicles are his real ornament.[46]

In her essay "If *Freud* Were *Phyllis*", Gloria Steinem shows how the same
kind of thinking could be applied to men's clothing, with no more justification, if women were the upper sex: "When left to dress themselves, they
seldom could get beyond an envy of wombs and female genitals, which
restricted them to an endless succession of female sexual symbols. Thus, the
open button-to-neck 'V' of men's jackets was a well-known recapitulation
of the 'V' of female genitalia; the knot in men's ties replicated the clitoris,
while the long ends of the tie were clearly meant to represent the labia. As
for men's bow ties, they were the clitoris *erecta* in all its glory. All these were,
to use Phyllis Freud's technical term, 'representations'."[47] It is particularly
interesting that her "symbolic explanation" covers not only the shapes of
male dress, but its monotony, which both Freudians and masculine-egali-
tarian feminists regard as proof that "masculine" dress is better.

The theory of women's natural inferiority explains why refusing to adorn
ourselves won't help; if we really were inferior, we still would be whether
we "overcompensated" or not, so people who believe we are won't change
their minds just because we change our clothes. We won't even stop sexual
harassment; this must be stressed, because some feminists believe we will.
To the harasser, whatever we do is justification. George Orwell gives an

example in *A Clergyman's Daughter* (1935): "when a man wants a little casual amusement, he usually picks out a girl who is not *too* pretty. Pretty girls (so he reasons) are spoilt and therefore capricious; but plain girls are easy game."[48] Similarly, well-dressed women look as if taking them out would be expensive, and I think this is why I have had more wolf-whistles and attempted pick-ups when I haven't bothered with dress than when I have. Every book on sexual harassment I have ever seen confirms this; harassers plead either that the woman was only too grateful, or that the incident never happened and she made it up because she wished it had (just as Freud thought girls invented incest).

Although some rapists and their defending counsel cite the women's attractiveness as the reason for the rape, and their "provocative" red lipstick or false eyelashes as evidence of wanting it[49] (why, if men dislike cosmetics?), some rapists regard unattractiveness as challenging. Ray Wyre, a psychologist working with sex offenders, reports that some men go on what they call "grot runs", competing to see who can prove his potency by having intercourse with the ugliest woman.[50] Arguing that certain fashions encourage rape, therefore, is playing the male chauvinist's own game by parroting rapists and their apologists. It is no different from saying women invite rape by going out alone at night, but an anonymous member of the group Women Against Violence Against Women, who objected to a curfew even when Peter Sutcliffe, the "Yorkshire Ripper", was at large, wrote: "It is not an accident that men wear practical clothes while women are incapacitated in tight clothes which restrict movement. Our strength to fight back is undermined . . . It is possible to forget your body in loose comfortable clothing. This is not so in tight jeans and a flimsy blouse, for these emphasise our vulnerability. You have to be careful you are not showing too much flesh. These clothes also mark us as targets for attack . . . FASHION = CONTROL = VIOLENCE AGAINST WOMEN."[51]

This conflates several different questions. Nobody can deny that tight clothes can impede movement and therefore resistance to attack, but loose ones can be difficult to fight in too. The question of showing flesh, moreover, has nothing to do with physical vulnerability, only with the attitude of the person who sees it, and that is what needs to change. (The only time I have ever been seriously molested was when wearing a long, though admittedly low-cut, evening dress.) Why should women have to dress to show an invulnerability which is more apparent than real, since the only clothing that will really stop a rapist is armour?

Germaine Greer's *The Madwoman's Underclothes* should be called *The*

Madwoman's Lack of Underclothes: "many women's liberationists have eschewed the skirt for the boiler suit, claiming that skirts mean immobility and availability. Now I know boys who are more intrigued by a front zipper than anything else. A woman in a boiler suit is like a hermit crab, you must wonder and fantasize about her shape . . . clothes do not actually influence availability. If all that stands between a male chauvinist and the accomplishment of his desires is a knicker, then you've had it. On the other hand, if you know karate, it doesn't much matter whether you're wearing pants or not."[52]

Rebecca West wrote in 1912: "There is even an idea that women should regulate their dress acording to men's lack of self-control, rather than their own comfort."[53] It isn't only comfort which is at stake, as she knew: she herself dressed decoratively and must have wanted to be free to do so. Moralists of both sexes have blamed women and their adornments for men's sexual excesses ever since antiquity (see Juvenal and Tertullian) though Margot Asquith, an anti-suffragist, astonishingly remarked: "Allurement has never been considered a sin."[54] Jane O'Reilly recalls that in her pre-feminist girlhood she "attended, along with most of the Catholic schoolgirls in St Louis, the organizing rally of . . . Students for a Decent Society . . . we would never wear strapless evening gowns. Those indecent creations, we were assured, provoked occasions of sin, *for the boys*".[55] Teachers at Germaine Greer's convent school predicted similar consequences "if we did so much as bare the top part of our arms . . . they were too innocent to realise that there are a lot of men out there who have lascivious thoughts when they see school uniforms";[56] such uniforms regularly appear in sex shops. Other attempts at harassment-proof clothing have been equally self-defeating, as I shall later show. Robin Morgan writes: "There is always the basic Every Woman Loves a Rapist/All Women Want to Be Raped/Good Girls Never Get Raped/It's Always the Woman's Fault cliché . . .Thus, if she wears slacks, that's obviously meant as a challenge; if a skirt, it's an incitement. If she glowers as she strides down the street, it's meant as an attention-getter; if she looks pleasant it's a come-on."[57] The conclusion should be clear: clothes and cosmetics don't make us sex objects for men. Men make us sex objects for men.

It can happen in reverse. In one of the rare cases of a man confessing to being harassed by a woman, "a 40–year-old school inspector" was interviewed in Sue Read's *Sexual Harassment at Work*: "A female worker had come up to him, and in front of a group of her female work colleagues she had stroked his chest and given him a big hug, saying, 'You look so sexy in that shirt and tie.' . . . he happened to be wearing the same shirt and tie when he visited the same school a few weeks later. The same woman came up and announced to her fellow-workers, 'Here he is, and he's wearing that sexy shirt and tie again, just for me.' And she hugged him again . . . he now made sure he never wore those clothes again when he went to visit that school."[58]

"A short skirt or a low neckline means display and fashion to women, a more specific invitation to men," wrote Helen Franks in British *Cosmopolitan* in September 1984. Women have been told that they shouldn't be conscious of wanting sex (if they were allowed to want it at all) or that if they did, they shouldn't ask for it directly, so anything which increases our sexual attraction is seen as an indirect or unconscious way of asking. Every woman knows it isn't always the former, but what about the latter? If the Freudians are right, if sex is everything and everything is sex, we might as well try to escape our own shadows. The modernist architect Adolf Loos said all art was based on sex; he also called ornament a crime, though he was something of a dandy. What is surprising is that so many feminists who criticise or even reject Freud's view of women don't seem to move beyond the terms of the crudest popular Freudianism on this particular subject (Janet Radcliffe Richards is an exception). For instance, both Simone de Beauvoir and Theodor Reik quote Dorothy Parker's short story *The Lovely Leave* as an example of women's obsession with clothes. The protagonist buys a new dress to wear when her husband, serving in the Second World War, comes home on leave, at a price which will leave her in debt for months:

'Do you really like my dress?'

'Oh, yes,' he said. 'I always liked that dress on you.'

It was as if she turned to wood. 'This dress,' she said, enunciating with insulting distinctness, 'is brand new. I never had it on before in my life. In case you are interested, I bought it especially for this occasion.'

'I'm sorry, honey,' he said. 'Oh, sure, now I see it's not the other one at all. I think it's great. I like you in black.'

'At moments like this,' she said, 'I almost wish I were in it for another reason.'[59]

You can guess Reik's conclusion, but Beauvoir's is not very different. According to her, the woman needed appreciation of her dress in order to feel she existed, the implication being that if she had a stronger sense of self she wouldn't care. But suppose she had been a musician and had composed a new piece to play to her husband, and he had said "I always liked that piece", would anyone feel it necessary to invoke either penis envy or lack of selfhood in order to explain why she was upset? Probably not: some musicians are men.

The conventional explanation confuses desire for sex with desire for an audience. ("I can't take my eyes off those eyelashes of yours," said a teacher at my school to a girl wearing false ones, "but that's what you wear them for, isn't it?") One can of course argue, like Reik, that all display is sexual, but for him, what isn't? Why should it be seen as pandering to men's sexuality rather than expressing our own? Music and dance can be erotic, which is why some religious sects condemn them, but feminists don't say no woman should be a musician or dancer (though some feminist performers insist on all-female audiences). Someone once asked, "If a fashion model is a sex object, what's Mick Jagger?" Max Beerbohm's essay *The Badness of Amateur Acting* made the point that one can imagine a castaway on an island writing or painting, but not practising the "public art" of acting. This is also true of dressing up: people need someone to do it for. Children may appear not to, but they create an audience for themselves from their toys or their imaginations.

This answers Ainslie Meares's question as to why women dress up for other women. I read somewhere of a men's club debating whether to admit women, and one member protesting that they would spoil it by competing to be well-dressed. A movement founded with the aim of making life better for all women was bound to outlaw this kind of competition; but again, why take our motives at men's valuation? A man who thinks women hate each other will assume all our reactions are an expression of that hate, but is he any more to be believed than when he assumes our behaviour in his presence must be aimed at pleasing him?

Such men seem to have no idea that an atmosphere of knowledgeable and friendly encouragement can exist between women, just as it can in any group of people engaged in an activity that interests them; Lois Banner and Helen Franks have both noted it.[60] Jane Austen wrote, I think in a letter, "It is very hard that a pretty woman is never to be told she is so by any one of her own sex without that person's being suspected to be either her determined Enemy, or her professed Toadeater." I won't say competitiveness never happens, but I have never had any reason to believe that compliments on my clothes paid by women, including feminists, were actuated by anything except honest admiration, and the same is true of those paid by men (they exist) who are genuinely interested in the subject, unashamed to say so, and without ulterior motives.

Because women have always been in an inferior position, they have had

to get their own way by stealth or not at all. They have behaved like inferiors because they were treated as inferiors. It is all too easy to say "I must
have this because it's expected of me" rather than "I want it", especially
when we are financially dependent on someone else; it's the female equivalent of a man shrugging off responsibility for wearing a picturesque
uniform, and is reinforced by the idea that a woman should be selfless. If
she wants to spend money and time on her own pleasures, she may be reluctant to admit it even to herself, and certainly won't want to tell others. As
the *best* article already quoted put it: "The compulsion many women feel to
justify their spending seems to stem from an upbringing which teaches
them that a wife's duty is to be unselfish while the man has the right to
reward himself for his work with pocket money." Her work, of course, is
officially non-existent if she is at home, and unnecessary if not.

It isn't just a matter of individual men and women. Clothes and
cosmetics, for the vast majority of consumers, are provided by a male-dominated industry. Objectors to fashion always say that its followers are tamely
submitting to a conspiracy whose only purpose is making them spend more
than they need. Though we have seen that some of these objectors were
anything but feminist, feminists have often agreed.

It is worth examining the trade's motives more closely. We have already
seen that from the industrial revolution onwards, a moral code evolved
which was based on a mixture of materialism and puritanism: self-indulgence was bad, but capitalists wanted to promote buying. This was aimed
at both sexes (Vance Packard's 1957 study, *The Hidden Persuaders*, shows
that advertisers found slogans like "you owe it to yourself" more effective
than "treat yourself to it"), but especially at women, because they bought
household goods, and they were now the only sex to dress decoratively. This
clashed with the idea that they should be self-denying; they were supposed
to put themselves last, but at the same time to stimulate the economy by
buying luxuries. There was only one way to resolve this dilemma: to tell
them that buying was a way of serving others.

The industrial revolution meant that people could now "better themselves" by acquiring possessions which had been reserved for the upper
classes, but which could now be mass-produced. Fashions in clothing were
set by ladies whose housework was done by servants. If women who needed
to work, whether in or out of their homes, could not dress fashionably
without inconvenience, that was their look-out. Hence the contradiction
between "women's work" and "feminine appearance". It was less of a
problem when working-class women could only afford to take trouble with

their dress on rare occasions, and even the most modest middle-class household had at least one maid. Feminists have frequently pointed out the unfairness of expecting women with jobs to maintain standards of housekeeping set by full-time housewives. The modern housewife is herself a conflation of two earlier types: the woman who ran a home and the lady who didn't. She is supposed to be the first while looking like the second, maintaining an impeccable appearance while doing housework and cooking and caring for children (see television commercials for household goods, for instance). Feminists from Charlotte Perkins Gilman in *Women and Economics* (1898) to Michael Korda in *Male Chauvinism: How It Works* (1974) have noted that the "dainty" sex has to do dirty jobs; a man once advised my mother, "Never let your husband see you looking dirty or untidy," and I was amazed to hear he was married with children.

Barbara Ehrenreich and Deirdre English's *For Her Own Good* explains: "Commercial prosperity now [after the First World War] *required* that people attempted to gratify themselves through individual consumption . . . The new emphasis on personal enjoyment was inevitably fatal to feminism . . . the female individuality which would be developed in the 'age of enjoyment' would be . . . relentlessly domestic", because the last thing men wanted was to lose their housekeepers. They also wanted their wives to like sex: "the experts were not only acknowledging female sexuality, but welcoming it . . . But there was also a hint of a threat to women in the new insistence on marital joy. At no time was a woman to 'let herself go' in terms of grooming or dress – lest she cease to be 'feminine.' . . . Even as a consumer she worked in other people's interests" and in the fifties, the era of permissive child-rearing, "By some curious asymmetry in the permissive ideology, everyone else in the family lived for themselves, and she lived for *them*."[61] This kind of buyer is ideal from the capitalists' point of view, because she is the most likely to take whatever they hand out to her; no wonder they were scared of women finding out that Soviet women could live without cosmetics.

When Christian Dior launched his "New Look" in 1947, with its tight waists and long full skirts, it provoked riots in Paris, while in Britain Harold Wilson, then President of the Board of Trade, and Sir Stafford Cripps, Chancellor of the Exchequer, urged women to boycott the style and fashion reporters to discourage it; Alison Settle asked the latter if he had ever heard of King Canute.

The look caught on, at first for special occasions only, but disapproval ended when shortages were replaced by encouragement to consume and the trade found that "it could exist alongside, and enhance, the dutiful house-wife look".[62] The symbol of women's frivolous self-indulgence became part of their *rôle* as defined by magazines like *Housekeeping Monthly* on 13 May 1955: "Touch up your make-up, put a ribbon in your hair and be fresh-looking . . . Don't complain if he's late home for dinner or even if he stays out all night . . . Remember, he is the master of the house and as such will always exercise his will with fairness and truthfulness . . . A good wife always knows her place." An American book on marketing published in 1958 claims: "There are many women – and men – who still have what might be termed a Puritan heart . . . A kind of serious-mindedness makes it hard for them to look at pleasure bare – with no reason behind it . . . Also, women have a slight embarrassment about being too dressed up or having too large a wardrobe. This attitude seems to come from the growing alikeness and equality – and also from the present emphasis on family living. The family is coming first in all things and clothes are something that cannot be enjoyed by the family as a group. Clothes are purchased by an individual; they are a selfish purchase, so to speak – and they often come at the bottom of the list."[63]

The Feminine Mystique describes in detail the methods by which the trade attempted to break down the stereotype of the fashionably dressed woman as self-centred and wasteful, an especial problem for manufacturers of such items as furs, who laboured to persuade mothers that a properly brought-up girl should want them. (A study made in 1981 quotes a woman saying: "I think that women who spend a lot of time on makeup and clothes are selfish. I think they neglect their children."[64]) Betty Friedan asked adver-tising men why they didn't encourage women's careers, because women with jobs would have more needs and more money (people who disapprove of them always say, "You wouldn't need all those clothes if you stayed at home"). The answer was that career women were too critical.

Why? The more important a woman's career is, the more mentally alert she needs to be, the more she will think of herself as a person in her own right, and the more satisfactions she has besides shopping. She won't be so ready to buy for the sake of buying, only to find herself disappointed and, the manufacturer hopes, eager to buy again. She is more likely to insist on what she really wants, and to reject clothes or hairstyles which interfere with her ability to do her job. People who think they are acting for others' good can be manipulated, because they may feel obliged to ignore their own pref-erences ("I don't like this new look much, but a man in my husband's position must have a fashion-conscious wife"). People who know they are trying to please themselves will insist on real pleasure, and avoid anything that fails to give it.

Some feminists deny women are manipulated at all, saying that though they may be misled in specific cases, their consumption is the result of a conscious decision to placate the powerful male and make the best of a bad job. I don't altogether trust this. Saying women never make an unconsciously influenced decision is as doubtful as saying that they never make a conscious one. It amounts to denying that they are capable of human weakness, which, paradoxically, is another way of denying responsibility. It claims not only that it is not women's fault that they are second-class citizens, which is true, but that no individual woman ever does anything to make the situation worse, which could only be true if we were all incapable of being fooled. If so, why, two years after Britain introduced a National Lottery, did over ninety percent of the population gamble regularly at odds of nearly fourteen million to one, when a Gallup Poll in 1989 reported that over fifty percent never gambled at all?

Ellen Willis, for instance, challenged Vance Packard on the grounds that "buying habits are by and large a rational self-interested response to their limited alternatives within the system" and "the fashion, cosmetics and 'feminine hygiene' ads are aimed more at men than at women. They encourage men to expect women to sport all the trappings of sexual slavery – expectations women must then fulfill if they are to survive." She points out that men's cosmetics are "not *essential* to masculinity (as makeup is essential to femininity), only *compatible* with it . . . For women, buying and wearing clothes and beauty aids is not so much consumption as work".[65] This theory isn't as different as it looks from the "brainwashing" one; neither admits that a free woman might want these "trappings" for herself. Packard himself admitted: "Heine noted long ago that 'when a woman begins to think, her first thought is of a new dress.' For centuries women have craved for an excuse for a new dress, and so have become co-conspirators with the dress marketers."[66]

The trade's policy was short-sighted. Turning consumption into work made the next generation rebel against it. "There are a hundred ways of selling hair tint without making love depend upon it,"[67] wrote Marya Mannes, but that how it was sold, exploiting not so much desire for love as fear of missing it: the corollary of "you get your man with a new hair colour" is "you won't if you don't". Of course it wasn't put so crudely; in Betty Friedan's phrase, it seemed "less ridiculous and more insidious" in a magazine article rather than an advertisement (hence the coining of the word "aditorial"). A British example told teenage girls to spend money on their boyfriends rather than on make-up, but to avoid being seen without any.[68] Friedan, who attended the all-female university Smith College, described the women teachers there in 1959 thus: "the woman scholar was suspect . . . . In self-defense she sometimes adopted frilly blouses . . . (At psychoanalytic conventions, an observer once noted, the lady analysts camouflage themselves with pretty, flowery, smartly feminine hats that would make the casual suburban housewife look positively masculine.) M. D. or Ph.D., those hats and frilly blouses say, *let nobody question our femininity*."[69]

More recently, Maggie Scarf quotes the case of a research student who was called "not very feminine" by a male colleague and reacted by taking much more trouble with her appearance. Scarf, a supporter of the Brovermans' study quoted in chapter 1, notes: "She was being a good 'feminine' girl now. That offhand remark had shot straight to a vulnerable place in her psyche . . . a lack of great concern about appearance had been, on the profile of the 'healthy, competent adult', one of the earmarks of general psychological well-being."[70] This out-Brovermans the Brovermans, who called women's interest in their appearance one of the few ways in which femininity was "more desirable". Perhaps the student was depressed not because she was caring for her looks, but because she only did so to deflect criticism. Who could enjoy doing anything for that reason? Both commerce and the educational establishment were behaving like domestic tyrants such as the architect Berthold Lubetkin, who, his daughter writes, "insisted . . . that [his wife] wear lipstick at all times, his preferred shade being a strident and uncompromising fire-engine red. If for some reason she forgot to apply it, or if the previous application had smudged or faded, he would draw her attention to the fact, and she would drop whatever she happened to be doing at once, go to the mirror and dutifully repaint her lips for him."[71]

A feminist book on depression sums up: "It is possible to enjoy being found attractive and to enjoy feeling attractive, but we can only enjoy these feelings if we are in a position where we have some control."[72] That we lack control is certain. Leah Fritz, who picketed the Miss America contest, writes: "The most impressive aspect of the experience was not the demonstration itself, but the expressions of hostility by male bystanders. As I marched around and around in our exhausting picket-circle, I would hear, alternately, shouts of, 'Hey, Good-looking – watcha doing tonight?' and 'Boy, get a load of *that* one. What a dog!' The men acted as if *we* were conducting a beauty contest! I had been to other demonstrations where we were heckled – even by Nazis in full, obscene regalia – but I never before had such a feeling of humiliation, of being *spat* upon. Thus I learned, with a terrifying immediacy, the meaning of the new term 'sex object,' and how, henceforth, to regard both the physical flattery and the physical insults of men. From that moment, I have never smiled back at a flirting construction worker or truck driver, nor given a damn about the way I appear, physically, in the eyes of men."[73] (Does that include her husband, whose "endurance and generosity" she praises?)

But if we reject what men like simply because they like it, we are letting men dominate us just as much as if we obeyed them. "The Puritan hated bear-baiting", said Lord Macaulay, "not because it gave pain to the bear, but because it gave pleasure to the spectators". This is not behaving like adults, but like children who automatically rebel against whatever their parents advocate; as one of H. G. Wells's characters said, "it lets the other side choose the battlefield". It is still marching to their tune, but deliberately out of time to it, not even cutting off our noses to spite our faces but to spite theirs.

Gloria Steinem has said that "women who 'ooh' and 'aah' about clothes and make a great fuss about them are playing into the image so many men like to have of us – of 'fluffy little things.' To play into that role is actually to help in the dehumanizing of women, and we should stop it."[74] I didn't become a feminist to live by what men think. Even if I could give them a better opinion of women in general and myself in particular by pretending to think something doesn't deserve to be taken seriously when I believe it does, that isn't liberation. We should be asking not what opinion men have, but whether they are right to have it.

One way for every woman to clarify her own feelings is to ask herself how she would feel if men regarded female beauty and fashion as they have traditionally regarded female strength and intelligence. Gabrielle Chanel believed that without men fashion would not exist; Ginette Spanier, *directrice* of the house of Balmain, said in a radio interview in 1980 that she believed it was something women did for themselves. How would you feel if you came across irrefutable evidence that what really attracted men was an unpainted face, short hair, flat shoes and dungarees? Would you choose to renounce dressing up or renounce men, assuming you haven't already done so? I would be more likely to do the latter; one of the reasons I stopped seeing a man I used to know was that he thought clothes a strange thing to care about (though even he cared more than he thought he did). If that was true, I concluded, he and I could have no future. The next question is: if we enjoy dressing up, should we? Is the game worth the candle?

6

DO APPEARANCES MATTER?

"I have no doubt you looked very charming: but should that delight you so very much?"

Anne Brontë   Agnes Grey

Alas, for a doctrine which can find no believing pupils and no true teachers!

Anthony Trollope   Barchester Towers

Design isn't considered important except in the fashion world, where nothing else is.

Minna Thornton

Do women care what they wear and how they look? You only need to look at any fashionable shopping street to know the answer. Yet it is widely believed that sensible ones don't. Can it be true, when all that time and money is spent on beautification, that it isn't thought important? But if it is important, why is it senseless to care about it?

Of the people expressing this view, some are feminist and some anti-feminist. Some say we shouldn't take a lot of trouble because men don't like it, and others that we shouldn't because they do. You may well wonder how they can all agree when their starting points are so different.

Read magazines and newspapers, and the plot thickens. The very publications that offer so much advice about appearance also have articles telling us not to care about it. As Jill Dawson puts it, "We may feel that we are being neurotic if we have a bad self-image, vain if we have a good one, or trivial to care at all . . . So to be concerned with fashion, to dress up and have fun with clothes, is to be stupid, even whilst every single day the fashion, advertising, and plastic surgery businesses (not to mention slimming ads, diet books, fitness centres, cosmetics industry) pump millions of pounds into all these things."[1] We have seen how conventional wisdom dictates that even the supposedly all-important man doesn't care either, and the better his character, the less he cares. I have seen that stated in a book on "marvellous men" produced by British *Cosmopolitan* with a slim, regular-featured, carefully dressed, groomed and painted woman on the front cover. French *Marie-Claire* followed a translation of an article by Susan Sontag on growing old gracefully, or at least naturally, with a feature on rejuvenating cream; similarly, articles on "fat liberation" regularly appear next to ones on slimming diets. Richard Hoggart wrote in *The Uses of Literacy* that the heroines of popular romantic fiction, supposed to reflect female fantasies, "are usually pretty (unless the burden is that even a plain girl can find a good husband)"[2] and for confirmation, select some Mills and Boon romances at random. Almost certainly, you will see a blurb like this: "Plain X was irresistibly attracted to dashing Y, but how could she hope he would look at her when there were girls like glamorous Z around?" You can guess the answer.

The *Observer* once printed an article by Mary Warnock asking for advice on fashion, among other things, for older women; the next week there was a response which said they should need none and if they did, they were suffering from "a serious case of arrested development", because a woman "knows what sort of clothes suit her and what she feels comfortable in . . . is aware of the folly and frivolity of slavishly following each new trend . . . it doesn't matter a jot what one wears".[3] This "I know what I like and you can't tell me anything I don't know" attitude would hardly seem conducive to success in Lady Warnock's profession of philosophy.

If it really doesn't matter, why was the writer so angry? Elizabeth Wilson wrote of anti-fashion letters in *The Guardian*, "These epistles attribute great power to fashion – it panders to female vanity, it entraps women as victims of sexual stereotyping, it is a capitalist plot to coerce us all into unnecessary consumption. Yet at the same time it is trivial and ridiculous."[4] Joyce Nicholson's *What Society Does to Girls* refers to "the whole horrible monstrosity of cosmetics advertizing".[5] A horrible monstrosity is no trifle.

I want to propose an alternative theory: in spite of those millions of pounds, what we have is not a society where beauty is too highly valued, but one where it isn't valued enough, and that this is the real source of much of the oppression which its pursuit is supposed to cause. I submit that what breaks women's spirit is not so much pursuing beauty as doing so while pretending that the object of the exercise isn't worth having.

This contradiction, like many others which afflict women, goes back a long way, as Wilkie Collins shows. In *The Moonstone*, tract-distributing Miss

Clack says of Rachel: "She looked pitiably small and thin in her deep mourning. If I attached any serious importance to such a perishable trifle as personal appearance, I might be inclined to add that hers was one of those unfortunate complexions which always suffer when not relieved by a border of white next the skin. But what are our complexions and our looks? Hindrances and pitfalls, dear girls, which beset us on our way to higher things!"

Books by ex-pupils of convent schools show how this attitude persists: in Antonia White's novel *Frost in May* "personal vanity was the most contemptible of all the sins" and "parts [in plays] which called for an attractive appearance were usually played by the most meek and mortified children of the school, while anyone suspected of thinking herself pretty was fairly sure to be cast for a hermit with prodigious wrinkles and a long beard."[6] Between the wars, Jane Trahey was constantly told girls didn't need the "pagan sign" of lipstick to be attractive, and for Clare Boylan "you made your first confession and your sin was taken away. Next came communion, when you got dressed up, like a bride, in tremendous acres of tulle and seed pearls and artificial flowers; but you got your sin back because the first thing you felt was *pride*."[7] Protestants were similar; in Scotland at the turn of the last century, Lavinia Derwent "thought it strange that Jesus always wore plain garments, yet we had to tosh ourselves up when we went to worship him" and in the post-war United States Nora Scott Kinzer's mother "used to tell me that it wasn't what a person looked like that mattered as long as that person had a 'beautiful soul'. But reality was another matter: my childhood preparations for Sunday school involved shiny, well-brushed shoes, white stockings, white gloves, flowered hat, and stiffly starched petticoat. God, cleanliness, fashion, and the latest fads were all intertwined."[8]

I have said that men's disdain for fashion closely resembles their attitude to other forms of "women's work", but there is a difference: the others can't be scrapped. Virginia Novarra has argued that the real difference between men's work and women's is that the former isn't vital and the latter is, and Mary Mellor agrees: "There is nothing essential about a woman's work that means a woman must do it, but somebody has to."[9] Somebody must bear children if the human race is to survive (there may be too many at present, but there must be some), and look after them until they can look after themselves. Shulamith Firestone and others have suggested that children's helplessness has been exaggerated, but it can't be denied altogether; self-sufficient teenagers might be a practical proposition, but not self-sufficient babies. A world of callous enough people might kill off everyone old, chronically sick or disabled (as the Nazis came close to doing) but not the next generation, or at least not all of it. Somebody must prepare food, maintain basic hygiene and safety in living quarters, and make and care for clothes.

Clothing is essential but fashion isn't. When a woman does anything regarded as feminine, men pounce on this as evidence that she is just a conventional woman at heart, as Theodor Reik did; Michael Korda calls it "a reflexive twitch of male chauvinist thinking".[10] If a man exults because he has caught a woman shopping for food, washing dishes or looking after her child, however, she can always retort that it must be done and there is no one else to do it. When one Sally Ward wrote to *The Guardian* in 1981 urging their women's page to "cut out all the sexist crap" of fashion and recipes, one of the many replies asked what radical feminists eat. When men refuse to share women's work, women struggle to overcome the refusal; when the work is unnecessary, the struggle is too.

Clothes are a popular choice for anyone who wants to make a gesture of protest. Styles of dress make an excellent Aunt Sally because changing them has immediately obvious results and isn't difficult, especially when it means simplifying them. Anyone who doesn't make the change runs the risk of being branded as a half-hearted protestor, which in turn means that anyone who doesn't want to be thought half-hearted has to make it. Objections can and will be met by the accusation of triviality, which is hard to counter. How can you argue with someone who points to the greater importance of rape, or even housework? But again, if it's so unimportant, how can expressions like Nicholson's "horrible monstrosity" be justified?

We still need to wear something. I remember reading of a poet who said, "I dress quite horribly to prove dress doesn't matter", but she still had to dress. Even if there were no social strictures on going naked, most climates wouldn't allow it, and the world is too crowded for us to live only in the ones that do. "Clothes never shut up",[11] say both Susan Brownmiller and Alison Lurie. Even if they did, bodies wouldn't. Leaving off clothes would only reveal more of them. Unlike other tasks, presenting an appearance can't be delegated or shared; the groups that enforced collective writing couldn't avoid each member having an individual body. If you live with someone whose domestic standards are higher than yours, you can say "If you care so much about the house or the meals, you see to them!" You might, in theory, find someone else to care for your skin and hair, choose your clothes, maintain them and dress you in them, but not wear them for you: the buck stops here. This is why that so-called trifle arouses so much passion. Marjorie Proops once wrote in her advice column: "If others are critical, you can shrug and say they can go to hell – and you can ignore their contempt. But when the contempt is of yourself, you cannot ignore it."[12] Disliking your own body hurts because it is more closely connected with you than anything else. It is your physical self, the source of your sexual identity (Elizabeth Wilson suggests this is why "gender-bending" fashions cause such outrage in some quarters) and you are never without it. Men who call appearance trivial are like men who call the issue of sharing housework trivial; they say it's meaningless because it means too much.

Failure in anything you want to do well can be devastating, but if you can't achieve the results you want in almost any other field, you can stop trying. At school you may be forced to study something you hate, but schooldays don't last for ever. As an adult you can at least try to earn a living in a way you enjoy, and even if you have to take an uncongenial job, you can do what you please outside working hours. You don't have to climb business or professional ladders if you prefer to stay at the bottom or change direction. You can say, "I want to do this well or not at all." Agatha Christie's autobiography explains why she abandoned her early ambition to be an opera singer: "there can be nothing more soul-destroying in life than to persist in trying to do a thing that you want desperately to do well, and to know you are at the best second-rate".[13] Modern technology helps: people who write illegibly can type almost everything except their signatures, poor mathematicians can use calculators, but nothing short of death will free you from your own body. Not only is it always there, but so is the possibility of comparison between it and others; when Emerson called conversation "the only art in which a man has all mankind for his competitors", he forgot appearance.

The same applies to the effects of age. Most of the words written about ageing beauties could apply just as well to ageing dancers, singers or athletes, but when the latter find their ability deteriorating with age, they can retire. Some, not only for financial reasons, prefer to go on till they drop, but the choice is theirs. You can't quit when you're ahead if your physical self is the arena; short of retiring to an uninhabited wilderness, which is becoming harder and harder to find, you can't stop being seen.

No wonder the fashion and beauty industries are popular. If we don't like how we look, they enable us to do something about it, and not having that option is one of the aspects of misfortune that make it hardest to bear. People in any kind of trouble, from the merely exasperating such as an overdue plumber to the tragedy of watching someone they love slowly dying, so often say "If only there were something I could do!" Doing something about what worries us is likely to be a more popular choice than just putting up with it.

But again, why do we worry, and who defines success and failure? Now we come to the feminists who want to reclaim women's culture. We have already seen that for them fashion isn't part of it, but part of the male idea of femininity which has been foisted on women. Their answer to the problem of our not liking our looks is that if it were not for men we should all like them. Not doing so is "unnatural", the result of "socially constructed standards", society being male. I shall come back to the issue of nature, but the question of what to wear still remains, so it is puzzling that none of the supporters of this theory seems to have explored an authentic "womanly" way of dressing, or if they have, it has made little impact. Feminists have tried to rediscover lost female rituals, but we have to decide what to wear for them. Part of the trouble is that in the modern world trousers are seen as masculine and skirts feminine, but there is no third possibility. Clothing which covers human legs is either divided between them or not; we must wear one or the other. Anti-fashion feminists have chosen trousers by an overwhelming majority, the only (fictional) exception I can think of being the protagonist of Fay Weldon's *The Fat Woman's Joke*: "Women should aspire to be as different as possible from men. You should wear a skirt as a matter of principle. There must be apartheid between the sexes."[14]

In real life separatist feminists don't wear skirts, and their exaltation of the natural woman makes it logical to reject cosmetics, which needless to say are also outlawed by masculine egalitarianism. In 1976 the pressure group Women in Media produced a pamphlet called *The Packaging of Women* which described cosmetics manufacturers, in terms worthy of John Seymour and Herbert Girardet, as giving "hope through a product rather than through self-realisation" and admitting to "peddling a confidence drug". Even those members of Women in Media who defended the products called them "a crutch", but a less harmful one than alcohol, nicotine or other drugs (what a generous concession!) Those against them objected to the advertisers' images of women and, when asked how they could sell a product designed to change people's appearance without showing any people, simply said that cosmetics were unnecessary. If, however, what they really object to is that some physical types are more widely admired than others, as their reference to images suggests, abolishing cosmetics wouldn't necessarily change that; it would merely emphasise the difference between those who match the ideal without artificial aid and those who don't. If they think it is only the existence of the cosmetics industry and its advertisements that prevents all women's faces from being seen as equally beautiful, why were they not so seen in periods when cosmetics were virtually outlawed?

We know that decorating oneself isn't regarded as doing anything. That is why it doesn't count as a form of "self-realisation", and that is why the contradictions in women's attitudes to adornment haven't been resolved. It's just too easy to say, "abandon it", like a male chauvinist doctor saying to a woman suffering from allergy to cosmetics, "Don't waste my time. If the stuff hurts you, stop wearing it," and scoffing if she answers "But I don't want to." Feminism was founded on the theory that nothing which made a difference to women's happiness was unimportant, and we have seen that feminists are more than willing to regard fashion as important when condemning it ("not just a trivial, insignificant area of women's lives", says the essay in *Women Against Violence Against Women*). We have also seen that they have found it hard to live up to their own dogma. Susan Brownmiller is one example, Joyce Nicholson another: "Why must a woman be so self-conscious if she is not perfect? . . . The more I know of conditioned women (and that includes myself) the more I despair of their need to conform to the given pattern . . . All that is necessary is a healthy and clean body, clean, shining hair and lots of exercise. A plain face is only plain until one becomes familiar with its expressions and the character behind it."[15] Then why does she despair, not only of others, but of herself? Another of her books provides the answer: "I can remember looking at my elder daughter when she was . . . about five, standing at a party in a white organdie frock I had made her, patterned with tiny blue flowers, and wearing a party cap with a silver star on her dark straight hair. She looked like a tiny fairy, and I can remember thinking she was the most beautiful creature I had ever seen."[16] The discrepancy between this and "all that is necessary" is clear. Such comments suggest the writers have to keep feeling the corpse of the supposedly dead ideal of beauty to make sure it's lying down. There can only be one reason: they are not sure it's dead.

They also suspect that nobody else is sure either. Since the issue affects everybody, no advice on it can be disinterested. Whatever the standard of beauty may be (another point I shall return to later), everybody either conforms to it or not, so people who tell you it's unimportant sound either like poor people saying money doesn't matter or like rich people saying it doesn't; Julie Burchill once observed that when ageing beauties say so, it's like being told money doesn't matter by a millionaire who's just gone bankrupt. If I knew anyone like George Eliot's Dorothea, I should find it hard not to suspect that her high-minded indifference to how she looked was based, however unconsciously, on the knowledge that she didn't need to worry. Eliot's descriptions of all her heroines show that the subject mattered to her if not to them.

Diagnosing a disease doesn't cure it, but it is an essential first step. We have seen that indifference to appearances is a cure that doesn't work for everybody, and feminism is supposed to be trying to reach all women. It works for some, like Gwen Raverat, and even she regarded it as making the best of a bad job: "I simply made up my mind that as I could not be good-looking or well-dressed, I would never again think about my appearance at all. I would have enough clothes to be decent, but I would try to be as nearly invisible as possible, and would live for the rest of my life like a sort of disembodied spirit. Of course I knew that this was not the best possible solution, but it was the only one that seemed to me practicable. And at any rate this decision did really set me free; I hardly ever thought about my clothes or my looks any more at all."[17] Of course? Feminists often seem to be recommending this as the best solution for everyone, always; the difference is that many of them would contest the phrase "I could not be good-looking". The concept of good looks, they would say, is one of the symbols of women's oppression. It is time to examine this claim in detail.

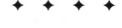

Hunt the Symbol

If you dislike a thing, you can make it out to be expressive of what you dislike. Lethaby dismissed Renaissance architecture as the "style of boredom", representing the High Priests, and as the art of scholars and courtiers; while praising Gothic as the art of hunters, craftsmen, and athletes. But all this tells us is that he preferred the latter classes of men to the former. The Parthenon no more expresses slavery or the City State than Beethoven's music expresses the petty German Courts of the early nineteenth century.

Reginald Turnor   The Smaller English House

An idea isn't responsible for the people who believe in it.

Don Marquis

If women's clothing and cosmetics symbolise women's oppression, is this because of their intrinsic character or just because they are what the oppressed sex wears? If the former, they should be abandoned. If not, there is no reason why they should; what needs to change is the oppression.

Symbolic meanings can be found not only in clothes, but gestures and even bodily functions; some theorists have thought women envy men because they urinate standing up, but in societies where men traditionally wore long robes, they squatted. The early nineteenth-century conductor Louis Jullien wore gloves when conducting Beethoven as a mark of respect, Wagner wore them when conducting works by Jewish composers in order, figuratively, to avoid soiling his hands. Women are supposed to walk in front of men in the West and behind them in Japan, and sexism exists in both. Orthodox Jewish married women shave their heads and wear wigs, but in the seventeenth and eighteenth centuries so did men; it was simply the fashion. Even where the phenomenon is the same, it can have different meanings for different beholders: the Virgin Mary has been described as an oppressive symbol by some feminists and a liberating one by others. Symbols are in the mind of the symboliser; as portraits and even photographs are said to do, they reveal more about their creators than about their subjects.

That being so, analogies between women's oppression and women's clothes need to be treated with caution. Even at their best, analogies are not facts. Opponents as well as supporters of feminism are only too fond of them. Freudians have taken little girls playing with hoses as evidence of penis envy; Simone de Beauvoir pointed out in *The Second Sex* that one could just as well say they liked penises because of their resemblance to hosepipes. *Media Sexploitation* by Wilson Bryan Key, an American anti-feminist, claimed that necklaces resembling those worn by Stone Age Brazilian Indians "established the wearer as the property of a man of wealth and power . . . North American women of affluence . . . were asked to briefly interpret the design's meaning . . . they simply did not know what the designs meant . . . overt meanings . . . were repressed behind conscious rationalisations such as, 'It's a good investment'; 'It brings out the real me'; 'It will go well with such and such new gown'; 'It's pretty.' The high price of this costume jewelry requires a strong purchase motivation – much stronger than such conscious rationalizations would support . . . how extraordinary it is that American women have no conscious idea of the symbolic meanings of even such simple decorative devices as the ribbon pinned snugly around their necks – a symbolic bondage collar".[18] He seems to assume that if an object had a certain meaning for the Caduveo Indians, it must have the same one for everyone everywhere, and anyone who denies it must be deceiving herself. What does he make of the fact that the modern Greek word for "yes" sounds like the Danish for "no", and that the Greeks, when they nod their heads, also mean "no"? More to the point, if women's collars mean bondage to men, what do male ones mean?

We have seen that the problem of skirts versus trousers is intractable, but many feminist parents avoid dressing girls in pink and boys in blue on the grounds that it's sexist. I don't deny that the distinction has consequences which lead to sexism, but the relation between the colours and the sex of their wearers is nothing like as straightforward as it seems. Letty Cottin Pogrebin writes: "whenever I'm even slightly attracted to something pink – say a frothy pink peignoir or a pink organdy bed canopy – I have a habit of remembering the dyed-to-match brainwashing . . . Actually, what I hate is what happens to pink when it's called into service to decorate a little girl's room or clothing. It colors ruffles that cannot be sat on, and lace that costs a fortune to clean . . . fabric that tears easily, thereby restricting girls' mobility and activity as effectively as shackles and chains. Pink is warm. But pink is suggestive of delicacy, of small, controlled motions in a small confined space."[19] Some anti-sexist parents have banned it: "one feminist mother went so far as to dye her daughter's whole layette a uniform black"[20] writes Sara Stein. More moderately, others asked "all of our relatives not to send pink, ruffles, lace or guns".[21] But Marjorie Garber quotes the *New York Times* as saying that "before World War I, boys wore pink ('a stronger, more decided color,' according to the promotional literature of the time) while girls wore blue (understood to be 'delicate' and 'dainty'.) Only after World War II, the *Times* reported, did the present alignment . . . come into being."[22] This does not seem to have been universally true; in *Good Wives* Jo explains that Meg's twins can be told apart because "Amy put a blue ribbon on the boy and a pink on the girl, French fashion". In Britain, boys in pink and girls in blue seem to have disappeared in about 1920, but are still found elsewhere, according to one report: "Several European countries, including Belgium, advocate pink for boys and blue for girls. Indeed, in Catholic countries there is a strong tendency to associate blue with girls, since that was the colour of the Virgin Mary's robe."[23]

I must add that I was dressed in blue, not because my parents wanted a boy (my mother wanted a girl and my father was neutral) but because my mother preferred blue as a colour and didn't care about convention. Pink doesn't mean femininity to me, it just means pink. A friend in her eighties commented revealingly, "You can dress a girl in blue but you can't dress a boy in pink," and *Woman* magazine had a correspondence on the same question in 1987. (One reader had seen a boy in a pink suit with BOY written on it in blue.) Colour therapists have claimed that independent people tend to prefer blue, but this might be because boys rather than girls are expected to be independent. If boys had gone on wearing pink and girls blue, wouldn't the experts claim that pink symbolised men's hotter blood and stronger sexuality, and wouldn't it be blue clothes and furnishings that were made in the delicate fabrics and pale shades that enforce "controlled motions in a small confined space"?

Attempts to find positive female symbols suffer from the same tendency to ignore whatever doesn't fit. American demonstrators' placards in the sixties carried a poem beginning:

Today at noon the moon,
Symbol of the female,
Rises to eclipse the sun,
Symbol of the male.[24]

The moon is the satellite of a satellite and borrows all its light from the sun. Do feminists want that image? Caroline Blackwood wrote of Greenham Common:

I saw my first web . . . It had been very cleverly woven, but it still seemed a bad peace symbol. Many people have a terrible fear of spiders. Webs are sticky and you can get caught in them. Once caught in a web, metaphorically you die. The peace women saw the webs as a symbol of strength . . . The explanation was all right, but as few people knew it, the web still seemed a very unfortunate peace sign.

The symbol of the snake, which was also beloved of the young girls of Greenham Common, disturbed me too. Why had they chosen such a stupidly frightening and poisonous symbol? . . . The snake, like the web, turned out to be a little better than it seemed, once it was explained. The snake sheds its skin and survives. It still seemed a great mistake when the peace women painted snakes on army trucks. The military couldn't be expected to understand the subtle symbolism.[25]

An essay by Angela Carter once suggested that a lipsticked mouth is a symbolic wound, as opposed to a Victorian woman's "rosebud mouth", but called the pale-mouthed look fashionable in the sixties "vulnerable"; the root of that word is the Latin for a wound, and pallor can be a sign of ill-health. I doubt if she thought women were more oppressed in the twentieth century than the nineteenth.[26] Besides, the Victorians didn't admire pale lips, except perhaps at the height of the vogue for pallor; in *Pendennis* the protagonist describes his first love's mouth as "of a staring red colour, with which the most brilliant geranium, sealing-wax or Guards-man's coat could not vie."

Muslim women sometimes wear veils to protest against anti-Islamic feeling, and some also claim that it protects them against sexual harassment (a point I shall return to later) and what Yasmin Alibhai-Brown called "the agony of living up to the dictates of fashion".[27] Her article was followed by correspondence in which someone called Western veiled brides "trussed-up"; apart from the fact that having a veil over one's face and being trussed up are not the same, bridal veils are not obligatory and only cover the face during the first part of the wedding ceremony, whereas an orthodox Muslim woman is supposed never to leave the house without one. Furthermore, in India it's bridegrooms who wear veils. The Egyptian writer Nawal El Saadawi, interviewed in *Sibyl*, said: "it is no different culturally from the postmodern veil of cosmetics and hair dyes that are forced on Western women by the media and beauty commercials". Apart from her assumption that nobody wears cosmetics voluntarily, there are two questions here: whether cosmetics are as restrictive as veils and whether they are equally compulsory. An article in the same issue of *Sibyl* reported: "Women athletes in Qatar must train wearing a full *hajib* over their tracksuits so they are unlikely to be in a position to compete equally on the rare day they are able to remove it."[28] A Saudi Arabian writes of the first time she was veiled: "I groped and stumbled . . . fearful of breaking an ankle or leg" and describes "sharp-eyed religious police patrolling the cities of Saudi Arabia, searching for uncovered women to strike with their sticks, or spray with red paint."[29] This applied, as a Japanese friend of mine who has lived in Saudi Arabia confirmed, to foreigners as well as Arab women.

The penultimate Shah of Iran forbade the *chador*; his son made it voluntary. "But in the late 1970s, as many Iranians turned away from what they saw as the corruption of the West, the *chador* became a symbol of the return to the purity of the Islamic tradition . . . After Khomeini took over, he began to order women . . . to wear the *hejab* . . . official films were censored so much that even women's bare arms were cut out . . . even just listening to music or the reading of poetry was suspect", writes one Iranian. Women were forbidden cosmetics, trousers and cycling: "Wearing make-up has become a feminist statement." Yasmin Alibhai-Brown adds: "Hundreds of women were imprisoned and beaten on the soles of their feet so they could not walk for months; some were hanged for transgressions of dress codes."[30] In Afghanistan, women risked torture by running secret beauty parlours.[31]

Decorative clothes and jewellery, according to several writers I have quoted, mean desire to seem weak and helpless but Paul Theroux writes that both sexes wear them in the remotest part of Tibet.[32] I can think of few people less weak and helpless than a Tibetan yak-herdsman.

Once we start thinking in terms of symbols, we are in danger of ending up like the man in an old joke who looked at all his food through a microscope and concluded that the only safe form of nourishment was boiled water. In practice, people outlaw aspects of culture which can be dispensed with while ignoring the possibly tainted origins of whatever is indispensable or even practically useful; a critic suggested that classicism in architecture should be banned forever because the Nazis liked it, but nobody suggests we should give up exercise because they recommended that. "I cannot enjoy reading works by people who treated women in their lives badly",[33] writes Pauline Bart, but what would she do if her life depended on an antibiotic discovered by a misogynist doctor? If she doesn't enjoy a book she is quite right to avoid it, but other people must be free to say, as I do, that since we can't eradicate the evil done by dead artists it is pointless to deprive ourselves of their art. It is also true that enjoying the art produced by the victims of evil is profiting from that evil as much as enjoying that produced by the evil-doers: since jazz was invented by slaves, everyone who enjoys it or any music influenced by it is benefiting from slavery in the same way as someone who lives in a city planned by slave-owners.

There is another danger in symbolic thinking: it leads to fighting the wrong enemy. People waste energy attacking not just the symptom rather than the disease, but something which may not even be a symptom. A friend told me that as a child, she loved reading aloud and felt frustrated when her English teacher passed her over in favour of poor readers. As it never occurred to her that they needed the practice, she kept thinking, "Miss X started with someone sitting near the window today, perhaps if I sit near it tomorrow she'll start with me." Much of the argument against "symbols of oppression" is on that level: for example, huntsmen thinking that changing the colour of their coats might give them a "better image", as if anti-hunting protesters hadn't made it clear that what they object to is killing animals. Worse, this kind of thinking can become an excuse for what would be called vandalism if done for any other reason. Sometimes it is vandalism in the strictest sense, as with Savonarola, Cromwell's Puritans, the Taliban and the Chinese during the Cultural Revolution when, according to Jung Chang, only Zhou Enlai's personal intervention saved the Forbidden City itself from destruction.[34] "How they must have enjoyed themselves!" said my father, looking at the images with smashed heads in Ely Cathedral. "How to behave like destructive small boys, *and* think you're saving your soul by doing it!" Karen Armstrong, a former nun, wrote of attempts to reform the dress of religious orders, "I can't help thinking that nuns are trying to find a new image, when what they want is a new reality."[35] Like huntsmen, the church isn't facing the root cause of the trouble: people are turning away from it because, rightly or wrongly, fewer and fewer of them believe in God.

Women have been, and are being, oppressed by men who liked dressing up and men who liked dressing down, men who liked women to dress up and men who liked them to dress down, men who wanted women's bodies hidden and men who wanted them exposed, men who cared passionately about art and men who gloried in their indifference to it. The roots of oppression must lie elsewhere.

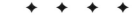

Caution – These Words Are Loaded!

Men talk of nature as an abstract thing, and lose sight of what is natural while they do so.

Charles Dickens   Nicholas Nickleby

Words can be dangerous. My mother, perhaps without meaning to, closed my mind for years to the debate about vivisection by saying: "If you have your tonsils out you're vivisected, but people don't call it that, they call it 'having an operation.'" Sheila Jeffreys approvingly quotes a separatist who "makes femininity sound quite brutal" with phrases such as "face masked with stinking, lurid chemicals".[36] Of course it sounds brutal put like that: what wouldn't? One could call music "bending our fingers around objects, forcing our breath through metal tubes, torturing our voices into unnatural noises". Words which arouse strong reactions keep occurring in feminist discussions without enough effort to define them accurately, with the result that they become virtually useless: all-purpose terms of praise or insult.

To begin with praise, "creative" is often used as if it were interchangeable with "good", which means that the user isn't really saying anything. When I say I don't like cooking, people often look surprised and say "But it's creative!" So is pottery, but I don't want to be a potter. Feminists have often queried, or even denied, the received wisdom about the joys of cook-ing (though some feminists do enjoy it) but the "creative equals good" equation can be found in feminist writing. Yet there is a creative element in clothing and adornment, so why isn't that seen as good? Many modern artists regard "found objects" as works of art, and if so, the act of assembling articles of dress is arguably in the same category. "Why should there be prizes for painting pictures, but not faces?"[37] asks Janet Radcliffe Richards. It may be objected that following fashions set by others is not creative, and obviously it is less so than inventing one's own styles, but it could be put in the same category as arts of interpretation such as dancing, acting, pro-ducing a play or performing music, all of which allow scope for some individuality. My mother's embroidery teacher once criticised her for copy-ing designs from Turkish pottery, which she wanted to do, instead of inventing them, which she didn't; I suggested reminding the teacher that Shakespeare borrowed all his plots. The anti-adornment feminists, however, deplore invented styles as well. More important still is the contradiction between creativity and another ideal which they invoke even more fre-quently and define even more vaguely: nature. My definition is: "natural" is whatever particular speakers or writers like, "unnatural" whatever they don't.

"Unnatural" is the stock adjective used by the detractors of fashion and cosmetics, which, says Adrienne Rich, make us "lie with our bodies".[38] But unless people who use cosmetics pretend not to (an attempt less likely to happen when they are socially acceptable than when they are not), where is the lie? As to clothes, all clothing is a form of disguise and so far as I know Rich is not advocating universal nudity. All civilisation is an attempt to improve on nature, so if we are trying to find out whether the improvement is genuine or not, nature won't do as a touchstone. It can even be argued that if nature includes human psychology (and how can it fail to?) the desire to change the status quo must be included too. When critics asked František Kupka why he painted abstracts instead of "from nature" he answered: "Whatever a human being does is part of nature." Many human activities are attempts to stretch natural limitations and even the most utilitarian clothes are examples of this. Carlyle pointed out in *Sartor Resartus* (1836) that we are not clothed animals but naked ones who put on clothes. The fact that our earliest human ancestors survived long enough to reproduce themselves shows that they were once able to withstand the weather condi-tions from which we now protect ourselves with clothing. We don't know how the change occurred, but we know it did. (It is said that a nineteenth-century Canadian Indian was asked how he could go naked in winter and answered "Me all face.")

Just as people now wear clothing instead of growing extra hair, they now enhance their sexual attractions by clothing instead of by physical modifications such as those of birds which grow more colourful feathers or sing during the mating season (nightingales, for instance, stop singing after nesting time). Unlike other species, we are always ready for sex, so it is natural for us to show it. As Wendy Chapkis asked, "what would functional clothing look like if our intended activity is sex?"[39] Besides, human aesthetics have extended into areas only indirectly connected with sex, if at all, which is why the fine arts exist. We saw in the last chapter that this is more complicated than it looks: if beauty simply means, in Elizabeth Wilson's words, "looks and appearance . . . defined as sexually alluring",[40] I don't understand her comment, supported by some of the men I have quoted, that elegance can be sexually inhibiting. Isn't elegance a form of beauty and if not why do women, and some men, try to be elegant? Again, classical ballet is intended to be beautiful, and if beauty always equals sex, why is it not considered a "manly" interest by the same men who read "sexy" magazines? (Such men went to the ballet more in the nineteenth century, but that was because it was almost the only way to see uncovered female legs.) Also, how could anyone be described as ugly but sexy?

The arguments against beauty culture could often apply equally to other fields in which they are seldom or never used. Once again, it helps to consider men; we have already seen that it wasn't a gross over-simplification to claim, as did a book on the fashion industry published in the sixties, that if it was natural for men to dress plainly no man behaved naturally until 1830.[41] Removing or even trimming beards interferes with nature just as much as some of the practices feminists object to. It would take a great many cosmetics to change a woman's face as much as shaving does that of a previously bearded man, though one friend told me his mother took ten years to notice his small moustache. Why should it be less acceptable for a woman to shave her legs and armpits than for a man to shave his chin?

Feminists reject the symbolic equation of hairiness with sexual potency (which contradicts the similar status given to baldness), and they had better: since hardly any women are as naturally hairy as most men, if the symbol accurately reflected reality feminism would be doomed. (A lesbian artist, Della Grace, led a campaign to make beards and moustaches acceptable for women. It didn't last, perhaps because few women could grow enough hair to look as if they were doing it deliberately.) Harriet Lyons and Rebecca W.

Rosenblatt write, "Man/woman is the only animal sexually active beyond the need to reproduce; the only animal that can experience orgasm at times when conception is impossible. We are both the most sex-driven and the least hairy of the animal kingdom, yet we persist in equating sexuality with furriness."[42] This would seem like an argument for shaving, but they encourage women not to. Presumably it is because of the association between hair and power that men don't like going bald; if being different from women were the issue, they would welcome it, because baldness is overwhelmingly male. It is a sign of ageing, but men are less worried by that than women, as innumerable feminists have observed, so they must care more about the aesthetic aspect of it than they think. (According to *Modern Woman: The Lost Sex* Eliza Burt Gamble wrote in 1893 that "Hairiness denotes a low stage of development", lack of it proving female superiority.)

Why, incidentally, do people speak of "wearing" beards, as if they were clothes? I suspect it may be an unconscious attempt to deny that men change their faces by implying, wrongly, that beards are not part of them: a clear case, if so, of twisting facts to fit a theory. Many aspects of beauty culture, including hair removal, have been criticised as "infantilising" women, but the same is true of returning a man's face to prepubescent smoothness (advertisements for razors and shaving creams stress "smooth-ness" and lack of "five o'clock shadow"). Italian men are said to shave their legs, though I haven't checked this, and any woman who walks alone down an Italian street knows how sexist they can be. Having seen Italian women strap-hanging in buses, I can testify that many have unshaved armpits, and a Dutchwoman once told my mother she left hers hairy to please men. (I once saw a newspaper poll on what men found attractive; the only man who liked hairy armpits also liked dirty feet.) The Taliban forced men to shave their armpits and pubic hair. Jean A. Rees, a writer of popular books on Christianity, tells how she was criticised for "unnatural" cosmetics and asked her critic why he shaved;[43] Harriet Beecher Stowe called shaving an "anti-patriarchal activity", and Sir Max Beerbohm described a moustache without a beard as a sign of levity. In late nineteenth-century France, according to one historian, this was becoming almost universal, whereas previously different kinds of beards and whiskers were signs of a man's profession, politics and class;[44] I am told waiters went on strike for the right to wear moustaches. Even now, some firms won't hire bearded men. Short haircuts also change nature, but many modern feminists have repeated William Prynne's argument that long hair "means" submission to men.

Whatever people are used to seems natural until they examine it closely, which is why so many theories turn out to be historically unsound. People observe the culture they grow up in before they learn about other times and places, and instinctively think of it as the norm, even if it hasn't been one for long: feminists have called secretarial work a "traditional" woman's job, though it was a man's from the dark ages until the twentieth century. Innumerable arguments against feminism can be reduced to "women have always been the second sex so they always will." Nor do feminists want to follow nature in all respects: one of their principal demands is freedom to use birth control, and most also defend abortion. If these practices are acceptable (which I am not disputing) and altering one's appearance isn't, the degree of interference with nature cannot be the criterion. Anja Meulenbelt has argued that if high heels were natural we should be born with them; Janet Radcliffe Richards, quoting a similar remark about bras, writes that this hardly differs from saying that if we were meant to fly we should be born with wings.[45] (The bra, invented by Herminie Cadolle in 1889, was less restrictive than contemporary corsets.) The moral would appear to be that it is permissible to alter nature for practical purposes, but not beautification: feminists cut their nails.

The apologists for unadorned bodies seem to have one unanswerable argument: damage to health. Beauty culture must be bad for women if it hurts. The problem with this philosophy is that almost anything can damage health in some circumstances, so it is almost as hard to avoid as unacceptable symbolism.

Some feminists celebrate the legendary Greek Amazons, who are supposed to have amputated their right breasts in order to handle bows freely. Mandy Merck writes that this is "notably absent from both Greek art and myth" suggesting it comes from αμαστος, which may mean "without a breast", one of the "folk etymologies invented by the Greeks in explanation of a name whose derivation was already lost".[46] Some of the Amazons' feminist admirers have taken the idea of amputation literally and not been put off, notably Benoîte Groult, who referred to the "rectification" of their breasts.[47] I can imagine her reaction if men used that word to describe cutting a woman's breast off. Feminists have enouraged women to participate in sport, but sport can injure and even kill; a BBC television newsreader reported on 22 June 1994 that in Britain a sports injury occurs every second. There have been feminist analyses of the risks and benefits of sport, but where is the rational discussion of the risks of beauty culture, whether they are worth taking and if so, how to minimise them? There is special pleading on both sides: members of the fashion and beauty industries make it all sound easy and painless, whereas feminists writing in opposition to it exaggerate just as much, or more, in the other direction. Wearing very high heels can certainly be uncomfortable and even dangerous, but when feminists liken it to Chinese foot-binding, no wonder they are accused of having no sense of proportion. Jung Chang describes the latter: "My grandmother's feet had been bound when she was two years old. Her mother . . . first wound a piece of white cloth about twenty feet long round her feet, bending all the toes except the big toe under the sole. Then she placed a large stone on top to crush the arch . . . My grandmother passed out repeatedly from the pain: "The process lasted several years. Even after the bones had been broken, the feet had to be bound day and night in thick cloth because the moment they were released they would try to recover . . . Men rarely saw naked bound feet, which were usually covered in rotting flesh and stank when the bindings were removed."[48] A girl with feet more than four inches long was considered unmarriageable and could be abandoned during her wedding ceremony.

Mary Daly rightly observes that Western scholars' language minimises the suffering involved: "One difference between footbound women and amputees is that the latter can, with prostheses, learn to walk, whereas perfectly footbound women could only fall from stump to stump and often had to be carried . . . [Vern Bullough's] choice of the bland term *effort* is deeply and subtly deceptive. If it conjures up any images at all, these are somewhere in the range of tight shoes, corns, bunions, or at worst a sprained ankle – hardly conveying the reduction of a woman's feet to putrescent three-inch stumps."[49] My great-uncle, travelling in China in 1875, saw women with feet no more than two or three inches long,[50] and some were still to be seen when I went there exactly a century later. Daly also points out that when foot-binding was forbidden and feet forcibly unbound, this produced more suffering, for once a woman's foot was broken it was easier for her to walk with bindings on than without them. The same applied to a Burmese woman's neck-rings: once her neck had been stretched by them, she might even die if they were taken off, as was sometimes done for a punishment. Feet, however, were unbound in the name of liberation.

Germaine Greer claims it is illogical for wearers not only of high heels but of bras, lipstick and nail varnish to object to female circumcision, but praises performance artists "like Orlan who carve the insignia of the stereotype into their own flesh",[51] which is far more painful. Never, in all the diatribes against high heels I have read, have I seen any definition of the point at which the danger level starts, as if there were no difference between five inches and two, wearing them all day and every day or for half an hour a month, or walking one mile or twenty in them; I have heard them condemned by five feminists of whom three were smoking at the time. David Kunzle described tight corsets as a source of pleasure in "body sculpture" rather than pain; maybe he exaggerated, but Angela Carter wrote that he made her rethink her assumption that "sexually specific clothing" made women "dupes of male fancy".[52] Cosmetics can cause allergies, but if we tried to ban everything in that category, not much would remain. Some people are allergic to distilled water. A Dr Ian White said on BBC Radio 4 on 16 December 1992 that cosmetic allergy affects one user in fifty, which means it is no more common in Britain than a household without a television set. Lyons and Rosenblatt call shaving "painful" because it hurts to use deodorant or swim in salt water immediately afterwards, and you can cut yourself if you do it in a hurry, and electrolysis "hazardous" because it needs to be done expertly; would they ban cars because driving can kill if done carelessly or immediately after drinking? Lee Comer called tweezers, depilatories and cosmetics "mutilation".[53] This reminds me of "temperance" advocates who write as if everyone who is not teetotal is an alcoholic, and of whom J. C. Furnas's history of American prohibition commented: "the moderate drinker was specially unpopular because he made Temperance propaganda look bad. The spewing drunk in the gutter was a fine Exhibit A, but not the well-tailored gentleman having a cool sherry-cobbler . . . and . . . none the worse for it".[54]

Feminists who take issue with the pro-nature theory, however, are sometimes equally reluctant to draw distinctions. They may be anxious to defend their own culture and fear being accused of prejudice, especially racism, if they criticise someone else's. "In designating types of dress," write Joanne B. Eicher and Mary Ellen Roach-Higgins, "writers frequently use ethnocentric, value-charged terms such as mutilation, deformation, decoration, ornament, and adornment." When using the last three "they are clearly making a value judgment regarding its merits as an aesthetically pleasing creation. Similarly, their calling a type of dress a mutilation or deformation indicates they have judged it to be nonacceptable."[55] Not necessarily: they may be saying it is meant to be aesthetically pleasing by the dresser, not that they themselves think the attempt is successful, just as calling wallpaper interior decoration doesn't necessarily imply liking it, and a picture is still a work of art if somebody, or even everybody, regards it as bad art. As to mutilation and deformation, whether any aspect of dress deserves these terms should depend on whether they do serious damage to the wearer, which can and should be evaluated. Lakoff and Scherr try to suggest that "our 'normal' enhancements of what is already there" are not so different as we think from other societies' practices such as scarification: "animals are not noted for redness of lip, curl and length of eyelash, opalescent blush of fingernail, or luxuriance of hair on the head" so, the book implies, we are going against nature by simulating them as much as if we scarred ourselves. True, these characteristics are not found in most animals (though some have manes) but they are found in *homo sapiens*, which means they are as natural to us as, say, scales to fish. The authors express doubts about frequent changes of clothing, but in this we do resemble other animals, who don't take their old coats out of storage, but grow new ones. They also appear to be in two minds about tattooing (I have seen a woman with a tattooed feminist symbol) and attempt to draw an analogy between the amount of pain caused by mutilation and the lifelong discomfort of restrictive clothes ("it evens out"). I find this more than dubious, especially as they extend it to financial discomfort; if buying expensive clothes and cosmetics were a form of masochism, those who can afford them most easily wouldn't buy them. Besides, the alterations to people's appearance practised in some other societies do cause long-term as well as short-term pain (foot-binding and neck-rings, for instance) and some of ours do the opposite; the growing popularity of cosmetic surgery as a substitute for dieting suggests the preference for short-term pain is increasing. The real trouble with the analogy, however, is this: how many years of shaving does it take to add up to the same amount of pain as scarification? (Tongue, navel and nipple piercing may be a fair comparison.)

Lakoff and Scherr quote women trying to distinguish between cosmetics "that merely enhanced what was already there, and those that actually changed appearance." How can you enhance without changing? "In the first category . . . were perfume, eyeliner, colourless nail polish; in the second, hair dye, lipstick, mascara." Why is painting a line round one's eyes in a different category from painting the lashes? There could hardly be a clearer indication of the difficulty of deciding where "nature" begins and ends, and the authors seem to be as confused as anyone; they say of the myth of Narcissus changed into a flower, "it waits to be plucked, its highest purpose is being appreciated. But in fact we cannot speak reasonably of a flower's 'purpose.' As an inanimate object, it cannot have one. Its function is purely in the eye of its beholder."[56] This would be true of an artificial flower, but Narcissus became a real one, the reproductive organ of a living plant.

Flowering plants can be just as tough as others, and women who object to being likened to them don't know their botany.

Rebelling against accepted standards of beauty can do as much damage as conforming. Robin Morgan describes a woman who "taxes her heart with her extreme weight; the mere exertion of walking along the street brings a fine mist of perspiration to her face; it is her defense against being objectified."[57] Could objectification hurt her more than she is hurting herself?

One reason why following nature appeals so strongly to people trying to formulate guidelines is that the desire for anything defined as "unnatural" can be written off as the result of social influences. It is too easily forgotten that societies are made up of people. Denial by the person with the desires in question proves nothing, as it can be attributed to one of two popular psychological ideas: conditioning and the subconscious. Certainly both exist, but both can be made an excuse for ignoring any evidence which doesn't fit the speaker's or writer's theory. This reflects the so-called "nature-nurture problem" of working out what is caused by biology and what by the environment, which is insoluble because neither can be isolated: you can't do experiments with some subjects who have only an environment and others who have only biology when every living creature has both by definition. It's far too easy to say "You don't really want that, you only think you do because you've been conditioned, and subconsciously you know I'm right." Not only feminists do this, as Wilson Bryan Key shows; one of the anti-feminists' main arguments is that women only want equality because they have been conditioned to do so.

This is a very easy argument to use about our dissatisfaction with our own appearance; as Rosie Boycott put it, other animals are satisfied with theirs.[58] There are two answers to this: one is that animals lack the human capacity for thought and the other is that though they like themselves they can be savage towards others who are different. For instance, birds mob other birds, which should make us think twice about idealising nature. There is a clear parallel between this and racists who distrust everyone with differently coloured skin. The Chinese have been quoted as an example of a society which for many centuries had no desire to change its traditions. Hugh Baker, Professor of Chinese at the University of London, explains why: "Chinese culture and Chinese society embodied all that was civilised and superior . . . foreign policy since time immemorial had consisted of keeping the rest of the world at bay."[59] There was and still is a great deal of racism in China.

The alternative is admitting that other ways of doing things might be better, which in turn means at least the possibility of the dissatisfaction with our lot which, when it applies to our looks, is so deplored by feminists. (Examples are innumerable: children play at being grown up, adults idealise childhood, country-dwellers the town and town-dwellers the country. The reason is that when you consider someone else's life, you can pick out the parts you like and ignore the rest, which you can't do with your own.) Why do women always want to be different? Because the only woman who never does is the one who thinks nothing could possibly be better than the way she is already: this is an accurate description of some of the most chauvinistic men, and is at the root of their confidence that how they look doesn't matter.

One of the founding principles of women's liberation was that every woman is an expert on her own life; granted that her feelings may have been distorted by outside influence, if we don't use them as a starting point, what do we use? If we do, then our feelings that our appearance can be improved and that we may enjoy doing so should be taken into account. Nancy Friday's *The Power of Beauty* describes very young children preferring symmetrical features (although some of their social conditioning tells them they shouldn't) and Germaine Greer has written: "Most societies reject the grossly deformed. All societies have notions of beauty and fitness to which they aspire."[60] With fitness, at least, it would be anything but natural not to do so, because it would contradict the instinct for self-preservation. Symmetrical features have nothing to do with health, but symmetrical bodies do, so it is easy to see why the two may be associated. Nature has no mercy on the unfit, which makes health care and the idea of disabled people's rights unnatural. The criterion of fitness suggests a reason for preferring youth: a young body is at the height of its physical powers, an older one has passed it. Veblen claimed that the desire for objects to appear unused is a manifestation of his theory that useless objects have the highest status, but one could argue the opposite: an unused object has all its useful life before it. Feminists have championed the healthy body, preserved from being "mutilated" by fashion, but if health is the ideal, that implies it is better to be healthy than not, and, other things being equal, being young means being fitter. Health also being likely to have healthy children, and Nancy Etcoff claims beauty standards arise from the characteristics desirable for evolution.[61] At least some feminists sympathise with sufferers from acne, because it is a disease, and can be painful (I have had spots which hurt when the wind blew on them). Ann Oakley suggested: "The day when . . .

women's hair is obviously greasy and neglected, might portend some actual, rather than mythical, liberation"[62] but neglected greasy hair itches (again I speak from experience). I fail to see that tolerating an itching scalp to prove you are a feminist is any improvement on wearing uncomfortable shoes to prove you are a woman. One feminist I met called it "aesthetically prejudiced" to find people who "dare to be maimed" less beautiful, but beauty is by definition something which makes the beholder think "this is how things ought to be" and who, if only for practical reasons, wouldn't prefer not to be maimed? If being maimed is just as good as being whole, then good health is no better than bad, so why should feminists promote it? If being maimed is all right, why should saying fashion maims women be any condemnation of it? An author whose name I forget summed up the "natural" argument by saying only two generalisations are true of nature: it contains a wide variety of types and they adapt to changing circumstances. Finally, I have a private, unproveable theory that clothes and even cosmetics are our attempt to find a substitute for other animals' expressive tail language, which was lost to us when we shed our tails. If so, nothing could be more natural.

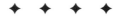

He used to say that nothing makes misery harder to bear than not having the right to it acknowledged.

Monica Stirling   Something to Write Home About

Nous avons tous assez de force pour supporter les maux d'autrui.

La Rochefoucauld[63]

No man ever got his soul saved while he had toothache.

General William Booth, founder of the Salvation Army

Some readers may object that feminist criticism isn't directed to decorative clothes or cosmetics as such, but only to an excess of them. This isn't true of, for instance, the passage from Andrea Dworkin's *Woman Hating* quoted in chapter 1, but even if it were, so what? Telling people they may do something provided they don't do it too much, without further guidelines, just leaves them worrying about whether they should be worried. Nobody would call anything "too much" unless it were better to have less of it. Anything which permanently damages health is a legitimate target, but that is as far as one can go without reaching the areas where no two people agree. This is what I call extremism and water, and many of the authors who have tried to solve the "beauty problem" haven't produced anything more.[64]

I suspect this argument results from attempts to mediate between those who disapprove of all fashion and beauty culture and those who don't, and like most compromises it pleases nobody. It also leads to the kind of half-hearted puritanism which says it's all right to do something provided you don't do it as though you meant it. This strongly resembles the view that it's acceptable for women to have careers, provided they are not as successful as men's.

All these exhortations not to be troubled by other people's standards ignore our own. "If you think a part of yourself is unacceptable, you must say why. Not 'Because it doesn't look good' – why doesn't it? Who said that?" writes Kaz Cooke, and Jane Cousins-Mills that asymmetrical breasts "shouldn't really matter"[65] because we shouldn't feel under pressure to keep up with "people's" standards of perfection. What if you are the one who isn't satisfied, and you find it easier to try to solve the problem than to ignore it? Pursuing excellence in any other sphere is seen as reasonable by most people; in beauty culture it's hard to find anyone who stands up for it without feeling the need for special pleading.

Not taking people's desires or worries seriously is insulting them, and it happens even to people who are seriously disfigured, of whom Doreen Frust writes: "we affront them and all the known rules of justice and fair play by telling them that they haven't really got a problem!"[66] Diane Coyle "was well on the way to being utterly disfigured by a growth above my right eye . . . I spent a quarter of a century with my life dominated by having a face that strangers would stare at then turn away from" until she had cosmetic surgery, to which she offered "a hymn of praise . . . Not just . . . for 'deserving' cases like mine" (it affected her vision as well as her appearance) "but for anybody unhappy about how their body looks . . . the surgeon is the liberator, not the oppressor . . . The surgery was gruesome and painful, and I would do it again in a trice if I needed to."[67] Gloria Steinem writes of a "teenage boy . . . whose face was ravaged by smallpox and acne, whose fundamentalist parents would not let him erase this evidence of 'God's punishment'" and who was also refused permission for cosmetic surgery by a judge. A surgeon, Leslie Gardiner, tells a similar story:

A factory overseer, who wanted me to alter the shape of his nose, had two fingers of one hand missing. Noticing this, I sympathized. 'I'm glad it happened,' he replied.

'Glad it happened?' I looked at him, he was a serious man and he had uttered the words seriously.

'I lost them in an accident,' he explained, 'and got compensation, so I'm using some of my compensation money to have my nose put right. I've learned to do without the fingers, the nose is much more important to me and I've suffered with it all my life.' He had a very ugly nose and he had, in a flash, revealed to me the true depth of his feelings about it.[68]

It must have been ugly, in his view at least, if it disfigured him more than two missing fingers.

It is often said that happy people don't care how ugly they are; this is tautologous, because the only happy ugly people are the ones who don't. Karen DeCrow wrote in a book for teenagers: "The idiocy of all this is obvious. First of all, it turns every female human being into an object; what is appropriate for a woman who wants to go on the stage (and who is, incidentally, born with classic features) is a big waste of time for other women . . . Any human being who values herself will not spend thousands of hours to change the texture of an elbow, to alter the color of her hair, to narrow the width of an ankle. And she certainly will not undergo major surgery to pin back ears, to shorten a nose, to enlarge breasts."[69] A man I know, of normal appearance, said of a television programme on cosmetic dentistry that he couldn't understand the mentality of anyone other than a professional model who had it; I asked him if he could understand the mentality of people who took music lessons when they were not trying to be professional musicians. He saw the point; would DeCrow? I can guess how she would be answered if she made similar remarks to a woman who wanted infertility treatment, but fertility is just as much a genetic accident as looks.

Letty Cottin Pogrebin compares cosmetic surgery to home improvement:

> my husband and I . . . made a purely aesthetic judgement. Why shouldn't I do the same thing when it came to self-improvement? . . . People are criticized for 'using' their looks but not for 'using' their God-given voices or other inborn talent. Furthermore, if self-improvement is a reasonable rationale for voice lessons that might help a person sing better, why shouldn't self-improvement be a reasonable motivation for surgery that might help a person look better?

. . .We complain because looks count so much to others, yet we can't seem to admit to ourselves that looks count to us, too . . . We know from experience that looks become less important the more people know or love each other, yet most of us still make an effort to look good for our friends and loved ones . . . If looks don't matter – if inner beauty is what counts – why do they [her children] notice and why do we care? We teach our children that looks don't matter . . .

Not much has changed since *Agnes Grey*. Why not? She seems to me to have put her finger on it: "we're not sure attractiveness is a legitimate value."[70] I am.

I repeat that I don't mean it's more important than character or intellect or a substitute for them, any more than ability to sing is. It can lead to discrimination, but so does, for instance, the even more personal matter of whether I like someone's sense of humour. If someone's idea of a joke isn't mine, it isn't that person's fault but I still won't be amused.

I believe it's the unwillingness to admit that looks matter to some of us that makes people confuse them with other things which undeniably matter more. If more people could admit that good looks were good intrinsically and that they care about them in themselves and others, they wouldn't be so likely to convince themselves that they were responding to character when really responding to appearance, which can cause real damage.

The same logic governs the judgment of attempts to improve on raw material as judgment of the material itself. Either such improvements are acceptable or they are not. If people are going to be allowed to make them, they must be allowed to make enough of them to provide the satisfaction which is their only point. It may be worth doing something badly if that is the only way you can do it; it is not worth doing it less well than you need to in order to enjoy it, especially when it is something which need not be done at all. A leaking roof is better than none and junk food better than starvation, but pleasures that don't please are pointless (as the novelist Angela Thirkell put it, "Never economise on luxuries") and allowing them is like letting people use machinery provided it doesn't work. The criterion is the same for both: fitness for purpose. Nobody, however, claims a machine that doesn't work is as good as one that does, so what this attitude leads to is the tyranny of practical values over all others. It also leads to an unfair advantage being given to the sort of luxuries which have similar criteria to practical matters, like sport. Although we don't need, say, football any more than we need frilly petticoats, sport has a pseudo-practical aura not only because it is a form of exercise (which we do need) but because the standard is clear: either you can run faster, jump higher, hit the ball harder than the next person or you can't. Sport also benefits from being associated with males, as does technology, though this too can be used for activities of no practical use such as computer games. Yet if we are going to permit useless values and pursuits at all, people must be allowed to decide for themselves how important they are and how much effort to put into them.

Treating other people's wishes with respect enables them to make up their own minds about whether or not the price of what they want is too high; if not, they may disagree just to prove who's boss. The most helpful attitude to cosmetic surgery I know of is that of a (male) friend of mine who said: "I don't think you need this operation, but if you decide you do, remember I'm still on your side, because it's *your* nose." Or as one of my cousins said when other family members criticised my parents for wanting to buy a house they thought unnecessarily expensive: "What's it worth to them?"

7

THE ULTIMATE ATTACK: FASHION AS PORNOGRAPHY

Porn is rape.

Graffito, York

When I first planned this book I had no idea that I should have to include anything about pornography, but I soon found that it was impossible to discuss feminist attitudes to fashion, or almost anything else, without confronting it. If there is one issue which has blown the idea of universal sisterly agreement out of existence, this is it. What is pornography? Is it violence? Where does it begin and end? Has it infiltrated fashion? Is all fashion pornographic? Are all aesthetics pornographic?

That last question, which has been asked in all seriousness and not always been given the same answer, shows why this must be discussed. If porn is rape and fashion is porn, it matters. If, as Michael Korda asserts, "every time we make an anti-Semitic remark we shake hands with the Nazis, however unconsciously",[1] are we shaking hands with Jack the Ripper every time we dress up? Some feminists would say yes, others emphatically deny it; some demand a legal ban on what others demand the right to enjoy.

Debates tend to polarise, and the poles in this one are frightening: either you are against all sexuality, or you are in favour of all its manifestations and images, the latter being what concerns us here. Either you condemn everything or nothing. News coverage doesn't help, as the American writer Wendy Kaminer points out: "Analysis, much less judiciousness, is dismissed as equivocation. In any case, it's not good TV. 'We're looking for a good debate,' the producer will say, and her vision of a debate is one person saying 'Is too!' and the other responding 'Is not!'"[2]

After examining the evidence, I conclude that not only do those involved have more in common than one might suppose (they could hardly have less) but that the real division is not so much between them as between the moderates and the extremists on both sides. The ultra-libertarian and the ultra-pornophobe share one opinion: that it is almost, if not quite, impossible to distinguish between what is pornography and what isn't. The only difference is that one likes it and the other doesn't.

Moderates in both camps unite in objecting to a certain kind of pornography; what they disagree on is whether censoring it will do more good than harm or more harm than good, and where to draw the line between it and what is tolerable or even desirable. This entails making distinctions, sometimes subtle ones, which is just what polarisation discourages. It also entails finding a way to handle disagreement between those who draw the line at different points. They are all afraid of throwing out the baby with the bathwater, but can't agree on which is the bathwater and which is the baby. For one side the baby is freedom of speech, artistic expression and sexuality, for the other it's the protection of women: from what?

About actual harm such as rape and assault, there is no dispute whatever. The difficulty starts with two claims whose validity can't be proved, despite repeated efforts: that porn provokes violence, and that it is a form of violence in itself. If real proof were found, the argument would end, and this chapter would not need to be written. I suggest the first step in clarifying the different shades of opinion is their holders' terminology.

One side proudly calls itself anti-pornography; its most famous representatives are Andrea Dworkin and Catharine MacKinnon, and its members have no hesitation in calling their opponents pro-pornography. Most of the latter dislike this, but there are obvious disadvantages to "anti-anti-pornography." Two other terms are "pro-sex" and "anti-censorship". The trouble with the first is that it pre-empts the discussion by labelling everyone who disagrees "anti-sex" by implication, just as anti-abortionists who call themselves "pro-life" imply that everyone else is pro-death; the trouble with the second is that not everyone who is against pornography is in favour of censorship. I propose to use Carole Vance's term "sex radical" as "radical feminist" is used by members of both sides, though both insist that only theirs is truly radical; this results in considerable confusion and plainly shows how much we need unambiguous language.

I think a slight digression is necessary here to distinguish between different feminist groups, in order to be clear about who said what. The most widely acknowledged division is between "radicals" and "socialists", the difference being, roughly, that radicals consider the cause of women's oppression to be male supremacy while socialists also accuse the capitalist system. Both, if taken to extremes, are apt to come round full circle to something not very different from anti-feminism. Socialism doesn't explain why male domination has existed in all societies of which we have any records, long before capitalism was invented, and seeing feminism as part of a "wider" socialist strategy can lead to its being swallowed up or put off until "after the revolution", which in practice means for ever. One reason for the resurgence of feminism in the sixties was that women who had thought the left was against all forms of oppression found that "working together for the revolution" meant the men on the barricades and the women making coffee. A Marxist feminist, Dee Ann Pappas, has argued that not only are received ideas of male and female nature fallacies, but so is human corruptibility: "systems not men create oppression in the world."[3] Who, if not people, made the systems?

Radicals, on the other hand, see themselves as attacking the problem at the root (which is what "radical" means), the root being male supremacy. This can easily change from an attack on male supremacy to an attack on men and belief in an innate female superiority, a philosophy of which feminists are frequently accused by their enemies. If it is true, the search for sex equality must be hopeless, as supporters of this view argue, advocating a retreat from men into a women-only alternative society; this brings us back to two sexes with fundamentally different natures, occupying separate spheres. Pornography belongs to the evil male culture (including that of the male left). Whereas socialist feminists, to use Olive M. Banks's terms, tend to be masculine egalitarians, supporters of separatism are anything but.

Even some feminist theorists, who should know better, tend to write as if every feminist either embraces socialism, or even Marxism, or rejects men altogether. Some socialist and other feminists claim that all radical feminists believe in a separate women's world, and the sex radicals claim that all anti-pornographers do so. They don't, which makes it important to find a term other than "radical" for those who do. Several exist, but they are inconsistently applied, the greatest confusion arising out of the various uses of "cultural feminist". This can mean a woman who wants a women-only culture, but it is also used by feminists who believe that aspects of culture which have been regarded as feminine are undervalued, but not necessarily unattainable by men. Helen Haste, for instance, uses "cultural feminist" in this sense; she believes that all radicals regard male nature as unchangeable, which is one reason why she doesn't call herself one. "Radical feminism", she says, "implies separatism and utopianism", which is exactly the radicals' definition of "cultural feminism".[4] An illustration from Gloria

Steinem's essay "If Men Could Menstruate" may help. "Radical feminists would add that the oppression of the nonmenstrual was the pattern for all other oppressions. ('Vampires were our first freedom fighters!') Cultural feminists would exalt a bloodless female imagery in art and literature. Socialist feminists would insist that, once capitalism and imperialism were overthrown, women would menstruate, too."[5] Other words indicating various "women only" positions are essentialist (meaning belief in immutable male and female essences), biological determinist (echoing the Freudian view that "anatomy is destiny"), separatist (meaning belief that men and women should live separately) and the umbrella term "difference feminist" which includes all these. I suggest the clear, though clumsy, term "cultural difference feminists" for advocates of women-only culture.

The slang use of the word "radical" as if it simply meant "extreme" (Mary Midgley and Judith Hughes, for instance, use it like this[6]) doesn't help, because it can be applied to an extreme version of anything; Helen Haste points out that it is sometimes used of Marxist feminists. This makes the phrase "moderate radical" sound like an oxymoron, which it isn't. It is perfectly possible to agree that the root of the specific disadvantages attached to being a woman is the belief that men are better, while not necessarily agreeing with all the evidence which some radicals present (just as one can be a socialist without being a communist) and it is in this light that I propose to examine that belief. "Liberal" is sometimes used for this category of feminism, but with even less precision.

To be fair, some of the radicals' more apocalyptic statements, taken out of context, do suggest essentialism. Robin Morgan's "pornography is the theory, rape is the practice" doesn't mean that every man who flicks through *Playboy* automatically becomes a rapist, and Susan Brownmiller's "every man is a potential rapist" doesn't mean that all men rape or even want to, just that women don't know they wouldn't, and are therefore intimidated. Similarly, Andrea Dworkin's "Women will know that they are free when pornography no longer exists" may only mean that in a truly free world it wouldn't (even some sex radicals like Ellen Willis, surprisingly, agree with that); but it does look as if what she said was that abolishing porn is all it takes to free all women. This naturally provokes comments like "what about equal pay?"

Another cause of confusion is that "cultural feminist" is used by the sex radicals about all radical feminists who disagree with them about pornography and sexual morality, reinforcing the belief that they are all essentialists. For instance, Alice Echols declared at the Barnard conference that radical feminists "attributed women's attachment to traditional morality not to the innately spiritual quality of women's sexuality, but rather to our socialization which encourages sexual alienation and guilt . . . Unlike radical feminists who attacked romantic love, cultural feminists apotheosize it."[7] In support of this she quotes not only some condemnations of all sex with men or even all sex, but also Dana Densmore's statement that "to make love to a man who despises you"[8] is worse than no sex at all. If you don't think any sex is better than none, you're anti-sex; if you defend any traditional "womanly" qualities, you must be retreating from a mixed-sex world, as if it were not possible, and even desirable, for men to adopt them too.

The 1969 Redstockings invented the "pro-woman line" as stated in their Principles, "We do not ask what is 'radical,' 'revolutionary,' 'reformist,' or 'moral' — we ask: is it good for women or bad for women?'"[9] and it was one of them, Carol Hanisch, who invented the slogan "the personal is political." If they didn't believe in going to the root of women's inferior status, who did? Another Redstocking called Brooke wrote an essay in *Feminist* called "The Retreat to Cultural Feminism" which in some ways anticipates Echols (it is noteworthy that Brooke is "speaking as a lesbian" herself) but it also contains unequivocal defences not only of heterosexuality, but of love, monogamy and marriage, as well as a section called "Building a Real Left". (Pornography isn't mentioned; the debate hadn't erupted when the book was written.) Some separatist lesbians, on the other hand, "believed that non-monogamy was essential to lesbian relationships".[10] Monogamy and romance are irrelevant to this book, but the point has to be made because so much writing by the sex radicals suggests that feminists divide neatly into two camps which can be labelled "pro-sex" and "anti-sex". They don't, but feminism isn't exempt from the tendency for parties in a debate to be dominated by their most extreme elements. Even some women who hate pornography, or at least some of it, are afraid of allowing any kind of ban, while others who are fearful of censorship feel that the most violent pornography must be stopped at any cost.

Surely it would be easy enough to do so without condemning fashion? Not all feminists think so. Adrienne Rich, in her afterword to the anthology *Take Back the Night: Women on Pornography*, writes "There is a continuum between the bridal mannequin, blank faced and sleepwalking in veil and train, in one store window, and the equally faceless mannequin in spike-heeled boots, chain jewelry, leather collar, and girdle, her body jerked awry as by the voltage of electric shock, in another . . . There is a continuum between the 'soft-focus' objectification of the pretty teenage model in the pages of 'women's magazines', 'fashion magazines,' or the daily papers, and the pipelines transporting young women runaways to sexual slavery . . . In between, there is the more elegant imagery purveyed by . . . *Vogue*".[11] This is the crux of the matter: where does actual harm begin?

The concept of the continuum isn't very helpful, because you could equally well say that a person dying of starvation, one dying of over-eating and one in between are on a continuum. The anti-censorship faction have great fun with this. Elizabeth Wilson has pointed out that some psychopaths have claimed to be turned on by pictures of women knitting, and Harriett Gilbert that paedophiles have said the same of choirboys on television; writing about Andrea Dworkin's novel *Mercy*, she adds that Dworkin "must know as well as anyone that descriptions of torture, whatever their intention, are found sexually arousing by many and, by some, are read for precisely that reason."[12]

Pornographers themselves sometimes pretend that, like Dworkin, they are writing for reasons of moral indignation: for examples, see any tabloid newspaper, with rape stories carefully placed next to nearly-nude pin-ups, and headlines like "Shocking Sex Scandal! Read All About It!" Richard Hoggart called this "best-of-both-worlds sexy".[13]

Writing like Dworkin's could be described as meeting the author's own criteria for pornography as defined by the ordinance which she and Catharine MacKinnon have repeatedly tried to make into an American law:

> the graphic sexually explicit sexual subordination of women through pictures and/or words, that also includes one or more of the following: Women are presented dehumanized as sexual objects, things, or commodities . . . as sexual objects who enjoy pain or humiliation . . . as sexual objects who experience sexual pleasure in being raped . . . as sexual objects tied up or cut up or mutilated or bruised or physically hurt . . . in postures of sexual submission, servility, or display; or women's body parts – including but not limited to vaginas, breasts or buttocks – are exhibited, such that women are reduced to those parts; or women are presented as whores by nature . . . being penetrated by objects or animals . . . in scenarios of degradation, injury, torture, shown as filthy or inferior, bleeding, bruised, or hurt in a context that makes these conditions sexual.

If men or children are substituted for women, adds the next paragraph, it is still pornography.

When this ordinance first appeared, Andrea Dworkin challenged objectors: "It needs to be better? Help us make it better. It needs to be clearer? Help us make it clearer. If anybody is concerned about the way this idea can be misused, help us to get it right."[14] There has been no shortage of concerned people, but little clarification, as Liz Kelly laments: "Few discussions took place on whether an amended version of the ordinance might produce a broader consensus – one had to be for or against it . . . What I would like to see is some critical but constructive discussion of the actual content of the ordinance, along with a serious debate of precisely what forms of restrictions on speech are acceptable. We know that some forms of speech represent a threat to someone's or some group's basic human rights – rights to survival, safety, equality, democracy and dignity. It is not a basic right to make a profit, exploit others or speak/act with total disregard of the consequences."[15]

Criticism of the ordinance's content has focused particularly on the concepts of degradation, servility and display which, as the critics said, could mean almost anything an anti-pornographer didn't like. This need not mean a feminist anti-pornographer. There are, as the sex radicals never tire of pointing out, pornophobes on the anti-feminist right (the far right consists almost entirely of them) and once a law authorising censorship was passed, their opinion would count as much as a feminist's: a democratic government is supposed to give equal weight to all its citizens' views. It is unjust to say Dworkin and MacKinnon's position is the same as that of a member of the American Bible Belt or its British equivalent (like the late Mary Whitehouse), but a law trying to ban anything as vaguely defined as degradation might well benefit Bible Belters more than feminists. This is why some passionate opponents of pornography also oppose censorship, as Robin Morgan does: "I abhor censorship in any form . . . I'm aware, too, that a phallocentric culture is more likely to begin its censorship purges with books on pelvic self-examination for women or books containing lyrical paeans to lesbianism than with *See Him Tear and Kill Her*. . . Nor do I place much trust in a male-run judiciary . . . Some feminists have suggested that a Cabinet-level woman in charge of Women's Affairs . . . might take pornography regulation into her portfolio. Others hark back to the idea of community control. Both approaches give me unease, the first because of the unlikeliness that a Cabinet-level woman appointee these days would have genuine feminist consciousness, or, if she did, have the power and autonomy . . . to act upon it; the second because communities can be as ignorant and totalitarian in censorship as individual tyrants."[18]

Supporters of the ordinance, on both sides of the Atlantic, deny that it would lead to censorship: it demands that people who feel they have been hurt by pornography should have the right to bring actions, which, they insist, is not the same. In practice, when legislation on similar grounds was passed in Canada, Morgan's warnings seem to have been fulfilled. Nadine Strossen, a lawyer and member of the American Civil Liberties Union, describes the results in her book *Defending Pornography*:[17] some of Dworkin's books, including *Woman Hating*, were seized, and so were a large amount of homosexual literature (male and female) and an exercise video. Not only that, but its seizure was defended by feminists on the grounds that it showed a woman in postures which could be construed as sexual (though this contradicts the criteria of the ordinance, which is supposed to cover only sexually explicit material). This brings us to one of the most obvious objections to it: is subordination of women unacceptable only when combined with sexual explicitness? Not, one might guess, to the authors of statements like that of Adrienne Rich; a dummy in a wedding dress isn't sexually explicit. But if the law is extended to cover all images of subordination or display, one might well say the sky was the limit. Strossen quotes objections to the exercise video on the grounds that it showed heavy breathing: how does one exercise vigorously without it? "Postures of subordination" could include, say, a picture of a woman sitting on the floor at her lover's feet, even if the only reason she was there was that she found sitting on floors comfortable and he didn't.

I made that example up, but here are some more of Strossen's: "In 1992, for example, the State of Washington passed a law banning the sale to minors of recordings containing 'erotic' lyrics . . . Frightening as it is to contemplate the wide-ranging 'erotic' lyrics – from country and western to opera – that would be off-limits to young people . . . it is yet more frightening to contemplate the devastating impact on music that might result . . . Susan McClary, a musicologist at the University of Minnesota, has described some classical music masterpieces as conveying the sort of sexually violent messages that would run afoul of the Dworkin-MacKinnon model law", one of them being the first movement of Beethoven's Ninth Symphony, which she describes as expressing "the throttling, murderous rage of a rapist." In visual art, "even images of nude or seminude bodies in wholly nonsexual contexts have been attacked", including a photograph of Ntozake Shange with bare shoulders (just like any Victorian lady in evening dress), a cast of the Venus de Milo and Goya's *Maja Desnuda*: "In 1992, Pennsylvania State University officials removed a reproduction of this acclaimed work from the front wall of a classroom following a complaint by English professor Nancy Stumhofer that it embarrassed her and made her female students 'uncomfortable.'" Similar incidents occurred at the University of Southampton, England, in 1995, and in the same year the City Fathers of Jerusalem turned down the offer of a replica of Michelangelo's David on the grounds of its nudity. An art collector who owned a Michelangelo drawing of a female nude told me that when he hung a photograph of it over his bed while serving in the army in the Second World War, his sergeant ordered him to take down that dirty picture. Similarly, photographs of naked children have been seized, as Polly Toynbee notes: "Even ads for nappies showing babies' bums have been censored . . . joyful family photos of young children in the bath [have been] pounced on at the chemist's . . . No doubt a paedophile will use any picture of a naked child . . . (Would someone into bestiality enjoy any picture of an animal?)"[18] Anti-paedophile American laws have made it criminal to photograph a naked seventeen-year old,[19] and in December 2002 councillors in Edinburgh restricted the showing of videos of school plays and sports.

It would seem that the attempt to legislate without censorship has had the same result as most compromises: the worst of both worlds. It throws away the one advantage of overt censorship, its clarity, by giving anybody who is offended at anything (and what isn't offensive to somebody?) a free hand to bring legal action. It makes every member of the population a potential protestor. The media won't sit around waiting to be sued; as Strossen shows, booksellers have revised their buying policy in a "safety first" direction rather than risk being put out of business, and the small, independent firms, those most likely to stock the feminist and other texts which strongly criticise society at large, are those most likely to suffer. E. M. Forster described the effect of the Incitement to Disaffection Act of 1935: "I know of a case in which some printers refused to print a pacifist children's story, on the ground that the story might fall into the hands of a soldier, and be held to have seduced him from his allegiance! The printers were over-timid. Yet this is what always happens and is intended to happen when a law of this type is passed. The public is vaguely intimidated, and determines to be on the safe side, and do less, say less, and think less than usual."[20]

Carole Vance has accused some partisans of censorship of "visual illiteracy and literal-minded overreaction".[21] Gill Saunders, a curator in the Department of Designs, Prints and Drawings at the Victoria and Albert Museum who mounted an exhibition of nude paintings there in 1989, can hardly be accused of the former. She wrote in the accompanying book, defining "objectification": "all images objectify; they make an object – a drawing, a painting, a photograph – of reality . . . because the majority of the images of the female nude which we see around us are expressive of the male view it does not necessarily follow that images of the female body are bad *per se* . . . The danger lies not in the objectifying of the body, an inevitable process of artistic practice but in certain images which encourage the viewer to read the body as an anonymous available object, images which degrade, exploit or mutilate the human body." She writes of a statue: "In this image . . . the body has been reduced to a torso . . . styled to be sexually provocative"[22] and elsewhere calls it "damaged and damaging". What statue? The Venus de Milo. Not only is "reduced to a torso" misleading because the Venus has legs, but Saunders must know that she has no arms not because the artist intended her not to have any but because they are missing. For all we know, if we found them, they might be making a gesture of defiance.

I doubt if she wanted this or other such images suppressed, but some feminists would. Alice Walker has experienced attempts at censorship (the film of *The Color Purple* was picketed because it claimed that some black men beat their wives, which I know to be true because I once had to share a flat with one who did), but she has condemned all statues of incomplete, therefore "mutilated" figures;[23] let me remind readers that plucked eyebrows have also been called mutilation. Marilyn French goes further: "I feel assaulted by twentieth-century abstract sculpture that resembles exaggerated female body parts, mainly breasts."[24] (Would this apply to any building with a dome and if not, why not? Couldn't spires and tower blocks be said to resemble exaggerated penises?) Fidelis Morgan warned in the introduction to her anthology of sexist quotations: "I do not want misogynist literature removed from anyone's shelves. There are appalling moves afoot to remove 'sexist' books from public libraries and to stop performing plays which display 'stereotypical attitudes to women' . . . Fleas swept under a carpet will merely multiply. Sweep them out into the light and you can deal with them."[25] Ironically, some of the sex radicals' insistence that pornography should not be considered on its own but as part of a whole spectrum of sexist images could encourage this: if porn is only part of the problem, why should protest stop there?

Moreover, some feminists advocate direct action. Ellen Willis, one of the most vocal, for whom a woman who enjoys porn "expresses a radical impulse"and who dismisses objections with "attempts to sort out good erotica from bad porn invariably come down to 'What turns me on is erotic; what turns you on is pornographic", thinks we should "acknowledge that some sexual images are offensive and others are not" (isn't that open to the same criticism: offensive to whom?), and adds: "Picketing an anti-woman movie, defacing an exploitative billboard, or boycotting a record company to protest its misogynist album covers conveys one kind of message, mass marches Against Pornography quite another."[26] I wonder where she stands on "Slasher Mary", the suffragette who scored Velasquez's "Rokeby Venus" in 1914 on the grounds that it degraded women, or on the following account by Zena Herbert:

Last year [1984] I was . . . rendered totally non-existent in the smashed sculptures affair that culminated in the Leeds trial of five women. The gory, inaccurate descriptions in newspapers mentioned that other sculptures were also damaged.

Nobody said those other pieces were made by a woman – me. Damaged means chipped or cracked. The truth was, 'smashed'. . .

The Dancer began mid-thigh because in the Atlas foothills, where the tents are low, women dance on their knees. I remembered women I had danced with, body jewellery shimmering, lamplit, free together. No arms: I saw no need. No legs: they would not show. Did I make a 'mutilated torso'? I made a velvet headdress with brass bezels and stranded bugle beads from the ears to the breasts. (Nipple and labia rings – and testicle rings for men – are traditional with Rif-Kabyle. I wear them from choice.) The brass half-skin fastened with beads and a single ring linked the labia. The Dancer was in a sexual situation and had chosen to close her body.

. . . some women tutors complained that my work was sexist and racist . . . The next day my women were in smithereens.

The horror of seeing another woman hammer faces and breasts, even clay ones, is indescribable. I felt sentenced, unheard, by a self-appointed executioner-judge. In the brouhaha perhaps someone saw the copper glint and thought it chains, but the shackles described so luridly in court were in the minds of those who saw something that did not exist. There were no manacles, no chains. I made my women free, not slaves. If clay women made from my photographs are obscene then I, by merely being female, must be obscene; and that is ludicrous.

. . . May we not depict woman other than dressed (nakedness, I was told, is undignified) standing (other postures are degrading) and alone (to be near another woman implies a sexual relationship)? . . . The field will be left to pornography, with the abused image of woman the only one made or shown.[27]

Her statues certainly showed an abused image after they were smashed, just as the Rokeby Venus with knife marks in her back did. If anything but standing is degrading, what about a seated monarch surrounded by standing courtiers? (As the actress Josephine Hull observed, "Playing Shakespeare is very tiring. You never get to sit down, unless you're a King.")

Accusations extend to content as well as form. Jane Caputi's *The Age of Sex Crime* comes close to accusing everyone who writes, say, a novel or an opera about Jack the Ripper of helping to legitimise his actions, regardless of its tone (does anyone know that "he" wasn't a woman? This would explain why the victims were not raped). You might begin to wonder whether any writing about violence is safe, but if it isn't reported, how are we to know about it? I can think of nothing more morally repulsive than the idea of people being titillated by accounts or pictures of the Holocaust, but the only way to prevent it is to suppress them, which will delight the Nazi apologists who insist it never happened.

Caputi quotes Susan Sontag: "To photograph people is to violate them"; does this mean that the practice must be abolished, and if not, what? Is seeing violation too? Caputi's views on fashion are not surprising: "If the doll – the perfect, plastic illusion of a woman – is clearly central to the masculine realm of pornography, so too is the doll – as mannequin – an elementary fixture of feminine fashion. Moreover, women are exhorted to make that mannequin their model in more ways than one. An article on master designer Christian Dior revealed that, 'The greatest of M. Dior's virtues is, of course, his burning desire to make all women beautiful. "My desire," he says, "is to save them from nature."' Who, however, will save us from M. Dior, for conforming to that pornographic ideal of 'beauty', often requires both the artificialization and the veritable mutilation of the natural female body."[28] Similarly, Susan Griffin calls lipstick a "pornographic mask" and Andrea Dworkin writes: "ordinary women wear makeup. Ordinary women attempt to change our [*sic*] bodies to resemble a pornographic ideal."[29]

Attempting to define violence in imagery is impossible when faced with statements like this. Lisa Jardine (who scouted the idea that political correctness led to "crass strait-jacketing") suggested, in a *Guardian* article entitled "It may be art, but is it violence?": "Perhaps it really is time we took down from the walls of our public buildings works of art, however sanctioned by the passage of time, which contain graphic representations of acts which violate, harm or humiliate *anybody*."[30]

Numerous letters followed asking what churches should do about cruci-
fixes, and contesting her claim that all such art invites the spectator to
identify with the perpetrator (just as Caputi and John Berger claim that all
images such as the Rokeby Venus and fashion photographs identify the
spectator with a supposedly misogynist male). No wonder Carole Vance
warned that, "Unless we advance in this area, we will be consigned to the
public display of the most homogenized 'positive' images and to sexual
representations that are the counterpart of socialist realist art."[31] It has been
claimed that anti-pornographers have actually prevented the showing of
pornography at feminist meetings convened in order to discuss it.

We are dealing not just with images, but sexuality itself. To feminists
who ask about sexual attraction, Sheila Jeffreys replies: "Fancying was, and
is, seen by many as objectifying, as based on rules about physical perfection which were deeply discriminatory, even sometimes racist and ableist
. . . It was felt that a simple and learned physical urge towards a stranger
was not a good way to begin relationships." That it is learned is taken for
granted, so apparently is the equation of any discrimination against any
degree of disability with racism. Quoting Margaret Nicholls, a lesbian
who expresses misgivings at the idea that politically correct sex must
always mean lying side by side, she asks "what is so very wrong with this
picture".[32] By itself, nothing: but is she saying they must never lie any
other way? Probably, judging by her reaction to a conference at Oxford on
safe sex of which Robin Gorna reports: "The consultation with the
Students Women's Committee was the most unnerving. The poster was
placed on the agenda after a discussion of their latest Campaign Against
Pornography (CAP) project . . . They objected that the use of the front –
and, indeed, any – photographic image was oppressive to women, and
suggested that a line drawing would be less objectifying . . . The sexual
explicitness was taken as oppressive. To integrate the women's comments,
we would have had to return to vague language avoiding any erotic feeling or description of specific sexual acts"[33] (when the conference's whole
purpose was telling people which sexual acts are safe and which are not).
Jeffreys comments: "Gorna accepts that safe sex education can only pro-
ceed through the medium of pornography."[34] Is a drawing of an
able-bodied woman "ableist" and one of a disabled one "mutilated"?
Jeffreys was one of the authors of the Leeds Revolutionary Feminists' pamphlet *Love Your Enemy?*. When it was published in book form, they added,
describing the "furore" that broke out, "we found it difficult to recognise
ourselves in some of the caricatures that emerged from the debate as

cadres, an elite, authoritarian" because they were "in no position to impose anything". It stated: "Men are the enemy. Heterosexual women are collaborators with the enemy" and likened them to collaborators with the Nazis."[35] (Is it coincidence that Zena Herbert's sculptures were smashed in Leeds?)

The words "degradation, exploitation, objectification, oppression" apply to what women do in private, with other women as well as men; if the personal is political, they must. Emma Healey reports, reluctantly: "One woman was criticised for touching her lover's breasts because this was deemed to be objectification."[36] Nobody, she claims, actually said "Thou shalt not enjoy lesbian sex." Who needed to?

This, inevitably, produced the same result as those anti-smoking militants who make non-smokers want to start smoking. An Australian writer, Catharine Lumby, contrasts "the Good Girls who exhibit fear and repulsion about pornography and the Bad Girls who get a kick out of being politically out of line".[37] Mary Stott has pointed out that "the one certain way to make a child read something is to say 'you mustn't'".[38] She could have added that the one way to prevent it is to say "You ought." However it is expressed, a request to put away that nasty porn and look at something nicer does what *Playboy* couldn't: it makes porn glamorous.

As so often happens, the reactors over-simplified almost if not quite as much as their opponents. Lynne Segal, for instance, freely admits that their views derive from the libertarian optimism of the sixties; she and many others worried about a reversion to the attitudes against which those libertarians rebelled, and which were highly sexist (though, as we have seen, so were some of the libertarians). It is worth quoting one, John Calder: "When we abolish all censorship pornography will almost completely disappear except for a small number of people who will find in it the only sexual satisfaction that is possible for them."[39] Another contributor to the same volume, Roger Manvell, was more cautious, pointing out that in Elizabethan times bear-baiting was regarded as respectable entertainment, and also citing the Nazis. Their name is much bandied about by both sides in the debate; pro-permissives have given it as an example of a repressive society, anti-pornographers as an instance of one where porn flourished. So it did, but mostly underground, except when disguised as race propaganda as in Julius Streicher's *Der Stürmer* (about which, according to a friend of my family who studied in Germany during the thirties, even some Nazis had misgivings). Streicher "revelled in pornography and was never seen in public without a whip".[40]

Again, it is rather naïve to assume that porn isn't sexist because it often shows dominant women: Melissa Benn, for instance, has asked why, if it leads men to attack women, it doesn't do the reverse as well.[41] The best answer to this is Linda Grant's: "The dominatrix may be an *image* of power but in the real world of prostitution it is the paying customer who calls the shots."[42] No man has to dial the number on the card reading "Naughty Boys Get Bottom Marks" or "Coloured Therapist Deals With All Unusual Perversions With Extreme Firmness" (actual examples) unless he likes, nor does he have to stay for all the time he has booked (I have heard, though only at fourth hand, that the majority don't). A man paying a dominatrix is like a mediæval monarch letting his jester tell him home truths, both knowing that if the jester told too many His Majesty would sack him.

The sex radicals' attitude has its contradictions too. If everything is relative, as Ellen Willis asserts, how can any image be a legitimate target for protest of any kind? If she sanctions protest she must have misgivings about the idea of limitless tolerance, and in practice, few of the sex radicals (I hesitate to say none) are happy about all pornography. Lynne Segal and Elizabeth Wilson both strongly criticised it, and Carole Vance, who coined "Vance's One-Third Rule: show any personally favored erotic image to a group of women, and one-third will find it disgusting, one-third will find it ridiculous, and one-third will find it hot", disapproves of the way women are expected to regard "quite horrid cartoons in *Hustler*" as "just a light-hearted joke".[43]

One of the few writers who attempt to put both sides of the case is Margaret Walters, who calls Catharine MacKinnon the mirror-image of Camille Paglia, self-styled "pornographer" and defender of prostitution: "It's hard to believe that she [Paglia] has looked at much hard-core pornography lately when she argues that it shows us . . . 'a pagan arena of beauty, vitality and brutality'" and Nadine Strossen "ignores the brutal nastiness of many freely available images, their sadism and their racism, and never considers their surely conceivable links with discrimination and violence."[44]

What are the "horrid" cartoons and hardcore like? Andrea Dworkin gives an example of the former: "*Hustler* magazine displays a cartoon called 'Chester the Molester' (part of a series depicting child molestation as humour), in which a man wearing a swastika on his arm hides behind a corner, holds a bat, and dangles a dollar bill on a wire to entice a little girl away from her parents. The child and her parents all wear yellow stars of David: each member of the family is drawn with the stereotypical hooked nose of anti-Semitic caricature."[45] Similar material appears in, of all places, Israel:

Israeli women call it 'Holocaust pornography.' The themes are fire, gas, trains, emaciation, death.

In the fashion layout, three women in swimsuits are posed as if they are looking at and running away from two men on motorcycles . . .Then the women . . . are shown running from the men . . . Their faces look frightened and frenzied . The men are physically grabbing them. Then the women . . . are sprawled on the ground, apparently dead, with parts of their bodies severed from them and scattered around as trains bear down on them . . .

Or a man is pouring gasoline into a woman's face . . .

Or two women, ribs showing, in scanty underwear, are posed in front of a stone wall, prisonlike, with a fire extinguisher on one side of them and a blazing oven open on the other. Their body postures replicate the body postures of naked concentration camp inmates in documentary photographs.

This is in "a left-liberal slick monthly for the intelligentsia and upper class. It has high production and aesthetic values. Israel's most distinguished writers and intellectuals publish in it" and similar pictures appear in a magazine "not unlike" the American *Ladies' Home Journal.* "For purists, there is an Israeli pornography magazine. The issue I saw had a front-page headline: ORGY AT YAD VASHEM. Yad Vashem is the memorial in Jerusalem to the victims of the Holocaust."[46]

Dworkin, some may object, is an extremist, but I don't see how else you could interpret what she describes. Serving on a jury at a pornography trial made one anti-censorship feminist reconsider her views:

All the books except one . . . were variations on a theme. That theme was the inextricable association of sex with brutality. Women . . . always raped, repeatedly, screamed with pain and then said 'thank you' to their violator. The message was clear: when women say no, they mean yes, the more you hurt them, the more they'll love it . . . Incest featured prominently, the settings varied, the most offensive being a concentration camp, and various accoutrements and instruments of torture were part and parcel of the sex act. This was presented as 'normal' – sex was never, ever, presented as an act of love or tenderness between two consenting beings, it was always indissociable from pain and degradation. These books were all united in their profound hatred of women and their urge to humiliate us. Interestingly, they were all imported from America. What made them all the more pernicious was the inclusion of an introduction, in pseudo-scientific language, by someone purporting to be an academic, presenting these books as 'normal' human behaviour. None of the books contained pictures . . . I wonder how many people who are so adamant about non-censorship have ever read one, or have any idea of the content. To be liberal about the sort of pornography with which I was confronted is as obscene as expecting a Black person to condone apartheid.[47]

Jane O'Reilly quotes Vincent Canby, in the *New York Times*, describing a film called *Ilsa, She-Wolf of the SS* as funny. It showed Nazis torturing people of both sexes, and children laughed at the trailer for it.[48] The pun is irresistible: can porn be corrupting? It can be.

Are lesbian pornography and sado-masochism, as practised by the lobby led by the American Pat Califia of the Samois Collective, somehow different? In *Feminist Review*, Spring 1990, Sara Dunn quotes Gayle Rubin's Barnard conference paper: "trying to find a middle-course between WAP [Women Against Pornography] and Samois . . . is a bit like saying that the truth about homosexuality lies somewhere between the positions of the Moral Majority and the gay movement", which Dunn calls "claiming a monopoly on virtue, (in this case by saying that to have *any* disagreements with Samois is *de facto* to be anti-gay)". Rubin's paper recognises only two schools of thought: conservatives opposed to all sex except for married couples trying to have children, and "dissidents" not opposed to anything. "Over and over women porn writers justify themselves in language as essentialist as those they most vehemently oppose," adds Dunn, asking why, if sex is inherently liberating, they "choose a vehicle that by its very nature *relies* on being illicit . . . Lesbian writers very often have a dishonest relationship with this illicitness . . . By styling themselves (and being styled) the illicit ones, the bad girls (as opposed to the good girls who don't like any sexual explicitness at all) these writers rely on the same sexual double-standards, the same sex-associated shame and guilt which they claim it is their mission to remove. The bad girls need the good girls to make them feel good (i.e., bad)."[49] This is simply inverted moralism.

In the same issue is an article by Margaret Hunt on the "ever-proliferating hit-list of sexual acts, styles of dress, and erotic reading preferences" which are condemned as "suggesting dominance and submission" and "Fascist regalia", and asks how the analogy with Nazis arose; the answer is that some (not all) sado-masochists dress up as, and play at being, Fascists and Nazis in the strictest sense of the words.

"By using racist scenarios such as mistress punishing slave, or fascist scenarios of Nazi punishing Jew in their sex play," writes Emma Healey, "SMers were eroticising power imbalance in ways that many women (both pro and anti-SM) found quite unacceptable." Sheila Jeffreys saw this as proof that they were Nazis themselves (Sara Dunn points out that Hitler tried to exterminate all homosexuals); they retaliated by calling the anti-SMers "fascists" for trying to dictate to them. "But the SM defence of SM sex is not always totally convincing either. The SM buzzwords, 'Love', 'Trust, and 'Consent' . . . can only fit into a fundamentally libertarian politics – a sort of 'anything goes as long as we consent to it' . . . I have heard some lesbians make great claims for SM as a cathartic experience . . . This is, I believe, something that only an individual lesbian can claim". Quoting a case of "a Jewish woman talking very powerfully and passionately of her right to use Nazi imagery in her lovemaking as a way of taking control of the fact that she had lost most of her family in the concentration camps", Healey adds that "it is hard to see how two white lesbians enacting a slave/master scenario could do the same. When lesbians were playing around with racist imagery and the power imbalances that racism creates, it was not their own history of oppression that they were playing with."[50]

Moreover, this imagery is seen in public. Lynne Segal has pointed out that "the most apparently 'violent' images of S & M pornography may be used in only the most consensual and consensual encounters between two people",[51] but pornography isn't confined to people's bedrooms; once something is on sale, even in restricted places, it's hard to make sure only consenting people see it, and not all of it is restricted (*Hustler* and the Israeli magazines are not). It is also fair to ask why people can't think of something better to do with their sexuality than imitate one of the most violent, sexist, racist and anti-homosexual régimes that ever existed, even if you draw the line at trying to prevent them doing so. You may feel disgust, as I do, at the idea of lovers who are not survivors of Nazism saying "Let's play at Nazis and Jews", but the only way to stop it altogether is to abolish personal privacy for everyone, as in *Nineteen-Eighty-Four*. (The same applies to people like the one in Nick Broomfield's 1997 film *Fetishes* who liked licking lavatories.) You may also ask why, if Califia is entirely happy about her practices, she tried to break herself of them, as she admits she did.[52]

What is the alternative to total acceptance of the gospel according to either Dworkin, MacKinnon and Jeffreys on the one hand (though they differ, because the first two are not lesbian separatists) or Califia, Paglia and Rubin on the other? It is doing what Gloria Steinem tried to do and what Ellen Willis and some anti-pornographers, for opposite reasons, declare to be impossible: define the difference between erotica and pornography. To do this, we have to ask not only where harm begins and ends, but what to do about disagreements. I can only make my own suggestion: in images as well as practices, we must separate inherent violence from violence which can be, but need not be, read into it. Does the material in question show it, or just remind someone of it (like Beethoven reminding someone of a rapist)?

First, there is the question of whether violence was used in making an image, as in the extreme case of snuff films, which purport to depict the murder of women. What matters here is whether the murders are real; it seems established that the first of the genre was not. Sex radicals often ask if anybody is sure snuff films really exist. I haven't examined the evidence in detail, but I think one should be wary of assuming they don't: the victims couldn't testify, and admitting to having made such a film would be tantamount to a confession of murder. Even with lesser crimes, it is too easy to assume that any film or picture which purports to show cruelty must have been faked. Maybe it wasn't. If not, the statement that "porn is rape" (or mayhem or even murder) is entirely justified.

What if no actual violence is used? There is still the possibility of its causing violence, and this is where opinion starts to divide. There have been repeated studies but as James Weaver explains, "any research protocol employing sexually abusive or violent behaviours as a response to viewing pornography cannot be sanctioned":[53] the only way you could be sure it caused rape would be to let some men who had seen it and some who hadn't loose on captive women and see which group raped more. Not only is this unthinkable (and the fact that it is shows there are limits to our world's allegedly boundless sexism) but no feminist would want it to be otherwise. But the sex radicals' optimism can go to extremes: I think this is because they are reluctant to say "I couldn't be corrupted by this, but *you* might." As Harriett Gilbert put it in *Sex Exposed*, "Surely she [Dworkin] cannot be saying that it is all right for *her* to travel this country, but too dangerous for lesser, less sophisticated people? This is certainly a common delusion among anti-pornography campaigners, whether they assess sophistication by sex, education or class."[54]

This comes close to suggesting that everyone is able to resist danger. Surveys on health suggest it would be truer that nobody is: "A survey published today [4 August 1997] by the recruitment agency, Reed Graduates, identifies students and recent graduates as 'the new high-risk group of persistent smokers' . . . Another . . . by the Health and Education Authority . . . blames editors of men's magazines and style titles . . . no amount of editorialising about the dangers of smoking could counter the damage done by seductive pictures of models with cigarettes, which are 'read' on an emotional level."[55] I have already mentioned the National

Lottery. But we don't all gamble or smoke even though everyone who isn't blind has seen advertisements, so some people must be more susceptible than others. Ellen Willis, we know, makes light of advertising's influence, but if pictures of happy smokers are so effective, why not pictures of happy, raped women?

Trickiest of all is the question of whether an image can be a form of violence in itself, irrespective of what it makes people do. I can't help thinking that at least some feminists fall back on this argument because they were getting nowhere with the previous one; the trouble with it is that it can so easily turn into a demand to ban everything that somebody somewhere dislikes. Worse, it can lead to equating imagery with rape itself: if this is what "porn is rape" means, it is not only wrong but dangerous, because it trivialises rape just as pornography does. Rape can leave a woman pregnant, infected with a fatal disease, or both. If it's violent enough, it can leave her dead. Images can't.

To untangle true from false claims, we need precisely what a polarised debate discourages: a sense of proportion.

This doesn't mean tolerating everything. Elizabeth Wilson warns: "Surely some pornography is still so deeply offensive, so violent and so degrading to women that its free circulation is something we should protest against. There is a moral point: that the very circulation of such material will in itself wear away any kind of standards of what is or is not acceptable. We are more and more in danger of believing that 'anything goes' — that there are no standards, that everything is relative."[56] It means knowing what is and isn't mutilation, what is and isn't rape. It means trying not to be illiterate, either visually or historically, as in Susanne Kappeler's analysis of Titian's picture of the rape of Lucretia which ends: "We are told we are seeing her consent."[57] Who are "we"? Not Titian's public. They knew that Tarquin took Lucretia by force, and that she then killed herself; classical history and mythology were the basis of their education. (I doubt if any Renaissance nobleman cared much if his pictures encouraged rape among his servants, but even they probably knew, from waiting at banquets where historical and mythological scenes were acted between courses.) Clive Bell wrote in his book *Art* that one reason people enjoy Titian's paintings is that they show women one would like to kiss looking as if they wanted to be kissed; should they be banned? I'd be surprised if someone didn't think so, given the examples above. Stephen Johnson reported in *The Independent* on 28 January 1998 that Mahler had been called pornographic for composing songs about children's deaths; on 28 January 1710 Isaac Bickerstaff wrote in the *Tatler* that "The *Prude* and *Coquet* (as different as they appear in their Behaviour) are in Reality the same Kind of Women . . . each of them has the Distinction of Sex in all her Thoughts, Words and Actions." Both, in Robin Morgan's phrase, put "the coarse before the heart."[58] As we saw in chapter 5, once people start looking for signs of oppression they find them everywhere; even Andrea Dworkin admitted to this when, after seeing pornography that showed hanged women, she found she couldn't see a doorway without imagining bodies hanging from it .[59] Opponents of sado-masochism praise "vanilla sex" but the New York *Tribune* in the 1850s referred to "ice cream drugged with passion-exciting vanilla".[60]

What, if anything, should be censored? Simply driving porn underground, which Susan Brownmiller recommended in *Take Back the Night*, is no solution because, as Wendy Kaminer points out, "working conditions in an illegal business are virtually impossible to police",[61] which makes violence more likely. If censorship does exist, Mary Stott suggests it should be "strictly limited" so that people know where they stand. If there is none, she adds, "to refuse to say, '*You* must not', doesn't let us off the hook of saying '*I* must not'".[62] I think censorship should at least be seriously considered for anything which portrays (rigorously defined) mutilation and torture, or even scatology, as trivial; this is a lie, and we have a duty not to let it stand. Anything else can be covered by saying, as a friend of mine did, "There's no law against it, but you don't have to like it."

Wherever lines, moral or physical, are drawn there is always an area only just on one side and one only just on the other; as Katharine Whitehorn wrote, "it is no good thinking that if you set [limits] in sensible places, the pressure will be off . . . I am not suggesting that the availability of child porn suddenly turns the whole nation into child molesters. But human beings have their dark side: different in each one of us. It is the job of civilisation to minimise it . . . not to whip it up and inflame it and give it new lurid dimensions, as the exploiters do."[63] A recent book by Valerie Bryson claims: "Opponents of censorship say that the damaging effects of pornographic material have been shown to be more than offset if an audience is 'de-briefed' by being provided with more accurate information about sexual violence"[64] which, if true, offers the best hope of long-term progress.

The best definition of pornography I know is Drusilla Cornell's: "(a) the portrayal of violence and coercion against women as the basis of heterosexual desire or (b) the graphic description of women's body as dismembered by her being reduced to her sex and stripped entirely of her personhood as she is portrayed in involvement in explicit sex acts."[65] It could also be used for men, children and homosexual desire. This is clearer than the Dworkin–MacKinnon definition and avoids at least some of its problems, though no definition is watertight and nor is any law; this could only happen in a perfect world, which would need no laws. I also accept Steinem's famous definition of erotica. She explicitly rejects "the confusion of *all* nonprocreative sex with pornography" and "the temptation of merely reversing the terms and declaring that *all* nonprocreative sex is good." Instead, "Pornography is about dominance and often pain. Erotica is about mutuality and always pleasure."[66] Kathy Myers adds that erotica doesn't equate all such pleasure with sexual availability.[67] This, I think, avoids what Vance and Segal, among others, are afraid of: insistence on a sexuality that is always gentle, the equivalent of John Betjeman's "ghastly good taste", banning all bright colours, loudness or energy. This is not to say that there is anything wrong with gentleness in itself, only with prohibiting anything else. Some would insist that such a prohibition doesn't spoil sex – Sheila Jeffreys, for instance; but there is nothing gentle about her own attitude to anyone who disagrees with her. Can it be that if the bad girls depend on the good girls, the good girls depend on the bad ones, and get their own kicks out of condemning other people's? Judging by the tone of their writing, I think they do.

It is worth emphasising that even if you abolished all imagery portraying human sexuality or even human beings, you wouldn't necessarily produce an egalitarian world. Islamic fundamentalists do condemn all such imagery, and women are far from equal in the societies they run. The Saudi Arabian woman I quoted earlier wrote of the long black cloak worn over her clothes that "Arab men barely glance at the child . . .but once she dons her veil and *abaaya* discreet glances come her way. Men now attempt to catch a glimpse of a forbidden, suddenly erotic ankle."[68] So much for veils freeing women from being sex objects! Similarly, a nun whose order had abandoned traditional dress told a reporter she was glad "to be rid of its embarrassing connotations of stifled sexuality . . . 'Many men find the nun's habit sexy,' she says, 'and I've had many approaches. When they brought in stripping nun-o-grams, I was very glad to be out of it.'"[69] Men watched transvestite entertainers like Vesta Tilley, and some even collected pictures of female miners in their working clothes, because their trousers showed more of their legs than contemporary female dress; one of the reasons bloomers were opposed was that they showed women's legs.[70] People might have standards of attractiveness even if they couldn't see: in H. G. Wells's story *The Country of the Blind* the inhabitants based theirs on touch and voice, and there are other forms of exploitation besides aesthetic ones. There is no substitute for respect for people as people, and no short cut to it.

Does this cover everything? Of course not. There are still, and probably always will be disagreements. Tolerating different viewpoints (and trying to convert the opposition by peaceful means) may be the best we can do here.

I have left one point to the last because it seems to me impossible to argue about it. Writing a book like this, which attempts to put across a point of view, is like underwater exploration: however deep you go, eventually you strike rock bottom. Rock bottom here is the theory advanced by Susanne Kappeler, and to some extent by Sheila Jeffreys. The latter's argument about "fancying" can be countered by pointing out that, in Mary Stott's words, "If you educate girls to *think* you cannot circumscribe their thinking"[71] and if people have an aesthetic sense that can't be circumscribed either. Janet Radcliffe Richards states that "beauty is the same sort of thing whether it is in paintings, sunsets or people",[72] which means those who care for the first two may care for the last. Susanne Kappeler states, however: "The concept of 'aesthetics' is fundamentally incompatible with feminist politics."[73]

Does this mean that all love of colours, shapes, sounds, movements, and presumably scents and tastes, is by definition evil? If it does, I can only repeat what I said of other intractable objections to fashion in chapter 1: if you agree, don't waste time reading this book.

8

Dress as Ritual

Dress should be handsome upon handsome occasions.

William Makepeace Thackeray   Sketches and Travels in London

Let us work when we work and play when we play.

Abba Gould Woolson, quoted in True Love and Perfect Union

People do need a carrot.

A former schoolmaster

We have had the ultimate attack; now comes the ultimate defence. If this book is in defence of the art of dress, this chapter is in defence of dressing up; and dressing up, in the sense in which I mean it, is the straw which breaks the progressive-minded camel's back.

Nothing more clearly illustrates fashion's low cultural status. For every feminist who says "down with art", there is another saying "that's not good enough." Feminist authors defend not only popular arts like rock music but Degas and Shakespeare, and such supposedly feminine ones as needlework.[1] There is widespread concern about whether live theatre or orchestral music will disappear because those who are ignorant of them don't know what they're missing, and what to do about it. Few people answer "nothing", but I have yet to see a whole-hearted defence of what is traditionally the pinnacle of the art of dressing. Efforts are made to stop folk costumes from disappearing, but even writers who don't believe that punks are the only liberated dressers draw the line at defending one form of dress which was taken for granted until the Second World War. It has gone into what may well be an irreversible decline and the almost universal reaction is: so what? The proof is that I actually feel nervous when typing the words for what I mean: formal evening dress.

What's so frightening? The same problem which dogs the whole subject of fashion, but in an aggravated form: it's seen as only for a privileged minority. Even raising the issue looks like giving ammunition to the critics who dismiss feminism as middle-class, which only brings us back, yet again, to the question of why fashion isn't seen as something which should be available to all. When élites are distrusted, the only way for a minority to be taken seriously is for it to be seen as persecuted, and where are frustrated wearers of evening dress on the "hierarchy of oppression?" But anything which makes women unhappy is supposed to be worth attention, and this problem is making this woman unhappy. Like housework, it's cumulative: on any one occasion dressing down rather than up may not seem a great sacrifice, but neither does washing all the dishes yourself.

If clothes, as Elizabeth Wilson has noted, have been more identified with upper-class status and its accompanying frivolity than any other luxuries, evening dress is more identified with it than any other clothes: we have to wear something, but we don't have to wear something special. That has made it an automatic target for socialists, and feminists sharing socialist goals. Deliberate informality has come to be seen as a way of keeping faith with progressive ideas, and not doing so, therefore, as a way of betraying them: Minna Thornton told me she had felt guilty about wearing a cock-tail dress. As long as what Liz Heron called the "basic shapes of serviceability" are preserved, feminists and socialists can feel they are, so to speak, living up to the principle of dressing down, in the spirit if not the letter. The difference between the practical and the impractical, however, does not lie so much in shape as fabric, and that was one of the aspects that was modified first. Though tails, the most formal clothes modern men wear except for special cases such as court dress and uniforms, derive from sports clothes, they have now acquired the equivalent status to a woman's long formal dress. Sir Victor Gollancz wrote that his friend John Strachey "showed me a card he had just discovered for one of his mother's parties at the turn of the century, with the word 'trousers' in the bottom left-hand corner: and he told me, when I looked blank, that it meant 'informal' – white tie and tails, but not knee-breeches."[2]

"At this time", writes Diana de Marly, "the question of correct dress for Socialist men came to the fore." Bernard Shaw "invented a one-piece outfit in brown knitted wool . . . On the first night of his *Widowers' Houses* in 1892, Shaw wore a silver-grey version in stockinet for the curtain call, as part of his campaign against evening clothes. Socialists argued that evening dress was a class livery",[3] preferring a black "working suit", perhaps because the theorists of socialism grew up when the effects of the masculine renunciation were at their height, and the only way for a man to dress colourfully or decoratively was to copy the costume of periods before socialism existed: just the example that the theorists wanted to avoid. Any attempt on the part of working-class people of either sex to dress up (as the newly rich proverbially do) could be written off as the effect of capitalist corruption, and sometimes still is. Seen in this light, the cult of informal dress begins to look like idealising the aspects of other people's lives that they themselves would like to escape, and also like a historical survival which might be reconsidered. It is certainly surviving, to the point of driving formality almost out of existence.

Does it matter? It does to me because I love it. Do I mean that literally? Yes. Women's evening dresses (or trousered equivalents) are the only ones where the designer doesn't have to take practicality into account, and can give free rein to the aesthetic side. Making them is like composing music for virtuosos rather than beginners: unless you ask for something totally impossible, there is no need to worry about whether your demands can be met. That doesn't mean such clothes are uncomfortable (Gwen Raverat's comment on crinolines applies here; long skirts are only a real nuisance if they are tight and have no slits). You couldn't go for a cross-country walk in them, but on festive occasions you don't have to (and as Women Against Violence Against Women pointed out, jeans can be tight too). They offer something unique, and if they were to disappear, the advantages of other kinds of clothing would not be a consolation for the same reason that, if Venice sinks, it won't help to say "You can still go to other places!"

When I was about six, I saw ball dresses in shop windows and pictures and fell in love with them, and said "When I'm grown up I want a dress like that" just as I said "When I'm grown up I want a house like that." I once tried, unsuccessfully, to persuade my parents to buy one and keep it for me until I grew into it. With dresses for immediate use I was more successful, only to be given invitations specifying "not party dress". Nothing has changed: I still fall in love with them, I still buy them, and then go through all kinds of manœuvres to find occasions to wear them. I once heard a teacher of historical dancing say, "Imagine you're in a beautiful castle wearing silks and satins!" Why not walk round the block and imagine you're dancing? I don't want to imagine, I want to do it. "It'll come back", some people say, though less frequently than they used to. When? Shall I still be alive? What is more, I know other people with similar tastes (though I've never met anyone quite as fanatical as I am), but the number of opportunities keeps on declining. "Freedom" in dress means freedom to wear anything except what I most want to wear, and if women who share my views don't make them clear, how is anyone to know we still exist?

We don't exist, says conventional wisdom, which amounts to a self-fulfilling prophecy. Admirers of Nicolas Ghesquière, the new designer at Balenciaga, praise him for making clothes in which women can go anywhere, rather than ones in which to make grand entrances, because "that old day-and-night thing is passé; women simply don't live like that".[4] "What is missing . . . is evening wear – because it's for grown-ups" runs a report on Calvin Klein's clothes for young people. "His theory: the young don't buy it" and another says of the Young Conservative Conference ball: "The problem is that most young people these days do not really want to go to events like this. Discos and dinner jackets do not go together. At least the leaflets advertising this year's bash did not bear the usual picture of a man and woman waltzing in evening dress."[5] That isn't the experience of universities: Oxford and Cambridge are most famous for giving balls, but they have also proved popular at the Universities of London and Sussex. Formal wear is compulsory for the American high school dances known as proms (increasingly imitated here).

Men's evening dress is regarded as slightly less frivolous than women's; the more formal the occasion, the greater the justification for the men's belief that their clothes are uninfluenced by fashion. Full dress is a uniform. There is only a little more leeway with the more recently invented dinner and morning suits, though there have been attempts to enliven the former.

A woman in evening dress, therefore, is the supreme example of the contradictory symbolism I mentioned earlier: she represents both the oppressed sex and the oppressing class. A music historian, Peter Gradenwitz, wrote that in the 1750s "many of them [musicians] wore lackeys' uniforms (as indeed musicians still do today, wearing the same uniform dress at concerts as do butlers and waiters)",[6] but a journalist has written that men's tails or dinner jackets symbolise authority while the female equivalent harks back to "when women led decorative lives." Heads men win, tails (no pun intended) women lose.

Once again, we need to look at the style's friends in order to understand its enemies. Helen Callaway explains that formal dress was used during British imperial rule as a way of asserting domination over subject races, coupled with insistence that Indians should take off their shoes in the presence of the British, while the latter were allowed to keep theirs on even in mosques and temples where religious law forbids wearing them.[7] But that is only half the story, because dressing for the evening was then a normal part of British life, at least for everyone above a certain social level; the Englishwoman whom Callaway quotes as stating that an officer dressed for dinner "not because he wishes to look nice, but because he is expected to live up to certain traditions" was unaccustomed to doing so herself, so I wonder how she knew.

It is worth reminding ourselves how normal evening dress was. It was regarded as something people automatically bought as soon as they could afford it. Gwen Raverat writes: "Right up to 1914 one always made some kind of change of dress for dinner, even if one were alone; and for quite a small party, full dress was usual."[8] Full dress for men meant tails; the reason that a dinner jacket is called a "smoking" in some languages is that men could neither wear one (except at home) nor smoke when ladies were present. An officer in the regular army who had served in the First World War told me many people thought white tie and tails wouldn't survive it, "but when we came back from the war, all the women we knew said, 'Oh, no you don't. *We* want to go on dressing up so *you've* got to'", which doesn't suggest submission to men. Tails did survive: in Margaret Kennedy's *The Fool of the Family* (1930) the hero is asked to a party:

> 'Is it a grand party?' asked Caryl nervously.
> Fenella said not . . . 'I mean is it white tie?' explained Caryl.
> 'Oh yes, of course it's white tie.'
> 'Then it is grand.'
> He had very little social sense . . . He thought a party was grand when people wore white ties and drank champagne.[9]

June and Doris Langley Moore's etiquette book (1933) gives the rules: "'Tails' are correct evening wear for any entertainment except an informal dinner. The dinner jacket *may* be worn, as our male adviser expresses it, 'at almost any place where you pay to go in'. Whether tails would be in better form than a dinner jacket at a theatre, a hotel dance, or a restaurant, cannot be decided without specific reference to the occasion. The dinner jacket indicates a casual attitude towards the entertainment for which it is worn, and this attitude is, naturally, sometimes quite the right one."[10]

Popular culture was led by Hollywood, where tails were worn (who thinks of Fred Astaire in anything else?) and dinner jackets still are. At an exhibition of 1940s fashions, I saw an evening dress loaned by a woman who had worn it to dinner at the college where she studied just before the war: it was compulsory on Saturday nights.[11] According to her house guests,

Naomi Mitchison, a lifelong socialist, dressed for dinner even in the eighties.[12] As to theatres, I quote Alison Settle: "Even in the heart of Paris in April you would find women going to the first night of a play in a little day suit . . . a London audience feels that it is due to the theatre and to itself to wear evening dress in the stalls. As for America, how can you expect women to enjoy real efforts to look smart in the evening when their men will not change from business suits?"[13] The dress circle in a theatre is called that because people dressed for it, as they did for at least some concerts; so much for Gradenwitz. When I told someone I knew that I regretted the change, she said she wanted going to the theatre to be an ordinary part of life, not something you had to wear special clothes for. I told her I wanted evening dress to be an ordinary part of life. She couldn't believe I was serious.

What happened? The Second World War and its disruption of civilian life. In the issue of *Woman* magazine coinciding with D-Day a letter to "Evelyn Home" 's problem page asked if turning evening dresses into day ones was a patriotic duty (only if she needed more day dresses, answered Peggy Makins, otherwise Evelyn Home). When the war ended, however, the practice did partly revive. The freedom of the better-off to dress every evening derived from employing poorer people to do manual work, but attending theatres, concert halls, hotels, restaurants or parties requires none. People tried to keep up the old traditions for these, as Gertrude Lawrence's husband describes: "She had seen England in battle dress, but she was confident that the khaki would be taken off and the white ties and tails brought out of the wardrobes when the war ended. The opening of *September Tide* will go down in London's theatre history as the first Gala First Night since the beginning of the war. It was completely in the pre-war tradition. The men had taken their white ties and tails out of storage and the ladies blossomed forth in dazzling new creations."[14] An interview with the conductor Anatole Fistoulari stated in 1946, "He likes to see both orchestra and audience in evening dress, because it has a psychological effect on the performance."[15] In a broadcast interview at the first Edinburgh Festival in 1947, Tam Dalyell described people who wore "our very best clothes as a treat", which in his case meant a kilt (he was a schoolboy), while men, "believe it or not" were in dinner jackets; now, "any clothes will do". Informal fancy dress is seen at Fringe events, but little or no formal dress anywhere. Where did the desire for it go?

Part of the trouble, I think, was that codes were enforced so rigidly. I have read of a journalist wanting to interview someone in a smart nightclub being refused admission even for a few minutes because she was in day clothes. Evening dress, once worn by wicked lords in melodramas, lost its last trace of aristocratic raffishness; it was what the establishment considered good for you, part of the ethos of the notoriously stuffy and anti-feminist fifties, ripe to be rebelled against by the next generation. What could be more likely to encourage the rebellious gesture of deliberately wearing the wrong clothes?

Brett Harvey remembers that in the United States, where soft fabrics were more easily obtainable than in Europe: "Fifties clothes were like armor",[16] much more so Dior's original New Look. This was when girls bought their first long dresses in a store's "Junior Miss Department": the name alone is enough to explain why teenage sub-cultures happened. There was no way young people could feel daring unless they became beatniks, whose culture could not have been more opposed to any sort of stylishness, let alone formality, in dress. Their successors were the mods and rockers of the sixties; mods were passionately interested in dress (one mod, interviewed in a newspaper, said his generation wanted "to stay smart for ever, not scruffy like our parents"). As their ideas became accepted into mainstream society, fashion grew more and more informal, but people didn't stop dressing up; no "dolly-bird" wanted to go to a party in the same clothes she had worn all day, even if what she changed into wasn't much like conventional evening dress. In fact, long dresses became commoner than they had been for some time on such occasions as were still formal. I think this was because of mini-skirts: when short skirts were so short that any impression of even diluted formality was impossible, there had to be another length for grand occasions, and if so it might as well be completely different.

All rules, however, were increasingly under attack. Twiggy, the most famous model of the period, wrote in a guide to fashion that she was disappointed when the Savoy Hotel allowed people to come in wearing jeans, which she feared would mean fewer and fewer came in anything else.[17] She may be right, as a girl of thirteen commented: "Everyone longs for days out of school uniform – those two or three days when you get to express your own individuality . . . We become engrossed in wondering what to wear, yet everyone's answer is the same: jeans! Blue jeans are the most popular, though occasionally there may be an adventurous soul who wears a black or green pair. So much for individuality."[18]

It was Twiggy and her contemporaries, however, who started the process. In a newspaper interview at the height of her career, she said "all those fancy couturiers are dead on ideas" and that she wore anything she wanted to. If so, she has no reasonable grounds for objecting if people decide that all they want to wear is jeans. When rules are removed, the practice to which they used to apply changes from an institution to a tradition, and while apathy protects the former, it destroys the latter. Changing an institution takes effort, which the apathetic won't make, but all that is needed to kill a tradition is lack of will to keep it alive. A rule will remain in force until someone abolishes it, and people who only dressed in a certain way in order to comply may find they like it. If there is no pressure, they may never find out. Physically, thanks to easy-care fabrics, dry cleaning and zip fasteners, dressing up has never been so easy, but changing is still more trouble than not changing. People resent their freedom of choice being limited by anything except practical considerations such as safety (and sometimes by those), but if there are no rules so many automatically take the easy option that eventually there is no other left to take: think how many people sincerely deplore the death of specialist shops, while doing all their own shopping at the supermarkets which put the specialists out of business.

This is where conformism comes in. Men's dress clothes, even more than their ordinary ones, illustrate the advantages of freedom from choice. A man seeing "white tie", "black tie", "morning dress" or "lounge suit" on an invitation knows exactly what is expected and can decide for himself whether the dress code puts him off accepting. A woman has much more freedom to exercise her preferences, but runs the risk of finding everybody else's are different; the wording of the invitation, however, gives some guidelines. One of my childhood memories is of hearing my parents arguing about whether the annual dinner of an academic society, on whose committee my father was serving, should be "black tie" or not. I thought I was solving the problem by saying, "Why not make it optional?" (I had only just learned the meaning of the word). "Oh no!" he answered, "that doesn't solve anything. All it means is people waste hours wondering whether they should dress up or whether they shouldn't, if they do will they be the only ones who did, if they don't will they be the only ones who didn't, and in the end all the people who've got dinner jackets and long dresses come in their ordinary clothes because they don't want to look ostentatious, and all the people who haven't rush off to hire them because they don't want to look poor." The trouble with telling people to do their own thing is that they don't; they do what they think will be everybody else's thing, and then feel resentful if it isn't.

Why? Dressing up is not just a public art but a social one; you need not only someone to do it for but someone to do it with. If misery loves company, so does formality. Party-goers look forward not only to wearing their own dress clothes but seeing other people's. Besides, their own clothes are seen together with the others and however sublime theirs may be, if not accompanied by a good sprinkling of others in the same style, they will be as out of place as a burst of song in a supermarket. The more stylised and removed from everyday life they are, the truer that is. The musical analogy is exact: wearing the wrong clothes is like joining in what you thought was a chorus and finding nobody else has, but with the further embarrassment that you can't stop. Being the odd one out is only enjoyable if it is deliberate. People don't like giving the impression that they were being deliberately rude when they were not, and the over-dressed, unlike the under-dressed, can't pretend they were short of money or time to change. They may be suspected of wanting to show off their wealth, and the "ladies' and gentlemen's" code of which formality is a part condemns showing off. Katharine Whitehorn once wrote: "It goes on being agony when you are dressed quite differently from all the others, and none the less so if they're all in jeans and you're in velvet." I worry less about being different from other people than almost anyone I know, but I've been the only one in velvet and don't recommend it.

For men, it makes matters worse that formal dress is a uniform: they look so conspicuous in the wrong one. Women who are not sure how formal an occasion will be can sit on the sartorial fence by wearing something which could pass as either a rather dressy day outfit or a rather undressy evening one; men can't. "Evening dress optional" (sometimes shortened, ambiguously, to "dress optional") leads to a lot of female fence-sitting, so that men are less willing to change, saying "Why should I, if what you're wearing looks all right with me in an ordinary suit?"

Inevitably, people tire of worrying and decide that if they run the risk of looking fools whatever they do, they might as well save trouble. Also, it's hard to care about one's own behaviour when nobody else does. Making something optional is almost a statement of indifference: it's tantamount to saying "We don't care if you do or you don't", which cools even genuine enthusiasm. (I once heard a man tell a woman who had dressed up for drinks with him that he would like her just as much if she didn't. She shouted "Swine!" and pretended to spit at him.) Again, people may go somewhere in a group, and if over-dressing is embarrassing, having persuaded someone else into it is worse. Hosts are reluctant to put pressure on guests, guests even more reluctant to put it on hosts, leading to dialogues like "Do we wear anything special?" "Not unless you want to." "What do *you* want?" "I don't mind, what about *you?*" This not only wastes time but can mean both sides miss an opportunity they wanted to take, because each one thinks the other doesn't.

Besides, you may be asking your friends to wear clothes they don't have and can't afford to buy or hire. They might be too embarrassed to tell you so and run into debt. Organisers of public entertainments think of this too. It's a vicious circle: the fewer the occasions for evening dress, the less likely people are to buy it and the less willing others are to stipulate its wear. The less demand there is for it the more expensive it becomes and fewer items are sold secondhand, restricting a cheap source of supply. Professional fashion advisers frequently write that evening dress is required so seldom that it's cheaper to hire it; this increases the likelihood that nobody will do so, not only because some people dislike hired clothes but because, to quote a businessman I once knew, "money spent on hiring is money down the drain." People who buy clothes are more likely to want to get their money's worth by frequent wear. The same advisers recommend "separates which you can wear with something else after the party's over" for women; this blurs the line between "special" and "ordinary", making it seem less worth crossing. I have heard women say, "When I see a lovely dress like that I wish I'd made more of an effort", but that won't happen if they never see such dresses being worn.

We know the result. William Ivey Long, a Broadway costume designer who sometimes designs wedding dresses, said: "What you find today is the bride all done up and the rest of the party rather casual. I wish people dressed up more, but I understand why they don't, because unless the whole crowd is going to play the game it's hard to get people into it."[19] (Male morning dress seems to be rarer in the United States than Britain. I think women put pressure on men to wear it for the reasons my First World War veteran acquaintance described; that explains why it's worn much less at funerals, which women can't have so much fun dressing for.) An article on men's fashion sums up: "The notion of a fashion democracy in which everyone dresses to suit himself may be appealing in the abstract, but the reality is otherwise . . . Left to their own devices, people will seek the lowest common denominator."[20] If you think that's exaggerated, ask yourself whether, on being invited to a party and told to wear whatever you liked, you would wear full evening dress.

You might if you like to shock ("if you don't know what to wear, wear something outrageous" a young women's magazine once urged) and you added some detail to show you weren't serious ("a ballgown with sneakers" in Minna Thornton's phrase) but what if you are not that sort of person and don't like jokey details? This kind of permissiveness is like saying it's all right to play Bach, but only in jazz arrangements. Half-hearted Puritanism again: you can do what you want provided you don't do it as if you meant it.

Advertisements for entertainments at National Trust properties have stated that dress is "entirely optional – T-shirts to tiaras!" It is significant that they spell it out. I wonder how many tiaras, or anything remotely like them, ever appear, and whether their number is maintained? As these events always seem to be inaccessible by public transport, I've never found out. In my experience, "optional" means that, just slowly enough for it not to be immediately obvious, the amount of evening dress goes down and down, until there are only a few elderly "Disgusted of Tunbridge Wells" types left. When they die, it will simply not occur to their survivors that the option still exists, and then it might as well be banned, except that a ban might encourage it. St Paul said that the man without scruples should give in to the man with scruples; the reverse happens in practice.

When the argument that "nobody's interested any more" is used about arts with élitist reputations, their defenders have sometimes called the pessimists' bluff. For example, "performances by Pavilion Opera Educational Trust have been rapturously received by children in schools from Brixton to Southall, Tower Hamlets to Cleveland . . . Pavilion's productions, unabridged and always in the original language, make no concessions to their young audiences . . . Freddie Stockdale, a Pavilion trustee, . . . claims that it is more often teachers who are resistant to opera. 'They say: "It's not what our children are interested in."' But Stockdale reckons that as long as he can get opera to inner-city audiences between the ages of eight and 14, the chances are that they will take to it."[21]

On 8 November 1999 *The Independent* reported: "Chris Smith, Secretary of State for Culture, has sought an assurance from the Royal Opera House that it will not have any more black-tie events after its reopening next month" because "this is meant to be the people's opera now and black-tie evenings send out the wrong signal." "When I took the job of chairman of the new Opéra-Bastille", Pierre Bergé told *The Gramophone* in August 2002, ". . . I wanted people to come in their jeans . . . I don't like these places where everybody feels they have to dress up in their tuxedos." He is Chief Executive Officer of Yves Saint-Laurent, famous for designing tuxedos for women. John Rosselli writes: "Outside Glyndebourne, Salzburg and one or two other such festive places, audiences no longer feel the old urge to dress up."[22] How does he know? Eight-year-olds in Brixton felt no urge to go to the opera until they saw it. This trend, he adds, "marks not so much a change in the social make-up of opera-goers as wider changes in dress habits" which explains a lot: objecting makes you look like a snob who wants to discourage social change.

Change is desired not only to encourage poor opera-lovers but to discourage patrons who only go for the snob value. (This applies to other performing arts, but opera is the best example because it is still the one for which people are most likely to dress. Oddly, they do so less for ballet, where visual as opposed to musical elements are more important.) Not only is it unjust that snobs should occupy seats which real enthusiasts long for, but they can be disruptive. Susanne Kappeler apparently disapproves of silent audiences (a question irrelevant to this book, but I want to put it on record that I totally disagree) and calls them "an invention of polite society";[23] if she is using the traditional class definition, this is quite wrong. Molière, Marivaux and Fanny Burney (a music critic's daughter and a dramatist as well as a novelist) all castigated the behaviour of aristocratic audiences, for instance in Burney's *Cecilia*: "the place she had happened to find vacant was next to a party of young ladies, who were so earnestly engaged in their own discourse, that they listened not to a note of the opera, and so infinitely diverted with their own witticisms, that their tittering and loquacity allowed no one in their vicinity to hear better than themselves".[24] "To disturb others who wish to listen is gross ill breeding" wrote "Censor" almost exactly a century later; "but, unfortunately, it is common with the very class who pretend to an exclusive share of good breeding" and there have been letters to that effect in the magazine *Opera*. Some of the class in question regarded the artists they patronised (in all senses of the word) as servants, which helped foster the view that real lovers of music, dance or drama don't care what they wear.

This is a perfect example of what logicians call the undistributed middle: "cows have legs, I have legs, therefore I am a cow." If those who go just to be seen dress up and you dress up, you only go to be seen. Books by lovers of the arts tell another story, as in the memoirs of Angela du Maurier: "It was in the early part of 1946 that I went to Covent Garden for the first time since 1939. The occasion was a performance of *The Sleeping Beauty* . . . I and the friend with whom I went naturally wore our best evening dresses . . . I think we were the only people 'dressed' . . . I *long* for a compulsory order that to sit in the stalls, boxes, stalls-circle, etc, at Covent Garden, one must be in evening dress"[25] and she wrote of the ballet itself, "Such beauty made me cry". Ida Cook, a typist earning £2 6s. (£2.30) a week, and her sister saved up for two years to visit America to hear their favourite opera singers, which cost them £100 each. Far from resenting the need for evening dress (Ida made theirs), she wrote:

> Which of us who saw the Met in the great days of the prosperity boom [1927] can ever forget . . . the display of dresses, furs, and jewelry?
>
> The Metropolitan and Covent Garden also looked then as opera houses should look. How I hate the drab austerity of an 'undressed' Covent Garden today! Opera is a festive art, and in my view, the audience should pay it the compliment of looking a little festive too. Pushing your way into the stalls of a great opera house in scruffy jeans and pullover brands you as either tiresomely common and insensitive, or rather pathetically exhibitionist.[26]

The Cooks were among the "ordinary" people whom successive governments and arts administrators have tried to convince that "culture is for them too". Are their modern equivalents so different? I wish someone would hold a survey on whether people would, given the opportunity, like to dress for performances at their local theatre or concert hall (or dinner at their local hotel), but I know of none; the evidence can, unfortunately, only be drawn from the places with a reputation for social exclusivity because there are no others where such clothes are worn. These places seem totally opposed to the spirit of "arts for all" which is the only possible justification for funding the arts with public money; how, when live performing art is fighting for its life, can anyone defend restricting people's access to it by discriminatory dress codes?

To answer one question with another: has abolishing such codes produced "arts for all"? Has it brought in that "new audience", has it stopped complaints about élitism or the poor paying for the rich to enjoy (I have heard this) "irrelevant rubbish"? We know it hasn't, any more than new liturgies have produced a religious revival; it hasn't stopped disruptive behaviour either. Nor are the reasons purely financial: I have read that many music students don't go to concerts even when tickets are free.[27] They of all people should know dress isn't formal. The Ballet Boyz claim young people are afraid of going to the ballet because they worry about what to wear.[28] Sir Colin Southgate, when Chairman of the Royal Opera House, was accused of pandering to "the snobbish elements of our society"[29] for saying he wouldn't want to sit next to someone whose clothes smelt. My suggestion will probably strike some readers as insane: might encouraging dressing up work better? Judging by the statistics, it can't work worse.

Although most social events are increasingly casual, even people who can ill afford it have formal weddings. The evolution of wedding dresses shows a desire to emphasise the uniqueness of the occasion. If they could be worn for anything else, they wouldn't be wedding dresses, which is why attempts to make "convertible" ones fail. A book on egalitarian marriage claims: "the penchant for Victorian gowns . . . no longer reflects an allegiance to the old code. Couples may still love to dress up and create a dramatic rite of passage for themselves, but as much as they crave a grand and solemn ceremony, no one buys into the symbolism."[30] Christmas decorations as we know them became popular at about the same time as conventional wedding dresses. They too cannot be suitable for anything else without ceasing to suggest Christmas, and they too are enjoyed by many people, including myself, who don't practise the religion they symbolise.

When I visited Sweden in 1989, I found Stockholm the most casually dressed capital city I have ever seen. It was normal to see men in the streets wearing denim cut-offs, trainers and nothing else, but a neighbour on the flight, who had married into a Swedish family, complained that they had insisted on his bringing morning dress and a top hat for a wedding. At the opera house at Drottningholm, there were postcards of the audience on sale (as a hint, perhaps) and there was only one man not wearing a dinner jacket apart from the king, who wore tails.

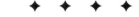

Case Study: One Festive Place

I propose to examine in detail the example of the one "festive place" I know well, because I go there regularly: Glyndebourne. Long ago I decided that I would rather pay for one evening a year there than many somewhere else, and if the sort of behaviour Fanny Burney described had happened, my first visit would have been my last. Nothing could appear more remote, at first glance, from the Pavilion Opera Trust, but it shares the same uncompromising philosophy and met similar resistance. When John Christie and his wife Audrey Mildmay founded a private opera house in 1934, even the first director thought it wouldn't last two years; sixty years later it had to be rebuilt because of the demand for tickets, and it has imitators. Christie's comment on audiences, who are "recommended" to wear evening dress, might have been made on purpose to annoy élite-haters: they must "touch their hats".[31] Spike Hughes's history of Glyndebourne says: "John Christie's frequently expressed determination to make his audience 'take trouble' by wearing evening dress has over the years proved to be, in fact, the least of the efforts the audience is expected to make – although one would not think so from the way some of the Press still moan about it after thirty years . . . The very fact that Glyndebourne is where it is, that performances begin when they do, that attendance involves a complete break with daily routine makes even the most experienced and frequent visitor 'take trouble' . . . You cannot 'drop in' on the spur of the moment as you can in Vienna or at Covent Garden"[32] and Gerald Coke, former Chairman of the Glyndebourne Arts Trust, wrote: "He [John Christie] was completely unsnobbish in the social sense and indeed had no use for those who went to Glyndebourne because it was considered the right thing to do."[33] So why did he encourage a practice which allegedly appeals to no-one else?

The allegation would seem to be false, though some critics would love to prove the contrary. In February 1991 Peter Conrad published an article in *Opera Now* asking, "What have clothes to do with the enjoyment of music? . . . [evening dress] bespeaks self-consciousness and self-advertisement" (just what Ida Cook said of its absence). I wrote a letter which they published the following June, saying: "If he can neither concentrate on music unless he is informally dressed, nor believe that anyone else can, clothes have everything to do with his [enjoyment]." Malcolm Hayes, reviewing the opening night of that year's Festival, wrote: "Contrary to myth, the general atmosphere of opera-going at Glyndebourne blends intelligence with informality, and is a world away from the pall of corporate stuffiness that now regularly envelops the stalls at Covent Garden. Yet Glyndebourne has helped to give itself a reputation for that same stuffiness by refusing to shed its penguin-suited image . . . This is ridiculous when formal dress is far from *de rigueur* even, for example, at the Vienna State Opera. Civilised resistance is called for; if I'm allowed back to Glyndebourne, it will be wearing an immaculate lounge suit."[34] He has also called concert performers' dress "inappropriate and ridiculous".[35] Critics without his bias agree about the audience: "*although* evening dress abounds, the audience includes many opera-lovers"[36] (my italics); "rich-philistine gibes are better aimed elsewhere . . . at Covent Garden, I was stuck behind a bunch of boneheads audibly mocking events on stage . . . you don't meet it at Glyndebourne, where the connoisseur-count is high."[37] This suggests Mr Christie was right in thinking that being expected to change actually keeps boneheads out. That it didn't in earlier periods is easily explained: no extra trouble was involved when everyone dressed for dinner as a matter of course.

A semi-professional singer friend wrote to me that "Mr Hayes . . . really should be allowed his secret wish not to attend any further performances at Glyndebourne. Once you have lost your sense of occasion it is difficult to get it back. However, as no doubt he will return, he should be allowed to wear an old tee shirt and jeans. After all what is egalitarianism if we can't all do what we like? He should beware however, the mundane begets the mundane." When the theatre was rebuilt, speculation came to a head; the *Sunday Times* critic Hugh Canning prophesied, "the audience will change, for the better, and the 'recommended' dress code will become irrelevant." Hugh Pearman, architecture critic of the same paper, wrote that "all dress codes are fundamentally stupid", adding that the real opera-lovers are in the cheap seats wearing jeans. (This from a man has said he thinks that going to the theatre should be a special occasion[38] and earns his living appreciating the visual qualities of buildings; evidently that doesn't extend to what Sir George Christie, the founders' son and second Chairman of the Festival, calls the "human wallpaper".) It referred specifically to Glyndebourne, and it's a howler: jeans and trainers are not allowed even in standing room. (I once saw canvas shoes worn with an evening dress.) I have seen a dress there which was almost exactly the same colour as the irises I had been admiring in the garden; why is it acceptable to enjoy it in a flower-bed but not on people, or in day clothes but not evening ones? Lovers of opera praise it as a synthesis of all the arts, including the costumes worn on stage, so why not what's worn off it?

The conductor Sir Andrew Davis told *The Daily Telegraph* "people can wear dark suits instead of evening dress and not feel awful, which I think is an advance"[39] and it sounds hard to argue that it isn't; but should people feel awful if they do wear evening dress? The leading article that day condemned legalising euthanasia because "patients would feel obliged to . . . exit early" and carers "would be tempted to relieve themselves of a burden". This isn't the place to discuss euthanasia, but if even in questions of life and death the easy option may become compulsory as soon as it stops being forbidden, what can you expect in other matters?

For two of the three nights after I read Canning's prophecy, I had nightmares (this is the literal truth). Feeling like my mother when someone damaged one of her favourite books and she told him he could keep it, I wrote to Sir George, and so evidently did others; the 1996 programme book reproduces many years' correspondence on the subject, giving both sides of the question including someone who called expecting people to change "even meaner and more despicable" than a colour bar (has he tried changing his colour?) and another who referred to "the vulgarities of conspicuous display" and "the absurd situation of travelling down in evening dress" , and did "not consider it necessary to wear a special uniform in order to listen". The phrase suggests yet another failure to see dress as a pleasure in its own right; it also ignores the fact that casual clothes can also be worn to impress, and that when everyone else is formally dressed it's the person who isn't who is conspicuous. Others pointed out that the Christies had a right to decide what was worn in their own house and that opera has a visual side, but none of those quoted asked how someone who can't see any fun in catching a train wearing evening dress and carrying a picnic basket enters into the spirit of a form of drama in which people sing when supposedly dying of lung disease. Opera and ballet take you into a world where what is normally unthinkable happens; ordinary clothes, however good, can't help with that. In 1997, the folders enclosing tickets contained this paragraph: "It has always been part of the tradition of a visit to Glyndebourne that the audience 'dress up' — evening dress (black tie/long or short dress) is customary. Patrons have expressed a wish for this tradition to be upheld and for members of the audience to dress accordingly."

Some people may suspect those patrons just wanted to keep the place exclusive. I don't, nor do my friends (not all middle class) who have been there. Sir George's reply to me pointed out that evening dress is not compulsory, but ended: "We will, nevertheless, turf people out if they fail to dress, in our view, to the occasion. I am anxious that the enjoyment of the majority should not be mucked up by a mal soigné minority."[40] I don't recommend compulsion, because at an arts event, unlike a party, the social side isn't the main purpose of the occasion and people shouldn't have to miss it because they can't afford dress clothes or have accidentally damaged them at the last minute. Not making the rule rigid also lessens the temptation to rebel for the sake of rebellion, as John Christie, having been a schoolmaster, was no doubt aware. Bernard Levin's book on music festivals defends him: "[he] said that all those involved in the production, from the conductor to the scene-shifters, were taking every possible care to ensure that the performance was as near to perfection as human beings can attain; in return, he asked those in the audience to respond similarly, in the only way open to them".[41] I don't see how you can gain the full benefit unless you do. None of the objectors suggests destroying the garden or forbidding the restaurant to serve gourmet meals so as to ensure people don't go just for the food or the flowers; attributing bad motives to the opposition is a game at which two can play and I can't help noticing that, in the garden and restaurant, someone else does all the work.

Another opera festival I have not visited, Wexford, is allegedly greeted with window displays in every shop, discussions in every pub, and offers to do voluntary work in the theatre in exchange for rehearsal passes. Evening dress is compulsory.

Finally, the Head of Education and Community Services at Glyndebourne has said that she found dressing up "wonderful" and young people were "thrilled" to do it.

Taking trouble can beget willingness to take more; if people have to make an effort, they may as well do more rather than less. If this willingness disappears completely, live art is doomed, just as all intellectually demanding arts are doomed unless people are willing to make mental efforts. Live performances can't compete in convenience with recorded and broadcast ones, whose audience needn't even get out of bed, and can change channels or switch off at the first hint of boredom. It is therefore worth emphasising what only a live event can give: sense of occasion.

"If he [Malcolm Hayes] is still unhappy because dressing-up as a penguin makes you bird-brained and liable to be stuffed," my friend's letter continues, "he wants to apply his radical thinking to what he is wearing." I wish men would. "It is interesting to note", Spike Hughes wrote, "that it is always men, never women, who complain about having to dress up, although it is a far longer and more laborious business for a woman than ever it is for a man."[42] Men have less to show for it. When they complain that a dinner suit is boring ("the most difficult costume for a man to look well in" wrote Somerset Maugham) and that we only want them to wear it as a background for our own finery, I have some sympathy, but why don't they invent something they like better? David Thomas described a transvestite ball he organised, at which both sexes dressed as women because the men were only too pleased to change but the women refused to.[43] Men generally assume that the only alternative is yet more informality; the words "colourful and casual" have become linked like "sweet and gentle". In May 2002 the Hallé Orchestra abandoned tails, and a year later the BBC Symphony Orchestra restricted them to occasions when royalty was present. Letters to newspapers suggesting that musicians and clergymen should dress more casually assume formal dress must be black, or black and white; but why shouldn't one orchestra wear blue and another red? Men in the London Mozart Players wear red cummerbunds. As to the clergy, it is sometimes canonical for them to wear colours; Monica Baldwin, a former nun, wrote in her autobiography that the ceremonial dress of Catholic priests resembled women's evening dress.[44] The word "uniform" keeps appearing, but John Masters described the Sandhurst June Ball as "probably the most colourful function in pre-war England . . . women would come in evening dress – white, if they had any sense . . . The cadets and the women acted as a backdrop for the brilliance of . . . scarlet and gold, chocolate and French grey, royal blue and silver, dark green and light blue, white and crimson; kilts and trews, sporrans and aiguillettes and shoulder chains – and then the naval officers in their boat cloaks! . . . How drab I would look, a twerp of a junior in dull dark blue with a minuscule red stripe down the sides of my trousers!"[45]

The dinner suit was a compromise from the moment it was invented. It only exists because men couldn't be bothered to put on tails which, according to my father, are more comfortable once on than lounge suits. This isn't surprising since they were designed for horsemen, and are popular with dancers and violinists. He was none of those, but once ran across Trafalgar Square in full evening dress chasing a taxi, and welcomed the freedom to move his arms; a male friend made similar comments on wearing Georgian costume for a fancy ball. Tails at least enable a man to experience something different even though they leave no room for individuality, while "black tie" means having to change without achieving either. Men have reduced dressing up to replacing a bluish, greenish, grey or brown sack suit with a black sack suit and a different tie, and then complain it isn't enjoyable; I can't help thinking of children breaking toys and then crying because they no longer like playing with them.

Some, however, make the most of their opportunities, like Bernard Levin: "I have seen a beautiful wine-red dinner-jacket . . . and am much minded to buy it. Arianna . . . has found . . . a black velvet evening suit, waistcoat and all. It is useless for me to protest that velvet wears badly, that I shall have to throw it away within a year, that it costs a monstrous sum, that I shall have to buy silk shirts to wear with it, at even more monstrous cost . . . as soon as I have seen it, I know I must have it . . . does this mean that I shall not be wanting the red jacket after all? It does; *something* is saved from the ruin of my finances."[46] I have seen a man at Glyndebourne in a purple and gold jacket. A friend asked me whether to wear a blue velvet

one for the dinner of the Friends of the Victoria and Albert Museum; I said
that as the then Director, Sir Roy Strong, had expressed a wish that men
would dress more colourfully, I couldn't think of a better place for it. He
asked if that was consistent with feminism. I told him I said it because I
was a feminist.

A book on party-giving said of white tie and tails: "the young adore
it".[47] In 1988, I served on the committee of a charity planning a fund-rais-
ing ball for which the invitation stated "White tie or uniform." We were
warned that the tickets wouldn't sell; they sold out, and many of the buy-
ers were in their twenties. Sir Elton John has held White Tie and Tiara
Balls every year since 1999. Claudia Brush Kidwell and Valerie Steele
have pointed out that a man in a tail-coat reveals his figure in the same
way as a formally dressed woman.[49] Bringing tails back does pose a problem, however: they must be made to measure or they just don't fit. In an
age without cheap labour, that makes the cost prohibitive for many
people, so there must be an alternative. Why not go back to earlier periods for inspiration, as designers for women often do? Swallow-tails and
penguin suits don't exhaust the possibilities. "Who Are the Slaves of
Fashion?" asked *The Penny Magazine* in 1906, the answer being men: "The
day of knee breeches and silk stockings has passed, never, alas! to be
revived . . . The King himself introduced brocaded silk dress waistcoats,
but very few of his subjects had courage enough to follow His Majesty's
lead." My mother was once told by her escort at a party that she looked
like a Dresden shepherdess; when shall I be able to tell mine he looks like
a Dresden shepherd? (Attempts were made in the sixties, but rather half-
heartedly.) The pianist Melvyn Tan, who dislikes playing in both tails and
dinner jackets, designed his own form of evening dress. When I attended
an evening class he taught, he said some early music specialists recommended copying the gestures made by musicians in contemporary
pictures; when he asked them about concerts in costume, they said that
would be frivolous (he disagreed). I answered that even if we were sure the
musicians really made those gestures (artists can take liberties) it might
have been because of their clothes: if they held their wrists in a certain way
to keep the ruffles on their sleeves away from their instruments, adopting
the posture when not wearing ruffles is as pointless as putting a candle-
snuffer on an electric lamp.

The explorer Sir Wilfred Thesiger liked wearing tails when in England
(preferring Arab dress in Africa) and his books described the Bedouin and
marsh Arabs, living in extreme poverty, dressing up for occasions such as

weddings.[49] His uncle, the actor Ernest Thesiger, who once led the Men's Dress Reform League, advocated more comfortable clothes for men, but wore jewellery. Elizabeth Hawes also suggested alternatives, including "black faille trousers and a waist length, rose colored coat, square cut on the chest and worn with a white stock" and regretted that "men have no formal or semi-formal evening relaxing garment except their pajamas".[50]

One of Emma Lathen's thrillers describes a party: "John Thatcher had been exposed to the domestic architecture of Regency England before and had admired its many excellences. Now he realised that there had always been a sense of incongruity, of gentle friction between dissonant elements. Those Adam ceilings, those swagged draperies, those crystal chandeliers had never been meant for men in business suits and women in tweed skirts. They had been designed as backgrounds for peacocks, and tonight the Arabs did them justice. As they ascended to the drawing room, their flowing robes and brilliant headdresses improvised unexpected harmonies with the cool celadon green of the panelled walls."[51]

A woman can wear something suggesting the period of the building she is going to or the play, opera or ballet she is seeing (someone, when I went to Tchaikovsky's *Onegin*, asked if I was in the audience or the cast). People have worn Tudor costumes to Shakespeare's reconstructed Globe Theatre, though there is no pressure to do so. Dressing, if not in period costume, at least in something designed with aesthetic rather than utilitarian priorities, gives opportunities for entering into the spirit of an occasion and the ambience of its surroundings; I remember, at a concert in a room full of eighteenth-century portraits, feeling they must be wondering what those barbarians were doing there.

John Taylor agrees with Sir Peter Hall that an opera production should "look like the music" (or a theatrical one like the drama) and notes that this is audience participation: "For to argue with Shakespeare, the play's not the *only* thing. As in any aspect of culture, enjoyment is heightened and sustained by several accessory facets . . . Acoustics can make or mar a musical rendering, lighting and framing can damn the enjoyment of a painting, background can detract from the effect of sculpture, and surroundings from the effect of architecture . . . Certainly an appreciation of good wine involves more than lying drunk in the gutter – and an audience which will not make its own contribution to its own entertainment by heightening a sense of occasion with the right clothes is simply lessening its chance of getting its own money's worth."[52] The new audience whom impresarios are trying with increasing desperation to attract might prefer this form of participation to "the sort of . . . radicalism epitomised by . . . author Irvine Welsh: he urged that young people should be allowed to . . . give voice to their feelings during a performance . . . No one should be afraid of saying that some art forms need quiet concentration. Nor need one apologise that some, such as opera and ballet, can benefit from a sense of grandeur in productions and surroundings."[53]

Another article, admittedly slightly facetious, offers confirmation: "opera-goers can take a tip from rock . . . affect Onegin-style tailcoats and thus more thoroughly relate to the performance . . . rock could learn from opera . . . no one shouted rude words during the quieter, less immediately-engaging bits, no one drowned out the good bits with their off-key efforts."[54] A survey in *Opera Now* (November 1990) showed that it was those under 35 who most wanted to dress up, and at about the same time Miranda Jackson, in the magazine *Classical Music*, pointed out that while Kennedy in punk clothes draws crowds, Pavarotti in tails draws bigger ones. People have been seen dancing in the arena in evening dress on Viennese nights at the BBC Proms, which have no dress code whatever, and evening dress was also worn at Sir Elton John's gala concert at the Royal Opera House on 1 December 2002. There was a "black tie" casino at the 2003 Glastonbury Festival, and the *Big Issue* reported: "For just a fiver, visitors were able to hire dinner dress . . . creating a dramatic atmosphere where it became impossible to distinguish between the performers and the punters."

At most pop concerts and clubs, this would be unthinkable, but what you wear matters; youth sub-cultures have dress codes. The rock impresario Malcolm McLaren has said "the visual looks of groups are more important than the music".[55] (Are there non-visual looks?) Being in a room full of well-dressed people might help to make a classical concert a more complete experience in the absence of such visual elements as the light shows at rock concerts (introducing these has been suggested, but not taken up with enthusiasm). McLaren's former partner Vivienne Westwood has produced numerous collections of dresses based on past styles, and the models wearing them were described as "evidently enjoying their first experience of truly charming clothes. They have grown up in a time of dressing down. They are delighted at dressing up".[56] In the same week that Wayne Sleep said he had founded a new dance company because "dance was too good for the dinner-jacket and sequin brigade" (at Covent Garden) the feminist fashion writer Naseem Khan wrote of "countless sequins" being sewn on for the Notting Hill Carnival in an article urging that it should be taken seriously.[57] Black church congregations are among the most formally dressed.

Competitive ballroom dancing doesn't have an élitist image (Oxford and Cambridge practise it as a sport, but only started to quite recently) and requires full evening dress. That universities have taken it up at a time when social dancing is dominated by discos and the emergent clubbing culture suggests, like the popularity of line dancing, that younger people might wish to return to formal dance. A newspaper survey revealed that only 20 percent of young people go to discos;[58] I am willing to bet a higher percentage went to dances in the heyday of ballroom dancing between the wars.

Permissiveness in dancing, like permissiveness in dress, is more apparent than real. "I know someone with a philosophical objection to country dancing", said a friend who loves it, "because you do what the caller tells you. But go to a disco and people are all moving in the same way." Again, the heyday of the Palais de Danse was also that of the Picture Palace, and both were as lavishly decorated as their owners could afford (so, earlier still, were music halls). Such decorations in theatres have been attacked on grounds of élitism, but old-fashioned theatres are more popular than attempts at "democratic" ones. The Savoy Theatre was rebuilt in 1929 with multi-coloured seats: "It was not unknown . . . for female members of the audience to find out in advance the colour of their seat, and match their dress accordingly."[59] The revival of such practices might even make audiences more adventurous: they might be more willing to try something unfamiliar if they knew that even at the worst they would have had the pleasure of dressing for it.

A Spanish nobleman, criticising King Juan Carlos for not reviving traditional ceremony, told me: "the masses love it." Every royal occasion proves they do, although many socialists wish they wouldn't; this suggests that a republic would have to provide a substitute. I walked through Kensington Gardens at the height of the popular reaction to the death of Diana, Princess of Wales, among the innumerable flowers, hand-written messages, and photographs left by her admirers. Though there were many pictures of the "People's Princess" in casual clothes which they could have used, a large majority showed her in a ball dress and tiara. Katharine Whitehorn's etiquette book comments: "if you think formality is confined to the upper or toffee-nosed classes, just look at the pictures in your local paper of the Mayor and Corporation, none of them blue-blooded, opening the Dog's Graveyard in their robes. They love a bit of formality – and *why not?* They've as much right to it as the Queen of England, if that's what they want."[60]

When socialists "dress down" to show solidarity with the proletariat, the gesture can misfire. When Gordon Brown refused to wear evening dress to the Lord Mayor's banquet in 1997, he was condemned not only in the broadsheets but also in a letter to *The Sun*: "How churlish of Chancellor Gordon Brown to snub protocol by wearing a lounge suit . . .[it] stood out like a sore thumb, blighting his otherwise excellent speech."[61] It was also taking advantage of his privileged position as guest of honour, which meant he couldn't be refused admission. When Michael Foot wore a donkey jacket to lay a wreath on the Cenotaph, Katharine Whitehorn wrote: "if he thinks an ordinary working man wouldn't have attempted his Sunday best for such a ceremony, then he's crazy – and making the same mistake middle-class reformers have made for over a century. And that is to sentimentalise the toil of the toiler; to identify the working man with the working clothes; to brush aside the lace curtains and the shiny suit and the best teapot; and value everything about the poor – except their pride."[62]

They forget that the rougher your working clothes and environment are, the more likely you are to want something different when you go out to enjoy yourself, and formality can blur class distinctions as much as informality. A professional man of working-class origin told my father that a dinner jacket was one of the most democratic outfits men could wear, and I have heard a refuse collector express pleasure in wearing one.

Could dressing up be a sign of feminist values, Virginia Woolf's "private beauty", as opposed to the rituals she disliked so much where only holders of certain offices are allowed to wear certain clothes? Janet Radcliffe Richards suggests that fashion is part of women's culture, and in the nineteenth century women organised fashionable society functions. The link between these and attempts to return to a supposed matriarchy might seem tenuous, but here is one of Heide Göttner-Abendroth's "Principles of a Matriarchal Aesthetic", which she claims has survived in folk festivals (of which dress is certainly a part): "The ritual dance ceremony embraces music, song, poetry, movement, decoration, symbol, comedy and tragedy . . . the functions of daily life are necessarily involved."[63] This parallels the ethos of Glyndebourne or a formal dance. Feminists have wished there were a "rite of passage" for girls into adulthood; wearing their first long dresses at adult festivities used to be one. If this sounds frivolous, throughout history people have worn their best clothes for holidays, and the origin of "holiday" is "holy day"; if holiness means anything, what is holy is by definition better than what is not.

One reason evening dress is poor value for money is that it isn't worn often enough, and the solution is to wear it more. There is another way to offset the expense: when it suggests earlier periods, it doesn't date. A man in white tie and tails wears clothes differing very little from those he would have worn in the reign of William IV; if the monarchy survives he will probably be able to wear them in that of William V. The same goes for women wearing what used to be called "period gowns"; Ted Polhemus called this "anti-fashion",[64] like traditional folk costumes (which, at their most elaborate, were reserved for special occasions). Clothes which look centuries old when you buy them are no worse for looking older. If people can't mark a special occasion by formality, the only way to do so is to buy something new. Christmas decorations are timeless because they only appear once a year; many people complain that it no longer seems special because the build-up starts too early. British royal and military pageantry has been accused of fostering everything from backwardness to class distinctions, but it can't be said to foster planned obsolescence; ceremonial dress may be one way of squaring conflicting demands for variety in dress and ecology. Concern for the latter has led to reviving other things once dismissed as obsolete, from windmills to trams, and though conservationists are often derided for being in love with a past that never was, their opponents are sometimes in love with a future that never will be.

Lastly, if there were more occasions set aside for decorative dress, women might not wear it for everyday life when it hinders their activities or just looks silly, as feminists have often complained they do (wearing "gypsy" styles in glass and concrete offices, for instance). I am sure some of this results from waiting for a special event that never comes.

In the last resort, evening dress has only one justification: some of us want it to survive because we like it. We have to say so: there is no chance whatever of it reappearing at theatres, for instance, (especially subsidised ones) without public demand. I have heard of managements giving away tickets to patrons in evening dress; how I wish they would revive that! We shall be accused of selfishness, but this is always double-edged, because everyone has a self. If others don't want to wear something they dislike or to feel odd because they don't, why should we? If it inhibits their pleasure to dress formally, it inhibits ours not to. Jane Rule, a lesbian feminist whose book *A Hot-Eyed Moderate* refers to "something inherently silly about all seductiveness" and the "physical torture . . . of women's dress" (hot-eyed what?), admits: "I do dress up, rarely to please myself, usually simply to indicate that I respect special occasions, a dinner party, a concert."[65] Of course it isn't necessary; neither are the arts, whose supporters are also accused of selfishness, snobbery and hypocrisy (by that schoolboy I quoted in chapter 1, for instance). Finally, we have only limited opportunities for wearing what we like and they keep shrinking, while lovers of business or sports clothes can wear them every day.

Evening dress will only survive if it does something which day dress can't. It's not good enough to say "If only there were more occasions!" If we want them we must demand them, and if necessary make them. "If I can't dance in it, it's not my revolution" said the anarchist Emma Goldman, who believed in beautiful things for everyone. If I can't wear ball dresses in it, it isn't mine.

9

WHAT NEXT?

One can believe anything of the world's future.

Max Beerbohm   The Crime

The extreme view once was that all personal adornment was wrong, as seeking to excite the passions of men. This idea has happily passed away.

Elinor Glyn   Love: What I Think of It (1928)

When the sexual division of labor in the home melts away, so will the beauty problem.

Rhona Mahony   Kidding Ourselves (1995)

Books like this usually end by trying to predict the future. Like the architect who designed a bedroom for my mother with so many built-in cupboards there was no room for the bed, they nearly always forget something. It is more pertinent to ask what sort of future we want, and how we can encourage it.

I know what I want, but suppose I'm wrong? Suppose all fashion, all art, all notions of beauty are just by-products of sexism? They will disappear. What is against nature will die a natural death, and there is no need to kill it. We shall all wear our uniform boiler suits until they fall apart, the idea that some people are better-looking than others will go the same way as the idea that left-handed people are marked by the devil, and only historians will read this book.

If something really is part of human nature, however, it will be destroyed only if the human race is, and trying to kill it is throwing our efforts down a bottomless pit. If, therefore, the tendency to find some sights (and sounds, smells, tastes and forms of touch) more pleasing than others, even if there is no practical reason for it, is part of nature, it won't go away and we should be trying to enjoy its benefits and minimise its disadvantages as much as we can. The same is true of the appeal of novelty. If this is true for some people but not others, then we must recognise that both types exist and their views must be respected. So must whatever efforts they need to make to put them into practice.

We come here to a question which, though it goes far beyond the terms of this book, is highly relevant to it. What is beauty, in dress or people or anything else? Does it even exist? It is generally considered a truism that beauty is in the eye of the beholder; I think it more correct to call it, in Trollope's word, an untruism. There is disagreement and no proof, so what is to be done?

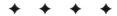

Nothing can permanently please, which does not contain in itself the reason why it is so, and not otherwise.

Samuel Taylor Coleridge

You can't try to do things right and not despise the people who do them wrong. How can I be indifferent? If that doesn't matter, then nothing matters.

Willa Cather   The Song of the Lark

Trifles make perfection, and perfection is no trifle.

Michelangelo

I have already discussed how feminist attempts to play down the importance of beauty fail to take the strength of people's feelings into account. The same goes for attempts to redefine its nature. Rita Freedman, pointing out that the definition of beauty has already been expanded to make room for different races, writes: "Our personal and social definitions of beauty can stretched to make room for the . . . plainer . . . and funny-faced among us."[1] Can they? Only at the cost of destroying their ability to serve the purpose for which they exist. Expanding the meaning of beauty to include people defined as plain is like expanding the meaning of musicianship to include people who sing flat or the meaning of honesty to include shoplifters. In this instance it is impossible to claim that "different" doesn't necessarily mean "inferior" (as one can with races) because "plain" is only a milder version of ugly, the opposite of beautiful. It is a word for an aesthetic judgment and nothing else, and either it means something or it doesn't.

This is what the would-be destroyers of unrealistic ideals won't face; this is where they themselves are unrealistic. They want to redefine an idea with no meaning except in terms of its opposite (just as bigness has no meaning if smallness doesn't) so that the opposite ceases to exist. This is like the remark quoted by the French feminist author Françoise Parturier: women are not inferior, but men are superior.[2] Their ideal could only be achieved if all colours and shapes were equally satisfying to all human beings, which they aren't; furthermore, if they were, words like "plain" and "beautiful" would be meaningless by definition. If Rita Freedman thinks that, why does she use them? As Janet Radcliffe Richards put it, "we cannot alter our standards to the extent of making everyone beautiful without getting rid of ideas of beauty altogether".[3]

Some theorists would say that this has already been disproved, and that all women will be beautiful when that universal scapegoat, our sexist society, is overthrown. Alice Walker cites China as an example: "Everyone wears essentially the same thing: trousers and shirt. And everyone is neat, clean, and adequately dressed. No one wears make-up or jewelry. At first, faces look dull, as a natural tree would look if Christmas trees were the norm. But soon one becomes conscious of the wonderful honesty natural faces convey. An honesty more interesting than any ornament. And a vulnerability that make-up and jewelry would mask."[4] The word "vulnerability" is interesting, considering how many feminists have said women look vulnerable with make-up ("I had always felt exposed by it", writes Jane Rule[5]). This description comes very close to the theory that everyone is naturally beautiful. I have two comments: one is that I have visited China and it didn't have that effect on me, and the other is that uniforms and paintlessness were imposed by force.

The Marxist ideal is set forth in Joseph Hansen and Evelyn Reed's *Cosmetics, Fashions and the Exploitation of Women*, which records a controversy in the American Socialist Workers' party in 1954. When women members criticised a pseudonymous anti-cosmetic article by Hansen on the grounds that not only was a smart appearance a social necessity but that some of them actually liked having one, he made it clear that they were not toeing the party line: "Lovers of beauty in the new society will feel no need, I believe, to decorate lilies . . . we ourselves touch such forms of beauty, I think, in a one-sided way in the admiration and love we feel for our comrades in the socialist struggle. It is their *character* that attracts us, not the smoothness of their complexion, the regularity of their features, their age, or the color of their skin. And character, as we all know, is determined by action, that is by the deeds we perform. That is where a revolutionary socialist looks for beauty in people." Aesthetics will disappear, becoming indistinguishable from morals. Reed's vision of the future was slightly different: "I am not speaking against good clothes . . . Under socialism, the question of whether or not a woman wishes to paint and decorate her body will be of no more social consequence than when children today wish to paint up on Halloween and other festive occasions, or when actors paint up for the stage, or when clowns paint up for the circus. Some people may consider them more beautiful when they are painted. Some may not. But this will be a purely personal opinion and nothing more."[6] She seems to forget that Halloween painting is supposed to look funny and slightly frightening.

This ideal sounds like Andrea Dworkin's hope, quoted in chapter 1, for a "truly democratic" standard of beauty allowing for "honorable variety" of physical types and rejecting the "crap" of cosmetics (she is closer to Hansen than to Reed). Ann Oosthuizen wrote a novel about a woman's introduction to feminism: "She felt silly with the amount of make-up she had on. Her face felt stiff under it, she wanted to see if she looked like a clown to them, but when she went to the toilet to see, there was no mirror to check up on."[7] Anja Meulenbelt's autobiography waxes lyrical in describing an all-women camp in Denmark: "one by one all clothes are removed . . . At night we sing: women over forty, throw away your corsets and your rollers and your sleeping pills. Join us – with us you are beautiful." They do, however, "decorate each other with chains which we crochet, with shawls, with flowers" and on a later occasion "I make my eyes glisten by putting black Indian stuff around them".[8] Her account of her feelings when dancing with other women in the camp strikingly resembles descriptions of falling in love, and Elizabeth Wilson has called it "an embrace of all by all in which all individuality, all difference – all identity – is dissolved".[9] In both cases, feelings of euphoria make everyone and everything seem beautiful, but on Meulenbelt's own showing, it didn't last: after leaving the camp, she writes, "I have looked again in the mirror and discovered that I still have a peculiar nose and ugly teeth." (Of course you can forget that if you never look in a mirror, just as you may think you are a competent musician or pronounce a foreign language well until you hear a tape-recording.) In real life, euphoria wears off, which is why the German writer Frigga Haug dismisses this ideal as "abstract and sickly-sweet" Utopianism.[10]

A variant of it, more tolerant of artificial decoration, appeared in a letter to *Spare Rib* in response to an article defending fashion, which other correspondents had attacked: "In my opinion there are no 'ugly' women,

regardless of how they express themselves through clothes and/or make up.
OR BY REFUSING TO DO SO . . . (Growing up in Germany, and being Jewish
the still lingering principle of the Hitler era, that a 'German woman never
paints her face', led me to feel very comfortable with every made up face I
encountered: it seemed to reject the whole ideology!) . . . Everybody who
feels good about herself IS beautiful . . . Would an artist stop painting just
because she doesn't want to use her 'privilege' over the multitudes who
can't, (or won't)? Which isn't to say that everyone who's not strictly
Academy material should give up painting if it is something they enjoy
doing."[11] She doesn't say everyone who enjoys painting is a great painter.

I once said to someone who told me beauty is in the eye of the beholder,
"You might as well say literary merit is in the mind of the reader". Some
people would, but when I asked him if he thought everybody's taste in literature equally good, tellingly, he didn't. Neither did Andrea Dworkin:
"[Joanna Russ] seems to think that all books by 'wrong' people are created
equal and I don't . . . I think great books, as distinguished from all other
books, do exist."[12] That means drawing a distinction between those who
have written them and those who have not. "Mustn't we," asked Mary Scott,
"in abandoning the patriarchal approach to 'truth' or 'literary merit' find
some other system of assessing value to replace it?"[13]

I return to Letty Cottin Pogrebin:

> whose idea of 'better' are we talking about here? . . . if the will to improve
> on nature is strictly the result of commercial manipulation, how do we
> account for the elaborate face painting and body adornment found in some
> tribal societies 6,000 miles from Madison Avenue? . . . Since every culture
> responds to some well-defined beauty ideal, and the existence of an ideal is
> an anthropological fact of life, why single out the Western beauty standard
> for special criticism? Is it any more reprehensible that Western-trained eyes
> respond to Western standards of beauty than that Western-trained ears
> prefer harmony to dissonance?
>
> We're told that beauty is in the eye of the beholder, as if it were some
> quirky individualized perception, yet survey after survey shows a remarkable
> consensus among people of all ages and races about what makes a face attrac-
> tive . . . We claim to find a variety of faces appealing, including older faces,
> yet the vast majority of us have been found to respond most positively to
> faces that are young and conventionally pretty.[14]

There is evidence both for and against theories about a wide variety of
types being admired. One much-quoted example, the plates distending
Ubangi women's lips, is a red herring; women wore them to make them-

selves ugly, to avoid being carried off by members of more powerful tribes.[15] Admitting variety, however, doesn't solve the problem, for two reasons: first, wide doesn't necessarily mean infinite (however many types were considered beautiful there might still be some that were not) and secondly, there may be a hierarchy within each one. An English textbook encourages children to appreciate different kinds of poetry with the words, "We must beware of criticising a poodle for being a poor specimen of a bloodhound, or a bloodhound for being a poor specimen of a poodle."[16] True, but a blood-hound could still be a poor specimen of a bloodhound. (My working definition of bad art is that it does nothing that good art of the same type can't do better.)

"Judge with your eyes", said Le Corbusier to his pupils. If you really think every kind of personal appearance and every kind of clothing is as good aesthetically as any other and the conventions of beauty are unreal, it shouldn't bother you if other people fit them and you don't. If it does bother you, you don't really think so. Both Quentin Bell and Sara Maitland have defined bad art as what happens when artists start saying what they think they ought to;[17] I can't help suspecting supporters of Joseph Hansen's view that beauty consists wholly in character are doing so. The desire to make all women happy with their looks can produce exactly the same results as the desire to present positive images of people in oppressed groups: pretending something satisfies us when it doesn't. This is simply wishful thinking, and no matter how elevated the moral reasons for doing so, what it comes down to is telling ourselves lies: exactly what the women's move-ment was founded to escape.

Germaine Greer has written enthusiastically about singing in a choir, which she could not have done without training; she doesn't seem to think "all voices were created equal" (a statement I have seen in print). Andrea Dworkin admitted "the sheer beauty of the art that presumes woman, at her highest, as a beautiful object",[18] and Shulamith Firestone that "Sex objects *are* beautiful. An attack on them can be confused with an attack on beauty itself."[19] This suggests the old standard might not be easily replaced, especially if Nancy Etcoff is right in believing that it developed for evolu-tionary reasons: "The idea that beauty is unimportant or a cultural construct is the real beauty myth."[20]

Naomi Wolf claims women should not object to being told, "I think you're beautiful because I love you", but would she like someone to say, "I think your book is good because I love you?" I wouldn't. She continues: "Many writers have tried to deal with the problems of fantasy, pleasure and 'glamour', by evicting them from the female Utopia. But 'glamour' is merely a demonstration of the human capacity for being enchanted, and not in itself destructive. We need it, redefined. We cannot beat an exploitive religion by asceticism, or bad poetry by none at all. We can only combat painful pleasure with pure pleasure." She presumably thinks the term "bad poem" means something, and how does she define "pure pleasure"? A "reinterpretation of 'beauty' that is non-competitive, non-hierarchical and non-violent . . . A woman wins by giving herself and other women permission: to eat, to be sexual, to age, to wear a boiler suit or a paste tiara or a Balenciaga gown or a second-hand opera cloak or combat boots, to cover up or to go practically naked; to do whatever she chooses in following – or ignoring – her own aesthetic. A woman wins when she feels that what each free woman does – uncoerced, unpressured – with her own body is her own business . . . Can there be a pro-woman definition of beauty? Absolutely. What was missing was play. The beauty myth is harmful and pompous and grave because too much depends upon it. The pleasure of playfulness is that it does not matter . . . no levity, no real game . . . Who says we need a hierarchy? Where I see beauty may not be where you do. Some people are more attractive to me than they are to you. So what? My perception has no authority over yours. Why should beauty be exclusive? Admiration can include so much. Why is rareness impressive?"[21]

Several points are at issue here. First, if there is any difference at all between beauty and non-beauty, there is a hierarchy, unless you argue that pleasure is no better than the lack of it: to paraphrase Kingsley Amis's famous remark, that nice things are not nicer than nasty ones. If that were true, how could there be a human need to be enchanted? Non-enchantment would be just as good. Wolf's compatriots have a word for that: gobbledygook. On the same principle, you can only say that the difference doesn't matter if you don't care whether you enjoy yourself or not, which we all do. Stravinsky once said you shouldn't judge music by how it made you feel, but as a musically trained friend of mine objected, if you don't judge a human art by its effect on human beings, how do you judge it?

Secondly, there is the question of levity. Any lover of any recreational activity would correct Wolf's statement to "no seriousness, no real game." The whole point is lost if how you play it doesn't matter; short of cheating, the easiest way to make yourself unpopular in sporting circles is to say, "It's only a game." Letting ourselves seek satisfaction has to mean taking all the steps necessary to achieve it. Wolf chooses her examples to suggest it's all a matter of putting on one form of clothing rather than another, but suppose you can't achieve the standard that satisfies you without doing more than that, perhaps much more, like Leslie Gardiner's patient who hated his nose? I fail to see how anyone would succeed in playing any but the simplest game well or writing a book, let alone one likely to please a discerning reader, by applying that method; as Sheridan put it:

> You write with ease, to show your breeding;
> But easy writing's curst hard reading.

As to rarity, I agree with Wolf that it is not an intrinsic virtue. But suppose the qualities which make people say "how beautiful!", if not rare by definition, are rare in fact, because most of us don't have them? A German feminist who is in favour of beauty, Barbara Sichtermann, is uncompromising: "the tragic part of this situation is that the commodity in question, which every woman would like to be able to supply and every man enjoy, is in fact in very *short supply*. Beauty is as rare as a black swan. And an even more modest attractiveness, such as a pretty face or 'good figure' . . . does not distinguish the majority of women . . . *Beauty cannot be democratized*. That is the embarrassing fact for a culture and policy which find their justifications in making all the desirable commodities of this world accessible to all."[22]

If Sichtermann is right, the same could be said for any other natural attribute, from intelligence to muscles, but here there is no argument: I suspect that one reason why people support the "eye of the beholder" theory with such passion is that they simply can't say the same of the ability to understand mathematics or lift weights. Inequality in these fields can be proved, but you can't prove beauty isn't purely personal, if only because of the well-known difficulty of proving a negative.

This naturally endears the "beholder" theory to everyone who wants a society with as little discrimination as possible, because in practical matters, you can't always do without it. Midgley and Hughes point out that nobody objects to forbidding blind people to drive.[23] Psychological satisfaction doesn't have such clear criteria, but that doesn't make it unreal.

Next, if you and all the people whose taste you respect define you as ugly, you are unlikely to be comforted by someone else who doesn't. The same applies to any branch of aesthetics: if you write a poem and its only admirers are readers whose favourite poems you detest, how pleased will you be? Janet Radcliffe Richards adds: "It makes no difference to argue that standards change and that there is some standard which could make anyone beautiful: even if that were true (which it almost certainly is not) it is irrelevant. Even if you would have been beautiful according to the taste of five hundred years ago it is not much consolation for being thought ugly now."[24] Especially, she might have added, if you are the person thinking it; even a strictly personal hierarchy is still a hierarchy to that person. "I want the face and body nature gave me to be seen as beautiful in itself, not because I've spent a lot of time and money tarting it up",[25] says a woman interviewed in a history of the women's movement. The end without the means again.

"I have noticed that the statements of protest coming from many women against the pressure to look good sound so *cheerful*", writes Barbara Sichtermann.

> 'We old people', the old women say, 'show off our grey hair and our wrinkles: we think we are beautiful as we are'. 'We fat people' say the fat people, we couldn't give a damn about all this dieting and massage business, we're proud of being fat. Who says fat isn't beautiful?' 'We knock-kneed women', say the emancipated women with quite normal flaws, 'we women with breasts which are too big or too small, we women with fat bottoms and big noses, we accept ourselves as we are and think we're just fine as we are.' . . . I am impressed by this new self-confidence among unattractive and old women. But there must be that element of sorrow there if this kind of emancipation is to last, if it is to be more than just temporary euphoria . . . I cannot see that the feminist critics of the dictates of attractiveness or the members of the Old and Fat Movements are looking for ways of coming to terms at all. Instead they seem to be disputing the fact that it is necessary to do so by simply turning fatness and old age into acceptable varieties of attractiveness, or worse, by repressing their longing for beauty altogether. Emancipation on those terms cannot last. What we repress comes to the fore again sooner or later – that much we now know.

She made an effort: seeing a television interview with ageing film stars, "I made a spontaneous attempt to adopt the humane aesthetics of emancipation and to tell myself that the wrinkled, smiling faces of these one-time stars telling their life stories were 'beautiful' – perhaps even more beautiful than the clear faces of their youth . . . But I could not convince myself."[26] Gilles Lipovetsky notes similar tendencies in France: "'Fat is beautiful.' 'Ugly is beautiful.' Such are the new watchwords of minority demands, the ultimate democratic avatars of the quest for personality. So be it; but who actually makes such claims? Who believes them? The chances that such voices will move beyond the stage of dissident symptom look virtually nil . . . the passionate desire to be beautiful remains widespread."[27]

The word "passionate" is enough to show up the flaw in Wolf's theory of play. That is why the "eye of the beholder" argument is like the idea that the whole issue is unimportant: another doctrine with no believing pupils and no true teachers. I don't believe any art which ever appealed to anyone was produced in that spirit, and if fashion is a minor or even a frivolous art, that doesn't mean producing it is easy: ask any comedian.

Molière, who wrote, directed and starred in the most famous comedies in the French language, considered comedy harder to write than tragedy because it meant being funny as well as intelligent. In the play where he discusses this, *La Critique de l'Ecole des Femmes* (1663), all the fools condemn his previous play and all the sensible characters praise it. One of the latter, a man, claims that "on peut être habile avec un point de Venise et des plumes, aussi bien qu'avec une perruque courte et un petit rabat uni" and a woman, Uranie, significantly named after the muse of astronomical poetry, says: "Pour moi, quand je vois une comédie, je regarde seulement si les choses me touchent; et, lorsque je m'y suis bien divertie, je ne vais point demander si j'ai eu tort, et si les règles d'Aristote me défendaient de rire."[28] When something doesn't please me, I don't ask if the Ugly Movement or the champions of utilitarian clothing say it should.

Molière knew art is a means of communication, which means that there has to be somebody to communicate with. This is the final objection to the idea that it doesn't really matter. Artists want to put their message over; Wolf wants to put hers, which is still disputed. In Rebecca West's novel *The Fountain Overflows*, the narrator's mother, based on the author's, tells her daughters: "I am foolish to say that I am glad you will have sensible clothes, I hope you will have lots of clothes that are not just sensible." She is a pianist, and the idea of there being no definitive values in art would have horrified her: "In her playing there was a gospel and an evangelist who preached it, and that implied a church which worshipped a God not yet fully revealed but in the course of revelation. But when Cousin Jock played he created about him a world in which all was known, and in which art was not a discovery but a decoration. All was then trivial, and there was no meaning in art or in life."[29]

That sounds suspiciously like Wolf's ideal, and also like postmodern irony. I am not arguing that art should never be ironic, but art which is always so is limited to say the least. Non-stop irony is only a step away from non-stop joking, which quickly becomes boring (readers can check this in any saloon bar). I am tempted to call postmodernism the latest variant on the half-hearted Puritanism I have already mentioned, because a language in which you can't say anything without inverted commas is the opposite of whole-hearted. If a preoccupation is justified, it shouldn't always be necessary to be ironic about it; if not, it shouldn't be pursued at all. Encouraging the pursuit of beauty provided neither it nor disagreements about it are taken seriously is like watering a plant with one hand while uprooting it with the other.

Evangelists, artistic or otherwise, expound views which have no merit unless they are true; if two of them differ, at least one must be wrong. To take that element out of art seems to me to destroy the whole point of it: I am sure this is what Keats meant by "Beauty is truth, truth beauty".

Either there are definitive truths, aesthetic or otherwise, or there are not. If there are, we should be trying to find them; if not, one person's idea is as good as another, and that has to mean that the ideas which require a great deal of time, effort and money to put into practice are as worth while as those which don't. Forget that, and we know what happens: the tyranny of the practical and the lowest common denominator, not because that is what people want but because it saves trouble. Beauty may or may not be in the eye of the beholder; cheapness and convenience are not.

Sidney Harrison advised young musicians, "Practise to play very well. Do not be a perfectionist. Perfection is for the gods, and they will punish you with a nervous breakdown if you try to be perfect."[30] It also defeats its own purpose. Artists say every work of art requires two people: one to do the job, and one to stand by with a gun saying "Touch that again and I'll shoot!" Perfection doesn't exist outside pure logic and pure mathematics, but excellence does. It isn't the same as faultlessness, but its pursuit takes as much effort as it takes, which is why "reasonably attractive" dress is no solution. Was anyone ever satisfied with writing a reasonably good poem?

The advantages of making less than the maximum of effort are negative: saving time, energy, money. Those of not doing less, if the effort is successful, are positive. That's why people go on trying. Simone de Beauvoir noted dressing up could bring "joies positives" and that actresses enjoyed it more than most other women; it didn't seem to occur to her that this might be because they had an excuse to take it seriously.[31] So can these joys be rescued without jeopardising feminism? If fashion and beauty culture refuse to die and cannot be made wholly democratic, what should feminists do?

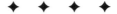

The feminist realization was that you don't get what you want . . . by pretending you don't want it. And you don't get what you want by pretending you already have it. You only get what you want by fighting for it.

Barbara Leon

I would like to say that the aesthetic side is as important as the purely functional.

Elizabeth Hawes   Men Can Take It

We want clothes in which we can dress ourselves quickly and comfortably . . . And we want to feel that in them we appear as charming, as chic and more entitled to self-respect than the ladies whose photographs today we admire.

Winifred Holtby   Fashions and Feminism (1927)

Young girl adolescents will not know that feminist thinkers acknowledge both the value of beauty and adornment if we continue to allow patriarchal sensibilities to inform the beauty industry . . . Rigid feminist dismissal of female longings for beauty has undermined feminist politics . . . Until feminists go back to the beauty industry, go back to fashion, and create an ongoing, sustained revolution we will not be free.

bell hooks   Feminism Is For Everybody (2000)

First, we must speak out and stop apologising. If we don't defend our point of view nobody else will. We must make it clear that we do believe beauty in dress exists (at least, it does for us), that we don't think the price we pay for it is wasted, that we intend to pursue it and oppose anyone who tries to stop us. We must also make it clear what we are defending: a pleasure, not a duty. A member of the Social Affairs Unit calls it a "moral transgression" to wear gym clothes to a supermarket.[32] Remarks like that give good grooming a bad name. What does it matter what people wear for a purely practical activity provided it is clean? I do agree that people have no right to endanger other people's health by abandoning hygiene (as some student radicals and their teachers have), nor to cause unnecessary offence to people's ideas of decency (as opposed to arguing that ideas you disagree with should be changed), nor to spoil other people's pleasure in social occasions that are important to them, but that is as far as duty goes.

"We can perhaps keep some elements of beauty in dress",[33] writes Janet Radcliffe Richards. That is not good enough. We want the highest standards possible in dress just as we do in, say, medicine or education.

We must confront the fear that care about fashion always leads to obsession, as expressed by the teenage narrator of a feminist novel: "What if I started sweating and it runs off my skin and right in front of somebody I change from my beautiful made-up self into my natural plainness, wouldn't that be worse than just being who I am?"[34] Phyllis Chesler writes that she isn't a Puritan but sounds very like one: "expensive or frequently changed costumes . . . seem to signify a growing passivity and dependence in men as well as women" and a book on consciousness-raising asks: "can women . . . without serious damage to themselves . . . alter the very essence of who they are?"[35] But appearance isn't essence. One journalist, Mary Davis Peters, answered claims that make-up "obliterated the personality" by saying that anyone whose personality is so easily obliterated has a problem far too serious to solve by either using make-up or leaving it off.

The solution is to develop our critical spirit. We must ask of any given style or practice: how much, if at all, does it interfere with other aspects of our lives? Is the result worth it? If it's a real nuisance, nobody will need ideological reasons for rejecting it; there might well be much less cosmetic surgery if people knew more about it, and if so, all that is needed is accurate information. If fashion writers don't dare offend advertisers by criticism, feminist ones might provide it. If not, we can still do so ourselves. The way to avoid being hamstrung by other people's standards is to define our own.

We must challenge terms like "slaves" and "victims" (crime novelist Mary Wings invented the term "fashion victor"), complaining about the work involved when we do it voluntarily, and pretending we are only wearing the latest look because the designer told us to, when we should be furious if there were no latest look to wear. If we behave like slaves, people will think we are slaves, which at least partially justifies their view that we are unfit to run the world. Simone de Beauvoir mentions that women's "slavery" to their dressmakers was used as an excuse to deny them the vote;[36] how would men like having their rights curtailed because of their "slavery" to sport, which also involves fashions (football supporters' replica shirts seem to change every year) and which isn't universal either? My father had no interest whatever in either sport or the other supposedly archetypal male passion, technology.

In 1951, Nancy Mitford described how French "femmes du monde" kept up couturiers' and hairdressers' standards: "Back goes the dress . . . back into the washtub goes the head, until the result is perfect."[37] I think that couture's decline into gimmicks is directly related to these clients' dying out, and it will only revive if a new clientèle with similar standards evolves. The mods of the sixties could not have been more different from those "femmes du monde" in background and tastes and rebelled against all they stood for, but Mary Quant's autobiography shows they resembled them in one way: "The young will not be dictated to. You can be publicized on the national network television programmes, be written up by the most famous of the fashion columnists and the garment still won't sell if the young don't like it."[38]

There will always be some people whose priority is saving as much time and effort as possible; some feminists mention this as an advantage of growing old. (A friend told me of a woman aged a hundred who was still interested in dressing fashionably; she herself wasn't, but, admired her spirit.) Sara Halprin begins her book on the philosophy of beauty by quoting a Chinese legend of a woman whose husband refuses to let her go on a pilgrimage because her beauty will lead to harassment from men. She disfigures herself and says in triumph, "Look at my ugly face!"[39] But why should she have to? "'You can be a sex object or you can be invisible' strikes me as a Hobson's choice",[40] writes Letty Cottin Pogrebin. Gloria Steinem has observed that the "wisdom of old age" is just another stereotype, frequently wrong. Moreover, in societies where old people hold authority, it's at younger people's expense: where the old are seen as wiser by defini- tion, the young are seen as less so. Do we want that?

Nor is it good enough to say, like one teenage feminist, "what I put on my face or feet or body has [nothing] to do with my politics".[41] If it is consis- tent with them it is part of them. Women whose achievements feminists praise cared about dress: the twelfth-century St Hildegard of Bingen (nuns in her convent wore enamelled crowns), Florence Nightingale (who renounced dressing fashionably to concentrate on her vocation, not because she disapproved of it), Josephine Butler, Colette, Dame Rose Macaulay, as her book *Personal Pleasures*[42] shows, and Dame Freya Stark.

Next, we must stop calling adornment "femininity". A man once asked me, "Can a woman look sexy in an equal society?" Only if a man can too. If fashion is a woman's right, it must also be a man's. "Femininity is a package deal for [Susan] Brownmiller", observes Wendy Chapkis, who feels that the package "of gender and wardrobe, identity and appearance, beauty and status" can be dismantled: "appearance can be a source of pleasure rather than anxiety . . . if it is firmly rooted in our own value independent of it".[43] The only way to break the link between "feminine" passivity and stupidity and "feminine" appearance is to make the latter available to men.

A non-sexist society can't have double standards. What makes some-thing sexist is its confinement to one sex; sequins are no more intrinsically sexist than striped pyjamas, and a world in which both sexes wore the former would be just as androgynous as the circles described by Melissa Benn: "She is in jeans and a fashionably baggy sweatshirt. He is in a stripy shirt and fashionably baggy shorts. Nearly everyone has short hair, the men's margin-ally more cropped."[44] She adds that they hadn't eliminated sexism. The designer Anne Tyrell once commented, "I do not think wanting to look glamorous, attractive to men is flying in the face of feminist ideals, it is just an element of life, and remains an important one for many women no matter how equal they may be in practical matters."[45] Unless men can be equal in impractical matters, I don't blame them for protesting: it suggests wanting equality and special "feminine" privileges as well. We have no right to object to a "glass ceiling" keeping down our opportunities at work, if we make one too; if we are defensive about our dress shops, no wonder men are defensive about their workplaces and clubs.

In Terence Rattigan's play *The Winslow Boy*, a male character accuses a suffragette wearing a "charming" hat of "trying to have the best of both worlds". Helen Franks heard a similar comment in 1984:

> 'It seems to me a very female as against feminist thing to do. Don't you see that as a compromise of your principles?'
> I said I thought it was a pity men didn't dress up so that they could realise the potential liberation and personal expression.[46]

The magazine *The Englishwoman* on 4 December 1909, suggested: "Woman's striving after the ideal may be a healthier sign than man's obsti-nate deference to established custom". Shere Hite agrees: "being more severe-looking has not made women as powerful as men . . . the way to equality may be just the opposite: let women retain all styles of dress as one of their options – and encourage men to take these options for themselves too."[47]

If men's clothes bore them why don't they invent alternatives, as women designers have (Chanel in the twenties, Mary Quant and others in the sixties)? Elizabeth Hawes quotes suggestions from male readers, including "innumerable" mentions of flared skirts. "For men to adopt feminine symbols would be to transgress, in the realm of appearance, the very essence of modern masculine identity", writes Lipovetsky. "We have not reached that point, and no sign of the times leads us to anticipate any shift in that direction. Despite the multiple forms of its democratization, fashion remains essentially inegalitarian, at least where gender is concerned. The masculine still occupies the inferior, stable position as opposed to the free, protean mobility of the feminine pole."[48] We know why: the "inferior" position saves trouble but enjoys higher status because "Boys Are Better." Feminism's task is to convince them they are not.

A word of warning, however: if men want to change, they must do it themselves. It will only put one more burden on women if men delegate all the work to them (many men already leave the choice as well as the care of their clothes to women). If they are genuinely interested, they won't want to. If they are not, let them keep their uniforms, like the numerous women who "always wear black" (or blue denim), but they will have no right to be jealous if people notice women's appearance and not theirs, or if fashion-conscious people prefer the company of those who share their interest. Sally Cline and Dale Spender write of making others feel good: "What is wrong is that women do it for men and men do not do it for women."[49] In *The Tenant of Wildfell Hall*, the hero's mother says (he disagrees): "it's your business to please yourself, and hers to please you," and as long as women and not men dress attractively, women appear to agree even if they don't.

I also think that fashion-conscious men would be more reasonable in what they expect of us, because they would know that, like athletes or artists, we need time and money to produce results. They would realise that dressing decoratively doesn't necessarily imply an ulterior motive. "Women's beauty, men reason, is designed to entrap them", writes Andrea Stuart. "They have no knowledge of our hidden world of play; they do not understand our delight as we plunder the dressing-up box and paint pictures with lipstick and powder."[50] Let them find out.

As to the man who feels any woman is lucky to have him, whatever he looks like and whatever he wears, I hope he will disappear, like the "gentleman" who thought it beneath his dignity to pay his debts, and the woman described by Vance Packard as wearing a colour which made her want to vomit because *Vogue* had said it was the coming fashion.[51]

Beautification would no longer be, as Lois Banner put it, "the most divisive, and ultimately the most 'oppressive' of all the aspects of women's separate culture"[52] if it were no longer separate. Frigga Haug describes "attempts to set ourselves apart from the slavegirl image, to repudiate any suggestion that we might be beautifying or displaying ourselves for the benefit of others, to defend our actions as sources of pleasure and self-confidence . . . what social relations . . . must prevail if we are to dismantle the edifice of domination, while at the same time rescuing its pleasures for ourselves?"[53] Barbara Sichtermann explains: "As far as the aesthetics of sexual attraction are concerned, reciprocity . . . that is with men 'joining in', would undoubtedly serve as a kind of liberation from elements of domination and submission. Both sexes would be looking and both sexes would be presenting themselves for inspection. The ideal of beauty would be bisexual. Attractiveness would no longer be synonymous with femininity and femininity would no longer be synonymous with efforts to be attractive. Instead, men could find out what it is like to show oneself off (homosexual men already know) and women could find out what it is like to dictate what constitutes beauty and to be onlookers. Between subject and object, between onlooker and object, between those enjoying the spectacle and those providing it, the bounds of gender would disappear."[54] Some feminists have coined the word "gynandry" because in "androgyny" the word for "man" comes first; this can be over-emphasised (when a word is made from two others, one has to be first) but I should like to see gynandry in dress.

Feminist Parenting mentions a girl who "loves the color pink, and lace, and ruffles . . . lipstick and lace have nothing whatever to do with muscle power and intellect" and a boy who longed for the "all the fun things like makeup and fingernail polish and swirly skirts".[55] A German writer, Marianne Grabrucker, wrote a diary of her daughter's first three years, and her struggles to give her a non-sexist upbringing: "I can't for the life of me understand why a twenty-one month old boy can't wear a smock . . . a girl may take to tools, but not a boy to make-up." At a party,

> boys . . . are wearing their everyday clothes, that is, track suit or jeans and pullover . . . I do want her to have a feeling for celebrations and beauty . . . I think that the choice that a girl has between trousers and skirt or dress is an advantage, one of the very few she has that men don't. Sometimes I wonder what is so awful about dresses that their sexist character has become the subject of so many theories . . . the fact that a dress . . . has become connected with a girl is one of the things against it . . . What seems to me questionable is that ideas of beauty that are linked to festive occasions require women to look feminine without any comparable changes being demanded of boys' behaviour in their development of aesthetic sensitivity. Boys go on wearing the colours reserved for them: dark blue, brown, grey and green. I pity them . . . I understand why boys have so little feeling for beauty. As long as boys are not able to dress in the same bright colours as girls, to adorn themselves as girls do, and this not only at home but also when they go 'out', then the pleasures of selection will, for women, continue to remain a duty.

A woman remains chained to her feminine beauty. But I don't think we should abandon it; we need more beauty and have to extend it to include boys and men. Let boys start wearing pink at last.[56]

Another writer on child-rearing, June Statham, mentions parents who "often discouraged particularly 'feminine' or frilly articles in girls"[57] but were less concerned about challenging stereotyped clothing in boys.

Susan Brownmiller criticised fashion in *Femininity* but was attacked for writing about it at all, and responded: "they said a feminist should not talk about clothes, but clothes are creative, wonderfully exhilarating and so can make-up be, but not when they are compensating for lack of opportunities, lack of equality, not when they are the tools for which we must fight for opportunities, status, men."[58] Germaine Greer, who has attacked other feminists' provocative dress, wrote in *The Female Eunuch*: "Most women would find it hard to abandon any interest in clothes and cosmetics, although many women's liberation movements urge them to transcend such servile fripperies. As far as cosmetics are used for adornment in a conscious and creative way, they are not emblems of inauthenticity". *The Madwoman's Underclothes* goes further: "It would greatly enhance our lives if everyone who lived inside a body was careful to keep it as pretty and sweet-smelling and attractive as possible"; she praises "the pleasing procedures of self-expression through adornment" and denounces men's "drab clothes which were neither loose and flowing enough to enhance nor tight enough to reveal the wearer's shape . . . It would be a great pity if the dazzling tradition of human body art were to perish in a waste of dreary conformity on the one hand and neurotic self-distortion on the other". She also demolishes the theory of "objectification" in five words: "the body is an object."

The Whole Woman seems wholly anti-fashion, but argues "for the recovery of women's culture . . . the creativity that makes everyday life balanced and elegant."[59] Fashion is part of that culture.

When Simone de Beauvoir dismissed the desire for pleasant surroundings as purely female, she ignored not only men like the brothers Adam and William Morris, but her compatriot Le Nôtre, who laid out the gardens at Versailles, and of whom she must have heard. This is the sexual division of labour again; when it's a highly-paid profession it's male, when it's unpaid and domestic it's female. We have seen that this particular split began in the nineteenth century, after the Adams's time, and Morris rebelled against it. Beauvoir's view of artists as people who create without knowing or caring whether their surroundings are ugly or beautiful is, like many of her statements, a generalisation; some do and some don't. Even if she were right, wouldn't it be desirable if somebody cared? (Among the categories in the Brovermans' study where the feminine was preferred was enjoyment of literature and art; if no men had those "feminine" interests, there would be no male artists, and how often someone says there's no female Michelangelo!)

Elizabeth Wilson, among others, looked back to the ideals of Morris's Aesthetic Movement: "This side of the 1970s women's movement has been forgotten or denied. The ugly stereotype of 'harridans in dungarees' is worse than merely inaccurate or sexist, for it effaces the desire for a harmonious life which underlay the whole atmosphere of 'struggle in which the women's movement was also steeped. We wanted work and home life, child care and other forms of creative endeavour to be integrated instead of parcelled up into separate times and places. Personal appearance and the kinds of interior in which this life was to be lived were equally the focus of feminist attention . . . It could be anti-consumerist without being puritanical, or rather could acknowledge that consumerism as a love of beautiful objects need not be wasteful."[60]

Quentin Bell hoped that fashion as we know it might die out and we should all simply find clothes that suited us and stick to them. I doubt that, because sooner or later people invent new styles and want to wear them, which means someone has to design and make the clothes. That is easy if, like Bell, you live in a community of artists and craft workers and can easily find someone to do the work for you or the leisure to do it yourself. Most of us must rely on mass-produced clothes. Prudence Glynn (the first fashion editor of *The Times*) wrote at about that time that when there are no trend-setters whose word is treated as law, "manufacturers on a large scale do not know what to make." If they are told to "do their own thing", she added, "they do fifty bits of other people's things, none of them well." No wonder: if their own thing didn't sell, they might go bankrupt.

That being so, we need designers. When, as Natasha Walter puts it, "the activities that result from narcissism" are no longer "the toys that women were given to distract themselves with as the men got on with running the world . . . The catwalk will . . . cease to be a symbol of our subordination and become a path to simple delight."[61]

Bernard Shaw, whose wife said he had no sense of beauty, might seem the last person to confirm my point of view, but he did so in *You Never Can Tell* (1897). An elderly man sees his daughter dressed as Columbine for a dance:

CRAMPTON: . . . Is this right? Would you blame my sister's family for objecting to it?

DOLLY [*flushing ominously*]: Have you begun again?

CRAMPTON [*propitiating her*]: No, no. It's perhaps natural at your age.

DOLLY [*obstinately*]: Never mind my age. Do you think it pretty?

CRAMPTON: Yes, dear, yes. [*He sits down in token of submission*].

DOLLY [*insistently*]: Do you like it?

CRAMPTON: My child: how can you expect me to like it or to approve of it?

DOLLY [*determined not to let him off*]: How can you think it pretty and not like it?

I cannot improve on Christian Dior's definition of fashion: "ephemeral architecture." What is ephemeral inevitably matters less than what is not, but both matter for the same reason: you can't avoid them, so you might as well enjoy them as much as possible. Dior had more in common than is usually thought with earlier designers like Poiret who had "no intention that fashions should change every year . . . The new look was turned into an edict by . . . the press . . . that a dressmaker should create a single female image and ignore the real women who would have to fit into it. It is the consequent misinterpretation of what Paris stands for that has led to the efforts to dislodge it"[62] and not just Paris but all fashion.

Janey Ironside, Professor of Fashion at the Royal College of Art, wrote that people who condemn its "slaves" are often slaves of an outworn fashion (a good description of conventional men) and the blurb of her book *A Fashion Alphabet* states: "fashion is one of the great living arts of civilisation and self-decoration one of the fundamental human urges."[63] The narrator of Anne Scott-James's autobiographical novel (1952) says:

The cosmetic industry . . . genuinely enhances beauty, promotes health and hygiene and prolongs youth . . . I don't pretend that fashion is a 'fine' art, but I would place it high among the decorative arts . . . The fine line of a dress, a perfect proportion or a superlative colour scheme can make me feel real emotion . . . Think of those self-righteous (and usually ill-written) letters which make a regular appearance in the daily papers. 'Sir, when will women learn that they are much more beautiful to us in the colours which nature gave them than painted up with hideous cosmetics?' . . . 'Sir, I have managed with two dresses and one apron for the past four years, and my husband says I am the best-dressed woman he knows.' . . . Sir, sir, sir, always protesting, hating, envying, with the same sort of destructive fury that slashes modern pictures and daubs unpopular statues.[64]

Letters from women who approve of burqas have exactly the same tone.

Mary Tuck's essay "Why be beautiful?" (1958) begins: "I am going to suggest that beauty care is compatible with good taste and is even a suitable preoccupation for an intelligent woman. Does this sound like a challenge? Unfortunately it is." She criticises both the lingering Victorian attitude that it was wrong to improve on nature and that of beauty writers: "The whole personality, capabilities, aims and actions, are subordinated to the imperative duty of appearing a beautiful object. No wonder the intelligent woman develops a suspicion that even to pay much attention to the shade of lipstick she wears immediately degrades her to the status of an object, a *thing* to be looked at and admired; not a person with genuine possibilities of initiating action and emotion. Look at men, the intelligent girl thinks enviously. None of this fuss about creating an elaborate artificial exterior. They simply *are* real by themselves without all this effort . . . But is it true that a man can completely escape this object status? Of course he can't! . . . All a man achieves by his refusal to admit this is an imprisonment in one fixed image of himself."[65]

Doris Langley Moore, among others, noted that "the inhabitants of Utopias almost always wear some kind of plain uniform garment . . . they are entirely educated in the fear of pleasure", though William Morris's Utopia was an exception. She enjoyed glossy magazines because of "the world they represent, that rarefied world where all women are graceful and beautiful, all men polite, all clothes clean and new, is so inviting a conception that recent utilitarian adaptations bringing the portrayal of the mode nearer to what is attainable in our daily lives, have diluted a very vivid feminine pleasure . . . Beauty, except of the rarest order, is so much enhanced by flattering apparel that good-looking women now enormously outnumber good-looking men, an undesirable situation for women and one which did not exist in the days when both sexes alike could indulge in the advantages of elaborate hairdressing, diversified colour and carefully chosen ornament." Elizabeth Hawes hoped that in future both sexes would wear uniforms for work, spending the money saved on "colorful and wonderful party clothes".[66]

Paula J. Caplan agrees: "It is not vain to want to create something that is more, rather than less, esthetically pleasing . . . It is not in women's interests either to adopt a standard because it has been applied to men or to reject one because men promote it . . . We must be free to decide what is good for us *apart from* what men traditionally believe."[67] Wendy Chapkis hoped "our wardrobe can expand to include elements beyond those appropriate to battle dress . . . rhinestone earrings and metal studs, leather ties, silver shoes, a strapped on dildo or a lacy bra, lipstick shining sensually on a mouth framed by a downy moustache, a brightly colored skirt worn comfortably over the hairy legs of either sex."[68] Shaving was too much for her, but Susie Orbach and Luise Eichenbaum reported that some members of women's groups found it possible "to be a strong, self-loving, competent woman who also shaved her legs".[69] In 1970, the year feminists disrupted the Miss World contest, Sally Medora Wood wrote: "I enjoy making myself attractive to both men and women, including myself. The process of objectification, by definition, originates in the perceiver and not the perceived . . . Every person has the right to decorate her or himself as she or he chooses."[70]

Altering our appearance isn't any stupider than suppressing traffic noise to listen to music. It's not that what we have isn't good enough, but that we like something else better. As a friend of mine said, "When you spend a lot of money on clothes, at least other people have the pleasure of looking at them. Some people spend just as much on hi-fi or camera equipment and give no pleasure to anyone but themselves." The revival of beauty culture has been called a perversion of feminism;[71] the real perversion was the idea that it should die.

Much of the world's folk music and literature was created by people trying to enliven monotonous work (the soldiers' songs of the First World War, for instance, many of them composed by the men in the trenches) but that doesn't mean that if you abolish war and drudgery people will no longer want music or stories. Robert Lynd wrote an essay beginning: "It is becoming more and more common to explain everything human beings do in terms of starvation or repression" and ending, "We might as well say that women and children who munch sweetmeats are starving. They're not."[72] But one can justify eating for pleasure and still have reservations about unlimited sweet-eating; some ways of pursuing pleasure may be better than others, and we should not be afraid to suggest it.

It shouldn't be necessary to "be crazy abut [*sic*] the kitsch and glorify the trashy"[73] in Elizabeth Wilson's words; as she pointed out, fashion has been condemned for sharing the same values as high art as well as for not sharing them. Quentin Bell asks, "can we in truth say more of a beautiful object than we feel it to be beautiful? . . . And yet a complete relativism seems equally unsatisfactory . . . when a work of fashion has stood the test of time we can judge it dispassionately."[74] I believe lasting values in art exist, but there is no short cut to them; attempts to create for posterity have never produced anything but failures, because it's lying: trying to use our successors' eyes instead of our own. We don't know what they will think and they won't necessarily be any more right than we are, but we do know they can't preserve what we have destroyed. If today's fashions are not worthy of us, let us have ones which are. If we want more practical or longer-lasting ones, we can have them; if not, we must admit it and then think how to solve the resulting ecological and economic problems. Dressing well is no more incompatible with being a serious person than having a sense of humour is.

I hope this book will help answer the accusations of snobbery, shallowness or collaboration with oppression which some feminists still make. Not answering them may mean seeing a potential source of joy disappear, perhaps for ever. We can avoid that if we have the courage. The solution is in our hands.

NOTES

Chapter 1 The Case Against Fashion

1   Betty Friedan, *The Feminine Mystique*, Victor Gollancz, 1963.
2   Adam Fergusson, *The Sack of Bath*, Compton Russell Publishing, Salisbury, 1973.
3   Jonathon Porritt (ed.), *Friends of the Earth Handbook*, Macdonald Optima, 1987.
4   Kathie Sarachild (ed.), *Feminist Revolution*, Random House, New York, 1978.
5   Yvonne Roberts, *Mad About Women: Can There Ever Be Fair Play Between the Sexes?*, Virago, 1992.
6   Andrea Dworkin, *Woman Hating*, Plume Books, New York and London, 1974.
7   Kirsty Dunseath (ed.), *A Second Skin: Women Write About Clothes*, The Women's Press, 1998.
8   Caroline Evans and Minna Thornton, *Women & Fashion: A New Look*, Quartet Books, 1989.
9   Joan Cassell, *A Group Called Women*, David McKay, New York, 1977.
10 Olive Banks, *Faces of Feminism*, Martin Robertson, 1981.
11 Letty Cottin Pogrebin, *Growing Up Free: Raising Your Child in the 80s*, McGraw-Hill Book Company, New York, 1980; Linda Tschirhart Sanford and Mary Ellen Donovan, *Women and Self-Esteem*, Anchor Press/Doubleday, New York, 1984; Penguin, Harmondsworth, 1993.
12 John Berger, *Ways of Seeing*, BBC and Pelican Books, London and Harmondsworth, 1972.
13 Elizabeth Wilson, *Adorned in Dreams*, Virago, 1985.
14 Michelene Wandor, *Once a Feminist: Stories of a Generation*, Virago, 1990.
15 Caroline Evans and Minna Thornton, *Women & Fashion: A New Look*, Quartet Books, London and New York, 1989.
16 Robin Morgan, *The Demon Lover: On the Sexuality of Terrorism*, Methuen, 1989; Susan Faludi, "I'm Not a Feminist, but I Play One on TV", *Ms.*, Volume V, No. 5, March/April 1995.
17 Patricia Aburdene and John Naisbitt, *Megatrends for Women*, Random House, 1993.
18 Susan Faludi, *Backlash: The Undeclared War Against Women*, Chatto & Windus, 1992.
19 Rosalind Coward, *Our Treacherous Hearts: Why Women Let Men Get Their Way*. Faber & Faber, 1992.

20 Germaine Greer, *The Female Eunuch*, McGibbon and Kee, 1970; *The Whole Woman*, Doubleday, 1999.
21 Natasha Walter, *The New Feminism*, Little, Brown, 1998.
22 Tara Kaufmann, "Oi! You! Where are your dungarees?", *Sibyl*, Issue 1, March/April 1998. Lucy O'Brien, "Bring back big bad boots", *ibid.*, Issue 2, May/June 1998.

Chapter 2   How Did We Get Here?

1 Margaret Leroy, *Pleasure: The Truth About Female Sexuality*, HarperCollins, 1993.
2 Lisa Tickner, *Spare Rib*, nos. 45–51.
3 Sheila Jeffreys, *The Lesbian Heresy: A Feminist Perspective on the Lesbian Sexual Revolution*, The Women's Press, 1993.
4 *Life*, Christmas 1956 issue, quoted in Betty Friedan, *The Feminine Mystique*, Victor Gollancz., 1963.
5 Rebecca West, *The Young Rebecca*, Macmillan, 1982.
6 Joseph Hansen and Evelyn Reed, *Cosmetics, Fashions, and the Exploitation of Women*, Pathfinder Press, New York, 1986.
7 Kathie Sarachild (ed.), *Feminist Revolution*, Random House, New York, 1978.
8 Gay Robins, *Women in Ancient Egypt*, British Museum Press, 1993.
9 Joyce Tyldesley, *Daughters of Isis*, Viking, New York and London, 1994.
10 Elizabeth Wilson, *Adorned in Dreams*, Virago, 1985.
11 Aline Rousselle, trs. Felicia Pheasant, *Porneia: On Desire and the Body in Antiquity*, Basil Blackwell, Oxford, 1988.
12 Jérôme Carcopino, *La Vie Quotidienne à Rome à l'Apogée de l'Empire*, Hachette, Paris, 1939.
13 Shelagh Brown, *The Art of Being a Single Woman*, Kingsway Publications, Eastbourne, 1989.
14 Elizabeth Dawes and Norman H. Baynes, *Three Byzantine Saints. Contemporary Biographies translated from the Greek*, Basil Blackwell, Oxford, 1948.
15 Aileen Ribeiro, *Dress and Morality*, Batsford, 1986.
16 Diana de Marly, *Fashion for Men*, Batsford, 1985.
17 Johan Huizinga, trs. F. Hopman, *The Waning of the Middle Ages*, Pelican, Harmondsworth, 1955.
18 A. W. Boardman, *The Battle of Towton*, Sutton Publishing, Strood, Gloucestershire, 1994.
19 Abu Muhammad al-Husain b. Mas'ud b. Muhammad al-Farra' (or Ibn al-Farra') al-Baghawi, trs. James Robson, *Mishkat Al-Masabih* ("The Niche of Lamps"), Vol. III, Sh. Muhammad Ashral, Lahore, 1964.
20 Ibn Battuta, *The Travels of Ibn Battuta*, Vol. IV, The Hakluyt Society, 1994.
21 Omar Bello, preface to Muhammad Bello, *The Concept of the Just Ruler*, MS forthcoming.
22 Margaret M. McGowan, lecture given at the Tower of London, 2 December 1989.

23 Giovanna Pezzuoli, *Prigioniera in Utopia*, Edizioni Il Formichiere, Milan, 1978.

24 Anne Campbell Dixon, *Country Life*, 28 July 1988.

25 "This heavy enlargement of doublets . . . these long effeminate tresses".

26 Reprinted in Ernest Rhys and Lloyd Vaughan (eds.), *A Century of English Essays*, J. M. Dent, 1939.

27 De Marly, *Fashion for Men*.

28 John Bunyan, *The Life and Death of Mr Badman*, 1680; J. M. Dent, London, 1928.

29 "And these great breeches like shackles, in which every morning one enslaves both one's legs, and in which we see these gallant gentlemen walking with their legs spread out like compasses".

    "without being unclean and grumpy as well".

    "I want headgear, in spite of the fashion, under which all my head can shelter comfortably; a fine long doublet, fastened as it should be, which keeps my stomach warm so that I can have a good digestion; breeches which fit my thighs exactly; shoes in which my feet are not tortured, according to the wise customs of my ancestors; and those who find me ugly can simply shut their eyes."

    "She must only dress up as much as the husband who possesses her may wish: he is the only one whom the care of her beauty concerns; and it must count for nothing if others find her ugly.

    "Far from her be the study of lively looks, these waters, whiteners and creams, and a thousand ingredients which give a flower-like complexion: every day these are deadly poison to honour, and care to look beautiful is seldom taken for husbands."

30 "A fatuous and ridiculous man . . . thinks at night about how and in what way he can be noticed next day. A philosopher lets his tailor dress him. It is as much a weakness to flee from the fashion as to affect it."

    ". . . he wears rouge, but rarely, he does not make a habit of it: it is also true that he wears breeches and a hat, and has neither earrings nor a pearl necklace; so I have not put him in the chapter on women."

31 Leslie E. Gardiner, *Faces, Figures and Feelings: A Cosmetic Plastic Surgeon Speaks*, Robert Hale, 1959.

32 Edmund Gosse, "The Whole Duty of Woman", *The Realm*, 1895; reprinted in *A Century of English Essays*.

33 Simon Sharp (ed.), *The Women's Sharp Revenge: Five Women's Pamphlets from the Renaissance*, Fourth Estate, 1985.

34 Rosamond Bayne-Powell, *English Country Life in the Eighteenth Century*, John Murray, 1935.

35 Wendy Frith, "Sex, Smallpox, and Seraglios: A Monument to Lady Mary Wortley Montagu", in Gill Perry and Michael Rossington (eds.), *Femininity and Masculinity in Eighteenth-Century Art and Culture*, Manchester University Press, Manchester, 1994.

36 Sarah Scott, *Millenium Hall*, 1762; Virago, 1986.

37 "You should know that women have all banded together to make themselves ugly, they will leave off slippers, and they are even talking of changing their dresses, of

wearing sacks, and putting their head-dresses on one side in order to displease you".

"My mother calls that a modest dress: so there is no modesty anywhere but here, since I see nobody but myself wrapped up like that; and so I am so childish, so curious! I don't wear ribbons; but what does my mother gain from it? that I feel excited when I see some."

38 James Upjohn, untitled MS in possession of the Clockmakers' Company, London, 1784.

39 William Hickey, *Memoirs*, ed. Peter Quennell, Century Publishing, 1975.

40 Robert Lynd, *Dr Johnson and Company*, Penguin, Harmondsworth, 1946.

41 W. M. Thackeray, *The English Humourists of the Eighteenth Century*, 1851.

42 Linda Walsh, "'Arms to be Kissed a Thousand Times': Reservations About Lust in Diderot's Art Criticism", in Perry and Rossington (eds.), *Femininity and Masculinity in Eighteenth-Century Art and Culture*.

43 Ralph M. Wardle, *Mary Wollstonecraft: A Critical Biography*, University of Kansas Press, Lawrence, Kansas, 1951.

Chapter 3   What Happened to Men?

1 Lois W. Banner, *American Beauty*, University of Chicago Press, Chicago and London, 1983.

2 Thorstein Veblen, *The Theory of the Leisure Class*, Macmillan, New York, 1899; Unwin Books, 1970.

3 Germaine Greer, *The Female Eunuch*, McGibbon and Kee Ltd., 1970

4 Elizabeth Wilson, *Adorned in Dreams*, Virago, 1985.

5 *Ibid.*

6 Juliet Ash, "Tarting Up Men", in Judy Attfield and Pat Kirkham (eds.), *A View from the Interior: Feminism, Women and Design*, The Women's Press, 1989.

7 James Laver, *Taste and Fashion from the French Revolution to the Present Day*, Harrap, 1931, revised 1945.

8 *Ibid.*

9 Caroline Evans and Minna Thornton, *Women & Fashion: A New Look*, Quartet Books, London and New York, 1989.

10 James Laver, *Children's Fashions of the XIXth Century*, Batsford, 1951.

11 Gwen Raverat, *Period Piece: A Cambridge Childhood*, Faber and Faber, 1952.

12 Bonnie G. Smith, *Ladies of the Leisure Class: The Bourgeoises of Northern France in the Nineteenth Century*, Princeton University Press, Princeton, New Jersey, 1981.

13 Ann Monsarrat, *And the Bride Wore . . . The Story of the White Wedding*, Coronet Books, Hodder and Stoughton, 1975.

14 Laver, *Children's Fashions of the XIXth Century*.

15 Alexander Woollcott, *The Letters of Alexander Woollcott*, Casssell, 1946.

16 Kimberley Reynolds and Nicola Humble, *Victorian Heroines: Representations of Femininity in Nineteenth-Century Literature and Art*, Hamish Hamilton, 1993.

17 Robin Tolmach Lakoff and Raquel L. Scherr, *Face Value: The Politics of Beauty*, Routledge Kegan Paul, 1984.

18 Gwen Raverat, *Period Piece: A Cambridge Childhood*, Faber and Faber, 1952.

19 Consuelo Vanderbilt Balsan, *The Glitter and the Gold*, George Mann, Maidstone, Kent, 1953.

20 Frankie Finn, preface to *Out on the Plain*, The Women's Press, 1984.

21 Quoted in Daphne du Maurier, *The Infernal World of Branwell Brontë*, Gollancz, 1960.

22 Roszika Parker, "Images of Men", *Spare Rib*, no. 90, November 1980. Reprinted in Feminist Anthology Collective (eds.), *No Turning Back: Writings from the Women's Liberation Movement, 1975–80*, The Women's Press, 1981.

23 Anna Walters, preface to Elizabeth Gaskell, *Four Short Stories*, Pandora Press, 1983.

24 Jennifer Uglow, *George Eliot*, Virago, 1987.

25 Joanna Russ, *How to Suppress Women's Writing*, University of Texas Press, Austin, Texas, 1983; The Women's Press, 1984.

26 A. R. Mills, *Two Victorian Ladies: further pages from the journals of Emily and Ellen Hall*, Frederick Muller, 1969.

27 Jane and Ann Taylor, *Little Ann, and Other Poems*, 1883.

28 Harriet Beecher Stowe, *The Chimney-Corner*, Sampson Low, Son, & Marston and Bell & Daldy, 1868.

29 T. DeWitt Talmage, D. D., *Marriage and Home Life*, Oliphant, Anderson and Ferrier, Edinburgh, 1892.

30 William Leach, *True Love and Perfect Union: The Feminist Reform of Sex and Society*, Basic Books, New York, 1980.

31 Gillian Kersley, *Darling Madame: Sarah Grand and Devoted Friend*, Virago, 1983.

32 Carol Farley Kessler (ed.), *Daring to Dream: Utopian Stories by United States Women: 1836–1919*, Pandora Press, 1984.

33 Phoebe Hesketh, *My Aunt Edith*, Peter Davies, 1966.

34 Gerd Brantenberg, trs. Gerd Brantenberg and Louis Mackay, *The Daughters of Egalia*, Journeyman Press Ltd., 1985; Esmé Dodderidge, *The New Gulliver*, The Women's Press, 1988.

35 Caroline Bird, *The Two-Paycheck Marriage: How Women at Work Are Changing Life in America*, Rawson, Wade Publishers Inc., New York, 1979.

36 Aileen Ribeiro, *Dress and Morality*, Batsford, 1986.

37 Joanne B. Eicher and Mary Ellen Roach-Higgins, "Definition and Classification of Dress: Implications for Analysis of Gender Roles", in Ruth Barnes and Joanne B. Eicher (eds.), *Dress and Gender: Making and Meaning*, Providence, Rhode Island and Oxford, 1992.

38 Letty Cottin Pogrebin, *Growing Up Free: Raising Your Child in the 80s*, McGraw-Hill Book Company, New York, 1980.

39 Mary L. Blanchard, "Boundaries and the Victorian Body: Aesthetic Fashion in Gilded Age America", *American Historical Review*, February 1995.

40 Anna Ford, *Men*, Weidenfeld and Nicolson, 1985.

41 Quentin Bell, *On Human Finery*, The Hogarth Press, 1976.

42 *Radio Times*, 2 March 1996.

43 Pogrebin, *Growing Up Free*.

44 Angela Phillips, *The Trouble With Boys*, Pandora Press, 1993.
45 Laver, *Children's Fashions of the XIXth Century*.
46 George Santayana, *The Last Puritan*, Charles Scribner's Sons, New York, 1936.
47 Elizabeth Hawes, *Men Can Take It*, Random House, New York, 1939.
48 Louise Chunn, "Can Clothes Damage Your Career?", British *Vogue*, May 1996.
49 *The Times*, 21 November 1992.
50 Deborah Laake, *Secret Ceremonies: A Mormon Woman's Intimate Diary of Marriage and Beyond*, William Morrow and Company, Inc., New York, 1993.
51 Philip Gibbs, *Crowded Company*, Allan Wingate, London and New York, 1949.
52 Virginia Woolf, *Three Guineas*, 1938; Oxford University Press, 1992.
53 Robin Morgan, *The Demon Lover: On the Sexuality of Terrorism*, Methuen, 1989.
54 Robin Morgan, *The Anatomy of Freedom*, Anchor Press/Doubleday, New York, 1982.
55 Carol Lee, *The Blind Side of Eden: The Sexes in Perspective*, Bloomsbury, 1989.

Chapter 4   Two Kinds of Freedom

1 Joyce Nicholson, *What Society Does to Girls*, Virago, 1977.
2 Carol Adams and Rae Lauriekitis, *The Gender Trap: A Closer Look at Sex Roles. Book 3: Messages and Images*. Virago, 1980.
3 Susan Bassnett, *Feminist Experiences: The Women's Movement in Four Cultures*. Allen and Unwin, 1986.
4 Elizabeth Janeway, *Man's World, Woman's Place*, 1971; Penguin, Harmondsworth, 1997.
5 Caroline Evans and Minna Thornton, *Women & Fashion: A New Look*, Quartet Books, London and New York, 1989.
6 Gloria Steinem, "Sex, Lies and Advertising", *Ms.*, September/October 1997; *Moving Beyond Words* Simon & Schuster, New York, 1994.
7 Reader Bullard, *The Camels Must Go*, Faber & Faber, 1961.
8 Nikolai Ostrovsky, *How the Steel Was Tempered*, trs. R. Prokofieva, Foreign Languages Publishing House, Moscow, 1952.
9 Francine du Plessix Gray, *Soviet Women: Walking the Tightrope*, Doubleday, New York, 1990.
10 Jung Chang, *Wild Swans: Three Daughters of China*, HarperCollins, 1991.
11 Paul Theroux, *Riding the Iron Rooster: By Train Through China*, Hamish Hamilton, 1998; Penguin, Harmondsworth, 1989.
12 Slavenka Drakulić, *How We Survived Communism and Even Laughed*, Hutchinson,1992.
13 Elizabeth Wilson, *Adorned in Dreams*, Virago, 1985.
14 Nicci Gerrard, *Into the Mainstream: How Feminism Has Changed Women's Writing*, Pandora, 1989.
15 Robin Morgan, *The Anatomy of Freedom*. Anchor Press/Doubleday, New York, 1982.
16 Evans and Thornton, *Women & Fashion*.

17 Sara Maitland, *Daughter of Jerusalem*, Blond and Briggs, 1978.

18 Kathy Davis, *Reshaping the Female Body: The Dilemma of Cosmetic Surgery*, Routledge, New York and London, 1995.

19 Gloria Steinem, *Revolution from Within, A Book of Self-Esteem*, Bloomsbury, 1992 .

20 Kenan Malik, "Football? I'd rather be at Sadler's Wells" and Nicholas Kenyon, "From where I stand", *Independent*, 17 October 1995.

21 Sarah Dunant (ed.), *The War of the Words: The Political Correctness Debate*, Virago, 1994.

22 It is infuriating when one misplaces references of this sort. Apologies to the reader.

23 Peter Vansittart, "A Novelist's View", in Peter Owen (ed.), *Publishing Now*, Peter Owen, 1993.

24 Carolyn Hart, "Children are obscene but not heard", *Independent*, 8 March 1995.

25 Bullard, *The Camels Must Go*.

26 Jonathan Kozol, *Free Schools*, Bantam Books, New York, 1972.

27 Anne Phillips, *Divided Loyalties: Dilemmas of Sex and Class*, Virago, 1987.

28 Naomi Wolf, *Fire With Fire*, Chatto & Windus, 1993.

29 Barbara Grizzuti Harrison, *Off Center*, Playboy Paperbacks, New York, 1980.

30 Rosie Boycott, *A Nice Girl Like Me, a Story of the Seventies*, Chatto & Windus/The Hogarth Press, 1984; Pan Books, 1985.

31 Tara Kaufman, "Oi! You! Where are your dungarees?", *Sibyl*, Issue 1.

32 Leah Fritz, *Dreamers & Dealers: An Intimate Appraisal of the Women's Movement*, Beacon Press, Boston, Massachusetts, 1979.

33 Marcia Cohen, *The Sisterhood: The Inside Story of the Women's Movement and the Leaders Who Made It Happen*, Simon and Schuster, New York, 1988.

34 Elizabeth Wilson, *Prisons of Glass*, Methuen, 1986.

35 Andrea Dworkin, *Letters From a War Zone: Writings 1976–88*, Secker & Warburg, 1988.

36 Rose Shapiro, "Prisoner of Revlon", *The Leveller*, no. 37, April 1980; reprinted in *No Turning Back*; Kathy Myers, *No Turning Back*.

37 Barbara Grizzuti Harrison, *Off Center*, Playboy Paperbacks, New York, 1980.

38 Catherine Itzin, "The art of non-fiction (or the social construction of aesthetic divisions)", in Gail Chester and Sigrid Nielsen (eds.), *In Other Words: Writing as a Feminist*, Hutchinson, 1987.

39 Elaine Hobby, *Virtue of Necessity: English Women's Writing 1649–88*, Virago, 1988.

40 *Independent*, 25 May 1994.

41 Paul McCann, "Losing a little spice", *Independent*, 7 October 1997.

42 Andrea Dworkin, *Right-Wing Women: The Politics of Domesticated Females*, The Women's Press, London, 1983; also in *Letters From a War Zone*; Esther Newton and Shirley Walton, "The Misunderstanding: Toward a More Precise Sexual Vocabulary" in Carole S. Vance (ed.), *Pleasure and Danger: Exploring Female Sexuality*, Pandora, 1992.

43 Evelyn Tension, "You don't need a degree to read the writing on the wall", *Catcall*, no. 7, January, 1978, reprinted in Feminist Anthology Collective (ed.), *No Turning Back*; Kozol, *Free Schools*.

44 Mary Evans, *A Good School: Life at a Girls' Grammar School in the 1950s*, The Women's Press, 1991.

45 Liz Heron, *Changes of Heart: Reflections on Women's Independence*, Pandora, 1986.

46 Amanda Sebestyen, "Sexual Assumptions in the Women's Movement", in Scarlet Friedman and Elizabeth Sarah (eds.), *On the Problem of Women*, The Women's Press, 1982.

47 Sheila Ernst and Marie Maguire (eds.), *Living with the Sphinx: Papers from the Women's Therapy Centre*, The Women's Press, 1987.

48 Anna Coote and Beatrix Campbell, *Sweet Freedom: The Struggle for Women's Liberation*, Basil Blackwell, Oxford, 1982; Susan Hemmings (ed.), *Girls Are Powerful: Young Women's Writings from Spare Rib*, Sheba Feminist Publishers, 1982.

49 June Burnett, *When the Singing Stops*, Hutchinson, 1988.

50 Caroline Blackwood, *On the Perimeter*, Heinemann, 1984.

51 Emma Healey, *Lesbian Sex Wars*, Virago, 1996.

52 Muriel Dimen, "Politically Correct? Politically Incorrect?" in Carole S. Vance (ed.), *Pleasure and Danger*; Sheila Rowbotham, *The Past Is Before Us: Feminism in Action Since the 1960s*, Pandora Press, 1989; Jane O'Reilly, *The Girl I Left Behind*, Collier Books, New York, 1980.

53 Joanna Russ, *Magic Mommas, Trembling Sisters, Puritans and Perverts*, Crossing Press, Trumansburg, New York, 1985.

Chapter 5   Who Are We Trying to Please?

1 John Robert Powers, *Secrets of Poise, Personality and Model Beauty*, Prentice-Hall Inc., New York, 1960.

2 Gayelord Hauser, *Mirror, Mirror on the Wall: An Invitation to Beauty*, Faber and Faber, 1961.

3 "Wives and Lovers", words by Hal David, music by Burt Bacharach, Famous Music Corporation USA/Famous Chappell Ltd., 1963.

4 Helen B. Andelin, *Fascinating Womanhood*, Bantam Books, New York, 1975.

5 Barbara Ehrenreich, Elizabeth Hess and Gloria Jacobs, *Re-Making Love: The Feminization of Sex*, Anchor Press/Doubleday, Garden City, New York, 1986; Fontana Paperbacks, 1987.

6 Marabel Morgan, *The Total Woman*, Fleming Revell, Old Tappan, New Jersey, 1973; Pocket Books, New York, 1975.

7 "J", *How to become The Sensuous Woman*, W. H. Allen, New York and London, 1970.

8 Barbara Cartland, *Barbara Cartland's Book of Etiquette*, Hutchinson, 1972.

9 Melissa Sadoff, *Woman as Chameleon or, How to be an Ideal Woman*, S. P. I. Inc., USA, and Quartet Books, 1987; Ellen Fein and Sherrie Schneider, *The Rules: Ten Time-Tested Secrets for Capturing the Heart of Mr Right*, Warner Books, New York, 1995; Thorsons, Wellingborough, Hampshire, 1995; *The Rules 2*, 1997.

10 Andrew Postman, "Big Fat Lies About Men", British *Cosmopolitan*, December 1996.

11 Dale Carnegie, *How to Win Friends and Influence People*, The World's Work (1915) Ltd., USA and Kingswood, Surrey, 1938.

12   A. S. Neill, *Neill! Neill! Orange Peel! A Personal Impression of Ninety Years*, Weidenfeld and Nicolson, 1973.

13   James Laver, *Style in Costume*, Oxford University Press, 1949.

14   Paul Tabori, *Dress and Undress*, New English Library, 1969.

15   Virginia Novarra, *Women's Work, Men's Work: The Ambivalence of Equality*, Marion Boyars, London and Boston, Massachusetts, 1980.

16   Paul Ableman, *The Doomed Rebellion*, Zomba Books, 1983.

17   Doris Langley Moore, *The Vulgar Heart: An Enquiry into the Sentimental Tendencies of Public Opinion*, Cassell and Co., 1945.

18   Clifford Longley, "Sexual symbolism at the altar", *Times*, 7 July 1986.

19   Terence McLaughlin, *The Gilded Lily*, Cookery Book Club, 1972.

20   Ainslie Meares, *The New Woman: Woman at the Crossroads of Social and Psychological Evolution*, Collins, 1974 .

21   Quoted in Shulamith Firestone, *The Dialectic of Sex: The Case for Feminist Revolution*, Jonathan Cape, 1971.

22   Mette Ejlersen, *I Accuse!*, trs. Marianne Kold Madsen, Universal-Tandem Co. Ltd., 1979.

23   Esther Vilar, *The Manipulated Man*, Farrar, Straus and Giroux, New York, 1972; Bantam Books, New York, 1974.

24   Ferdinand Lundberg and Marynia F. Farnham M. D., *Modern Woman: The Lost Sex*, Harper and Brothers, New York and London, 1947.

25   Art Buchwald, *How Much Is That in Dollars?*, World Publishing Co., New York, 1961.

26   A. P. Herbert, *Mild and Bitter*, Methuen, 1936.

27   John Brophy, *The Human Face*, Harrap, 1945.

28   Kenneth C. Barnes, *He and She*, Darwen Finlayson, 1958.

29   John Seymour and Herbert Girardet, *Blueprint for a Green Planet*, Dorling Kindersley, 1987.

30   Newby Hands, "Make-up? Break-up", *Harpers' & Queen*, August 1996.

31   Alison Settle, *Clothes Line*, Methuen, 1937.

32   Abioseh Nicol, "The Leopard Hunt", in *The Truly Married Woman and Other Stories*, Oxford University Press, 1965.

33   Doris Langley Moore, *The Technique of the Love Affair*, Gerald Howe, 1926.

34   Settle, *Clothes Line*.

35   Jean Rook, *Dress for Success*, Dent, 1968.

36   Rosalind Lowe, "Spend, Spend, Spend", *best*, 17 January 1991.

37   Mrs Humphry, *Manners for Women*, 1897; Webb and Bower, Exeter, 1979 .

38   Sally Cline and Dale Spender, *Reflecting Men at Twice Their Natural Size*, André Deutsch, 1987.

39   Settle, *Clothes Line*.

40   Herb Goldberg, *The New Male: From Self-Destruction to Self-Care*, Signet Books, New York, 1979 .

41   Paula J. Caplan, *The Myth of Women's Masochism*, E. P. Dutton, New York, 1985.

42   Martine Bourrillon, *Côté Cœur, C'est Pas le Pied*, Grasset et Fasquelle, Paris, 1984;

Eleanor Bailey, "Men Who Claim to be the Best Sex: Sexist and Proud of it", British *Marie-Claire*, March 1996.

43 Janet Radcliffe Richards, *The Sceptical Feminist: A Philosophical Enquiry*, Routledge & Kegan Paul, London, Boston and Henley, 1980.

44 Alison Lurie, *The Language of Clothes*, Heinemann, 1982.

45 Theodor Reik, *Sex in Man and Woman: the Emotional Variations*, Noonday Press Inc., New York, 1960.

46 Khushwant Singh, *Delhi: A Novel*, Penguin, New Delhi, 1990.

47 Gloria Steinem, *Moving Beyond Words*.

48 George Orwell, *A Clergyman's Daughter*, Gollancz, 1935; Penguin, Harmondsworth, 1990.

49 Sue Lees, *Carnal Knowledge: Rape on Trial*, Hamish Hamilton, 1996.

50 Ray Wyre, *Women, Men and Rape*, Perry Publications, Oxford, 1986.

51 Dusty Rhodes and Sandra McNeil (eds.), *Women Against Violence Against Women*, Onlywomen Press, 1985.

52 Germaine Greer, *The Madwoman's Underclothes: Essays and Occasional Writings 1968–1985*, Picador, 1986.

53 Rebecca West, *The Young Rebecca: Writings of Rebecca West 1911–17*, Macmillan, 1982.

54 Margot Asquith, *Lay Sermons*, Thornton Butterworth, 1927.

55 Jane O'Reilly, *The Girl I Left Behind*, Collier Books, New York, 1980.

56 Jackie Bennett and Rosemary Forgan (eds.), *There's Something About a Convent Girl*, Virago, 1991.

57 Robin Morgan, "Theory and Practice: Pornography and Rape" in *Going Too Far: The Personal Odyssey of a Feminist*, Vintage Books, New York, 1978; also in Laura Lederer (ed.), *Take Back the Night: Women on Pornography*, William Morrow and Company, New York, 1980, and *The Word of a Woman: Selected Prose 1968–1992*, Virago, 1993.

58 Sue Read, *Sexual Harassment at Work*, Hamlyn Paperbacks,1982.

59 Dorothy Parker, *The Penguin Dorothy Parker*, Penguin, Harmondsworth, 1977.

60 Banner, *American Beauty*, and Helen Franks, *Goodbye Tarzan: Men After Feminism*, George Allen and Unwin, 1984.

61 Barbara Ehrenreich and Deirdre English, *For Her Own Good: 150 years of the Experts' Advice to Women*, Anchor Press/Doubleday, Garden City, New York, 1978; Pluto Press, 1979.

62 Angela Partington, "Popular Fashion and Working-Class Affluence", Juliet Ash and Elizabeth Wilson (eds.), *Chic Thrills: A Fashion Reader*, Pandora Press, 1992.

63 Janet L. Wolff, *What Makes Women Buy: A Guide to Understanding and Influencing the New Woman of Today*, McGraw-Hill Book Co., New York, Toronto and London, 1958.

64 Elizabeth Nickles with Laura Ashcraft, *The Coming Matriarchy: How Women Will Gain the Balance of Power*, Seaview Books, New York, 1981.

65 Ellen Willis, "'Consumerism' and Women", in Leslie B. Tanner (ed.), *Voices from Women's Liberation*, Mentor Books, New York, 1971.

66   Packard, *The Waste Makers*, USA 1960; Longmans, Green, 1961; Pelican, Harmondsworth, 1963.

67   Marya Mannes, *But Will It Sell?*, Victor Gollancz, 1966.

68   Quoted in Barry Turner, *Equality for Some: The story of girls' education*, Ward Lock Educational, 1974.

69   Betty Friedan, *The Feminine Mystique*, Victor Gollancz, 1963.

70   Maggie Scarf, *Unfinished Business: Pressure Points in the Lives of Women*, Doubleday, New York, 1980.

71   Louise Kehoe, *In This Dark House*, Viking, 1996.

72   Kathy Nairne and Gerrilyn Smith, *Dealing with Depression*, The Women's Press, 1984; revised edition, 1985.

73   Leah Fritz, *Dreamers & Dealers: An Intimate Appraisal of the Women's Movement*, Beacon Press, Boston, Massachusetts, 1979.

74   Quoted in Nancy Friday, *The Power of Beauty*, HarperCollins, New York, 1996.

Chapter 6   Do Appearances Matter?

1   Jill Dawson, *How Do I Look?*, Virago, 1990.

2   Richard Hoggart, *The Uses of Literacy*, Chatto and Windus, 1957.

3   Barbara Leszczynsky, "Life After 50", *Observer*, 13 June 1982.

4   Elizabeth Wilson, "Fashion and the Meaning of Life", *Guardian*, 18 May 1992.

5   Joyce Nicholson, *What Society Does to Girls*, Virago, 1977.

6   Antonia White, *Frost in May*, 1933; Virago, 1978.

7   Jane Trahey, *Life with Mother Superior*, Michael Joseph, 1962; John Quinn (ed.), *A Portrait of the Artist as a Young Girl*, Methuen, 1986.

8   Lavinia Derwent, *A Breath of Border Air*, Hutchinson, 1975; Nora Scott Kinzer, *Put Down and Ripped Off: The American Woman and the Beauty Cult*, Thomas Y. Crowell, New York, 1977.

9   Mary Mellor, *Breaking the Boundaries: Towards a Feminist Green Socialism*, Virago, 1992.

10   Michael Korda, *Male Chauvinism: How It Works*, Barrie and Jenkins, 1974.

11   Susan Brownmiller, *Femininity*, Hamish Hamilton, 1984; Alison Lurie, *The Language of Clothes*, Heinemann, 1982.

12   Marjorie Proops, *Dear Marje . . .*, André Deutsch, 1976.

13   Agatha Christie, *An Autobiography*, William Collins, Glasgow, 1977.

14   Fay Weldon, *The Fat Woman's Joke*, McGibbon and Kee Ltd., 1967.

15   Nicholson, *What Society Does to Girls*.

16   Joyce Nicholson, *The Heartache of Motherhood*, Sheldon Press, 1977.

17   Gwen Raverat, *Period Piece: A Cambridge Childhood*, Faber and Faber, 1952.

18   Wilson Bryan Key, *Media Sexploitation*, Prentice-Hall Inc., New York, 1976.

19   Letty Cottin Pogrebin, *Growing Up Free: Raising Your Child in the 80s*, McGraw-Hill Book Company, New York, 1980.

20   Sara Stein, *Girls and Boys: The Limits of Non-Sexist Childrearing*, Chatto & Windus/Hogarth Press, 1984.

21 Dena Taylor (ed.), *Feminist Parenting: Triumphs, Struggles and Comic Interludes*, Crossing Press, Freedom, California, 1994.

22 Marjorie Garber, *Vested Interests: Cross-Dressing and Cultural Anxiety*, Routledge, New York and London, 1992.

23 William Hartston, *Independent*, 7 February 1994.

24 Charlotte Bunch-Weeks, in Joanne Cooke, Charlotte Bunch-Weeks and Robin Morgan (eds.), *The New Woman*, Fawcett Publications Inc., Greenwich, Connecticut, 1971.

25 Caroline Blackwood, *On the Perimeter*, Heinemman, 1984.

26 Angela Carter, "The Wound in the Face", *New Society*; reprinted in *Shaking a Leg: Collected Journalim and Writings*, Vintage, 1998.

27 Yasmin Alibhai-Brown, "Sex, veils and stereotypes", *Independent*, 22 December 1994.

28 Nawal El Saadawi, "Removing the veil" and Rosa Prince, "A robe is still a robe", *Sibyl*, Issue 3, July/August 1998.

29 Jean P. Sasson, *Princess*, Doubleday, London, 1992, Bantam Books, London, 1993; *Daughter of Arabia*, Doubleday, 1994.

30 Sousan Angadi with Angela Ferrante, *Out of Iran: One Woman's Escape from the Ayatollahs*, Macdonald, 1987; Yasmin Alibhai-Brown, "Muslim women's struggle to wear what they like", *Independent*, 23 June 2003.

31 Lindsey Hilsum, "Jeans and Mascara Under the Veil", *New Statesman*, 10 July 1998; Yasmin Alibhai-Brown, "The beauty secrets of Asian women", *Independent*, 26 November 2001.

32 Paul Theroux, *Riding the Iron Rooster: By Train through China*, Hamish Hamilton, 1998.

33 Pauline Bart, "The Banned Professor or, How Radical Feminism Saved Me from Men Trapped in Men's Bodies and Female Impersonators, with a Little Help from my Friends", in Diane Bell and Renate Klein (eds.), *Radically Speaking: Feminism Reclaimed*, Zed Books, 1996.

34 Jung Chang, *Wild Swans: Three Daughters of China*, HarperCollins, 1991.

35 *Independent*, 13 February 1993.

36 Jo, Bev, Strega, Linda and Ruston, *Dykes-Loving Dykes*, Battleaxe, Oakland, California, 1990, quoted in Sheila Jeffreys, *The Lesbian Heresy: A Feminist Perspective on the Lesbian Sexual Revolution*, The Women's Press, 1993.

37 Janet Radcliffe Richards, *The Sceptical Feminist: A Philosophical Enquiry*, Routledge & Kegan Paul, London, Boston and Henley, 1980.

38 Adrienne Rich, *On Lies, Secrets and Silence*, W. V. Norton, New York, 1979; Virago, 1980.

39 Wendy Chapkis, *Beauty Secrets: Women and the Politics of Appearance*, South End Press, Boston, Massachusetts, 1986.

40 Wilson, *Adorned in Dreams*.

41 Leonard Halliday, *The Fashion Makers*, Hodder and Stoughton, 1966.

42 Harriet Lyons and Rebecca W. Rosenblatt, "Body Hair: The Last Frontier", in Francine Klagsbrun (ed.), *The First Ms. Reader*, Warner Books, New York, 1973.

43   Jean A. Rees, *Danger – Saints Still at Work!*, Victory Press, 1972.

44   Anja Meulenbelt, Johanna's Daughter, *For Ourselves*, Sheba Feminist Publishers, 1981; Richards, *The Sceptical Feminist*.

45   Jacques Chastenet, *La Belle Epoque*, Arthème Fayard, Paris, 1949.

46   Mandy Merck, "The City's Achievements: The patriotic Amazonomachy and ancient Athens", in Susan Lipshitz (ed.), *Tearing the Veil: Essays on Femininity*, Routledge Kegan Paul, 1978.

47   Benoîte Groult, *Ainsi Soit-Elle*, Editions Grasset et Fasquelle, Paris, 1975.

48   Chang, *Wild Swans*.

49   Mary Daly, *Gyn/Ecology: The Metaethics of Radical Feminism*, The Women's Press, 1979.

50   Carolyn Beckingham, "A Traveller in Asia in the 1870s", *Asian Affairs*, October 1982.

51   Germaine Greer, *The Whole Woman*, Doubleday, London, New York, Toronto, Sydney and Auckland, 1999.

52   David Kunzle, *Fashion and Fetishism*, Rowman and Littlefield, Totowa, New Jersey, 1982; Angela Carter, *Shaking a Leg: Journalism and Writings*, Vintage, 1998.

53   Lee Comer, *Wedlocked Women*, Feminist Books, Leeds, 1974.

54   J. B. Furnas, *The Life and Times of the Late Demon Rum*, W. H. Allen, 1965.

55   Joanne B. Eicher and Mary Ellen Roach-Higgins, "Definition and Classification of Dress: Implications for Analysis of Gender Roles", in Ruth Barnes and Joanne B. Eicher (eds.), *Dress and Gender: Making and Meaning* (Cross Cultural Perspectives on Women Vol. 2), Berg Publishers Inc., Rhode Island and Oxford, 1992.

56   Robin Tolmach Lakoff and Raquel L. Scherr, *Face Value: The Politics of Beauty*, Routledge Kegan Paul, 1984.

57   Robin Morgan, *The Anatomy of Freedom*, Anchor Press/Doubleday, New York, 1982.

58   Rosie Boycott, "Looking at Looks", *Honey*, January 1981.

59   Hugh D. R. Baker, "The Myth of the Travelling Wok: The Overseas Chinese", lecture given to the Royal Society for Asian Affairs, 23 October 1996, reprinted in *Asian Affairs*, February 1997.

60   Nancy Friday, *The Power of Beauty*, HarperCollins, New York, 1996; Germaine Greer, *The Madwoman's Underclothes: Essays and Occasional Writings 1968–1985*, Picador,1986.

61   Nancy Etcoff, *The Survival of the Prettiest*, Little, Brown, 1999.

62   Ann Oakley, *Housewife*, Allen Lane, 1974; Penguin, Harmondsworth, 1976.

63   We all have enough strength to bear the troubles of other people.

64   Nancy C. Baker, *The Beauty Trap: How Every Woman Can Free Herself From It*, Judy Piatkus, 1986; Kaz Cooke, *Real Gorgeous*, Bloomsbury, 1995; Rita Freedman, *Beauty Bound: Why Women Strive for Physical Perfection*, Columbus Books, 1988; Rita Freedman, *Bodylove: Learning to Like Our Looks – and Ourselves, a Practical Guide for Women*, Harper and Row, New York, 1989.

65   Cooke, *Real Gorgeous*; Jane Cousins-Mills, *Make It Happy, Make It Safe*, Penguin, Harmondsworth, 1988 .

66 Doreen Frust, *Overcoming Disfigurement*, Thorsons, Wellingborough and New York, 1986.

67 Diane Coyle, "I was so ugly . . .", *Independent*, 5 March 1997.

68 Gloria Steinem, *Revolution from Within: A Book of Self-Esteem*, Bloomsbury, 1992; Leslie E. Gardiner, *Faces, Figures and Feelings: A Cosmetic Plastic Surgeon Speaks*, Robert Hale, 1959.

69 Karen DeCrow, *The Young Woman's Guide to Liberation: Alternatives to a Half-Life While the Choice Is Still Yours*, Pegasus, Indianapolis and New York, 1971.

70 Letty Cottin Pogrebin, *Getting Over Growing Older*, Little, Brown and Company, Boston, New York, Toronto and London, 1996.

Chapter 7 The Ultimate Attack: Fashion as Pornography

1 Michael Korda, *Male Chauvinism: How It Works*, Barrie and Jenkins, 1974.

2 Wendy Kaminer, *True Love Waits*, Addison-Wesley, Reading, Massachusetts, 1996.

3 Dee Ann Pappas, "On Being Natural", *Women: A Journal of Liberation*, Fall, 1969; reprinted in Sookie Stambler (ed.), *Women's Liberation: Blueprint for the Future*, Ace Books, New York, 1970; also in Leslie B. Tanner (ed.), *Voices from Women's Liberation*, Mentor Books, New York, 1970.

4 Helen Haste, *The Sexual Metaphor*, Harvester Wheatsheaf, Hemel Hempstead, Hertfordshire, 1993.

5 Gloria Steinem, *Outrageous Acts and Everyday Rebellions*, Henry Holt and Company, New York, 1995.

6 Mary Midgley and Judith Hughes, *Women's Choices: Philosophical Problems Facing Feminism* Weidenfeld and Nicolson, 1983.

7 Alice Echols, "The Taming of the Id: Feminist Sexual Politics, 1968–83", in Carole S. Vance (ed.), *Pleasure and Danger: Exploring Female Sexuality*, Pandora, 1992.

8 Dana Densmore, "On Celibacy", *No More Fun and Games*, No. 1, reprinted in Tanner (ed.), *Voices from Women's Liberation*.

9 Kathie Sarachild (ed.), *Feminist Revolution*, Random House, New York, 1978.

10 Emma Healey, *Lesbian Sex Wars*, Virago, 1996.

11 Adrienne Rich, Afterword to Laura Lederer (ed.), *Take Back the Night: Women on Pornography*, William Morrow and Company, New York, 1980.

12 Lynne Segal and Mary McIntosh (eds.), *Sex Exposed: Sexuality and the Pornography Debate*, Virago, 1992.

13 Richard Hoggart, *The Uses of Literacy*, Chatto and Windus, 1957.

14 Mary Kay Blakely, "Is One Woman's Sexuality Another Woman's Pornography?", *Ms.*, April 1985.

15 Liz Kelly, "The US ordinances: censorship or radical law reform?", in Gail Chester and Julienne Dickey (eds.), *Feminism and Censorship: The Current Debate*, Prism Press, Bridport, Dorset, 1988.

16 Robin Morgan, "Theory and Practice: Pornography and Rape" in *Going Too Far: The Personal Odyssey of a Feminist*, Vintage Books, New York, 1978

17   Nadine Strossen, *Defending Pornography: Free Speech, Sex, and the Fight for Women's Rights*, Abacus, 1996.

18   *Radio Times,* 23 August 1997.

19   Gayle Rubin, "Thinking Sex: Notes for a Radical Theory of the Politics of Sexuality", in *Pleasure and Danger*.

20   E. M. Forster, *Abinger Harvest*, Edward Arnold & Co., 1936.

21   Vance, *Pleasure and Danger*.

22   Gill Saunders, *The Nude: A New Perspective*, The Herbert Press, 1989.

23   Strossen, *Defending Pornography*.

24   Marilyn French, *The War Against Women*, Summit Books, New York, 1992; Hamish Hamilton, 1992.

25   Fidelis Morgan, *A Misogynist's Source Book*, Jonathan Cape, 1989.

26   Ellen Willis, "Feminism, Moralism, and Pornography,", in Ann Snitow, Christine Stansell, and Sharon Thompson (eds.), *Desire: The Politics of Sexuality*, Virago, 1984.

27   Zena Herbert, "*The Dancer* and *Heat*" in Hilary Robinson (ed.), *Visibly Female: An Anthology*, Camden Press, 1987.

28   Jane Caputi, *The Age of Sex Crime*, The Women's Press, 1988.

29   Susan Griffin, *Pornography and Silence*, The Women's Press, 1981; Andrea Dworkin, *Pornography: Men Possessing Women*, The Women's Press, 1981.

30   Lisa Jardine, "Is It Art Or Is It Violence?", *Guardian*, 2 December 1996.

31   Vance, *Pleasure and Danger*.

32   Sheila Jeffreys, *The Lesbian Heresy: A Feminist Perspective on the Lesbian Sexual Revolution*, The Women's Press, 1993.

33   Robin Gorna, "Delightful visions: from anti-porn to eroticizing safer sex", in Segal and Macintosh (eds.), *Sex Exposed: Sexuality and the Pornography Debate*, Virago, 1992.

34   Jeffreys, *The Lesbian Heresy*.

35   Lal Coveney, Tina Crockett, Al Garthwaite, Sheila Jeffreys and Valerie Sinclair, *Love Your Enemy? The Debate Between Heterosexual Feminism and Political Lesbianism*, Onlywomen Press, 1981.

36   Healey, *Lesbian Sex Wars*.

37   Catharine Lumby, *Bad Girls*, Allen & Unwin, St Leonards, Australia, 1997.

38   Mary Stott, *Forgetting's No Excuse*, Virago, 1975.

39   Christopher Macy (ed.), *The Arts in a Permissive Society*, Pemberton Books for Rationalist Press Association, 1971.

40   Alan Bullock, *Hitler: A Study in Tyranny*, Pelican Books, Harmondsworth, 1962.

41   Quoted in Sheila Rowbotham, *The Past Is Before Us: Feminism in Action Since the 1960s*, Pandora, 1989.

42   Linda Grant, "Cut and Thrust", *Guardian*, 5 February 1996.

43   Vance, *Pleasure and Danger*.

44   Margaret Walters, "American Gothic", in Ann Oakley and Judith Mitchell (eds.), *Who's Afraid of Feminism?*, Hamish Hamilton, 1997.

45   Griffin, *Pornography and Silence*.

46 Andrea Dworkin, *Life and Death: Unapologetic Writings on the Continuing War Against Women*, Virago, London, 1997.

47 Ros Schwartz, "A question of allegiance?" in Gail Chester and Julienne Dickey (eds.), *Feminism and Censorship: The Current Debate*, Prism Press, Bridport, Dorset, 1988.

48 Jane O'Reilly, *The Girl I Left Behind*, Collier Books, New York, 1980.

49 Sara Dunn, "Voyages of the Valkyries: Recent Lesbian Pornographic Writing" and Margaret Hunt, "The De-Eroticization of Women's Liberation: Social Purity Movements and the Revolutionary Feminism of Sheila Jeffreys", in *Feminist Review*, No. 34, Spring 1990.

50 Healey, *Lesbian Sex Wars*.

51 Lynne Segal, "False Promises – Anti-Pornography Feminism", in Mary Evans (ed.), *The Woman Question*, 2nd edition, Sage Publications, 1994.

52 Elizabeth Cowie, "Pornography and fantasy: Psychoanalytic perspectives", in Lynne Segal and Mary McIntosh (eds.), *Sex Exposed: Sexuality and the Pornography Debate*, Virago, 1992.

53 James Weaver, "The Social Science and Psychological Research Evidence: Perceptual and Behavioural Consequences of Exposure to Pornography", in Catherine Itzin (ed.), *Pornography: Women, Violence and Civil Liberties*, Oxford University Press, Oxford, 1993. The same point was made by E. Donnerstein at the United States Attorney General's Commission on Pornography, 1986, quoted in Carol Wehesser (ed.), *Feminism: Opposing Viewpoints*, Greenhaven Press, San Diego, California, 1995.

54 Harriett Gilbert, "So long as it's not sex and violence: Andrea Dworkin's *Mercy*", in *Sex Exposed*.

55 Clare Garner, *Independent*, 4 August 1997.

56 Elizabeth Wilson, *What Is To Be Done About Violence Against Women?*, Penguin in association with the Socialist Society, Harmondsworth, 1983.

57 Susanne Kappeler, *The Pornography of Representation*, Polity Press, Cambridge, 1986.

58 Robin Morgan, *The Anatomy of Freedom*, Anchor Press/Doubleday, New York, 1982.

59 Andrea Dworkin, *Letters From a War Zone: Writings 1976–88*, Secker & Warburg, 1988.

60 J. B. Furnas, *The Life and Times of the Late Demon Rum*, W. H. Allen, 1965.

61 Kaminer, *True Love Waits*.

62 Stott, *Forgetting's No Excuse*.

63 Katharine Whitehorn, "Porn free, but limits", *Observer*, 6 March 1988.

64 Valerie Bryson, *Feminist Debates: Issues of Theory and Political Practice*, Macmillan, 1999.

65 Drusilla Cornell, *The Imaginary Domain: Abortion, Pornography and Sexual Harassment*, Routledge, New York and London, 1995.

66 Gloria Steinem, "Erotica and Pornography: A Clear and Present Difference", in *Outrageous Acts and Everyday Rebellions*, also in *Take Back the Night*.

67 Kathy Myers, "Towards a Feminist Erotica", *Camerawork* 24, reprinted in *Visibly Female*, and Rosemary Betterton (ed.), *Looking On: Images of Femininity in the Visual Arts and Media*, Pandora, London, 1987 also *Visibly Female*.

68 Jean P. Sasson, *Princess*, Doubleday, London, 1992, Bantam Books, London, 1993.

69 Victoria McKee, "The Colour of Sanctity", *Independent*, 13 February 1993.

70 Kate Luck, "Trouble in Eden, Trouble with Eve: Women, Trousers and Utopian Socialism in Nineteenth-Century America", in Juliet Ash and Elizabeth Wilson (eds.), *Chic Thrills: A Fashion Reader*, Pandora Press, 1992.

71 Stott, *Forgetting's No Excuse.*

72 Janet Radcliffe Richards, *The Sceptical Feminist: A Philosophical Enquiry*, Routledge Kegan Paul, 1980.

73 Susanne Kappeler, *The Pornography of Representation*, Polity Press, Cambridge, 1986.

Chapter 8 Dress as Ritual

1 Richard Kendall and Griselda Pollock (eds.), *Dealing With Degas: Representations of Women and the Politics of Vision*, Pandora, 1992; Carol Rutter, *Clamorous Voices: Shakespeare's Women Today*, The Women's Press, 1988; Rozsika Parker, *The Subversive Stitch: Embroidery and the Making of the Feminine*, The Women's Press, 1984.

2 Victor Gollancz, *Journey Towards Music*, Gollancz, 1964.

3 Diana de Marly, *Fashion for Men*, Batsford, 1985.

4 *Independent*, 18 September 1999.

5 *Independent*, 14 April 1994 and 10 October 1997.

6 Peter Gradenwitz, in Hans-Hubert Schönzeler (ed.), *Of German Music: a Symposium*, Oswald Wolff, 1976.

7 Helen Callaway, "Dressing for Dinner in the Bush: Rituals of Self-Definition and British Imperial Authority", in Barnes and Eicher (eds.), *Dress and Gender: Making and Meaning.*

8 Gwen Raverat, *Period Piece: A Cambridge Childhood*, Faber and Faber, 1952.

9 Margaret Kennedy, *The Fool of the Family*, Heinemann, 1930.

10 June and Doris Langley Moore, *The Pleasure of Your Company: A Text-book of Hospitality*, Gerald Howe, 1933.

11 Caption of exhibit at exhibition at the Imperial War Museum, London, 1997.

12 Dea Birkett, *Independent*, 23 August 1997.

13 Settle, *Clothes Line.*

14 Richard Stoddart Aldrich, *Gertrude Lawrence as "Mrs A."*, Greystone Press, New York, 1954, Companion Book Club, 1956.

15 Donald Brook, *Conductors' Gallery*, Rockliff, 1946.

16 Brett Harvey, *The Fifties, A Women's Oral History*, HarperCollins, New York, 1993.

17 Twiggy (Lesley Hornby), *An Open Look*, Robson Books, 1985.

18 Sarah Barr, *Radio Times*, 11 March 1995.

19 *New Yorker*, 10 July 1989.

20 Anthony Gardner, "The Nineties Dress Code Crisis", *Harpers' & Queen*, October 1996.

21 *Independent*, 5 September 1996.

22 John Rosselli, "Opera as a Social Occasion", in *The Oxford History of Opera*, Oxford University Press, Oxford and London, 1994.

23 Susanne Kappeler, *The Pornography of Representation*, Polity Press, Cambridge, 1986.

24 Fanny Burney, *Cecilia, or the Memoirs of an Heiress*, 1782; Virago, 1986.

25 Angela du Maurier, *It's Only the Sister: An Autobiography*, Peter Davies, 1951.

26 Ida Cook, *We Followed Our Stars*, Harlequin-Mills & Boon, London, Toronto and Sydney, 1976.

27 Jane Pearson, "Talking 'Bout My Generation", *Classical Music*, 28 March 1998; letter, *ibid.*, 11 April 1998.

28 *Classic FM Magazine*, December 2001.

29 Ian Eccles, letter to *Opera Now*, May/June 1998.

30 Betty Carter and Joan K. Peters, *Love, Honor and Negotiate: Making Your Marriage Work*, Pocket Books, New York and London, 1996.

31 James Naughtie, BBC Radio 3, 27 May 1995.

32 Spike Hughes, *Glyndebourne: A History of the Festival Opera*, David & Charles, 1981.

33 Gerald Coke, Glyndebourne Festival Opera programme, 1976.

34 *Daily Telegraph*, 23 May, 1991.

35 *Independent*, 13 March 1996.

36 *Music & Musicians*, October 1981.

37 Michael Church, *Independent*, 19 May 1997.

38 BBC Radio 3, 22 May 1997.

39 *Daily Telegraph*, 24 June 1997.

40 Letter to the author from Sir George Christie, 18 April 1994.

41 Bernard Levin, *Conducted Tour*, Jonathan Cape, 1982; Coronet Books, 1982.

42 Hughes, *Glyndebourne*.

43 David Thomas, *Not Guilty: In Defence of Modern Man*, Weidenfeld & Nicolson, 1993.

44 Monica Baldwin, *I Leap Over the Wall*, Hamish Hamilton, 1949.

45 John Masters, *Bugles and a Tiger*, Michael Joseph, 1956 .

46 Bernard Levin, *Conducted Tour*.

47 Elizabeth Anson, *Lady Elizabeth Anson's Party Planners Book*, Weidenfeld & Nicolson, 1980.

48 Claudia Brush Kidwell and Valerie Steele, *Dressing the Part*, Smithsonian Press, Washington, 1989.

49 Wilfred Thesiger, *Arabian Sands*, Longmans, Green, London, 1959; *The Marsh Arabs*, Longmans, Green, 1964.

50 Elizabeth Hawes, *Men Can Take It*, Random House, New York, 1939.

51 Emma Lathen, *Double, Double, Oil and Trouble*, Simon & Schuster, New York, 1978.

52 Peter Hall, Glyndebourne Festival Opera programme, 1998; John Taylor, *It's a Small, Medium and Outsize World*, Hugh Evelyn, 1966.

53 David Lister, *Independent*, 30 March 1999.

54 David Belcher, "Exposed – A Rock Fan at the Opera", *Scottish Opera News*, April–July 1988.

55 Interview in *The Face*, quoted *New Statesman*, 3 June 1983.

56 Marion Hume, *Independent*, 14 October 1994.

57 *New Statesman*, 7 September 1984; Eithne Power, *Radio Times*, 1–7 September 1984.

58 *Independent*, 9 March 1996.

59 Michael Church, *Observer*, 30 May 1993.

60 Katharine Whitehorn, *Social Survival*, Magnum Books, 1980.

61 R. Higton, letter to *The Sun*, 18 June 1997.

62 Katharine Whitehorn, "Coat of Many Colours", *Observer*, 15 November 1981.

63 Richards, *The Sceptical Feminist*; Leonore Davidoff, *The Best Circles*, Century Hutchinson, 1986; Heide Göttner-Abendroth, "Nine Principles of a Matriarchal Aesthetic", in Gisela Ecker (ed.), *Feminist Aesthetics*, trs. Harriet Anderson, The Women's Press, 1985.

64 Jane Rule, *A Hot-Eyed Moderate*, Naiad Press, Tallahassee, Florida, 1985.

65 Ted Polhemus, *Fashion and Anti-Fashion*, Thames and Hudson, 1978.

Chapter 9 What Next?

1 Rita Freeman, *Bodylove: Learning to Like Our Looks – and Ourselves, a Practical Guide for Women*, Harper and Row, New York, 1989.

2 Françoise Parturier, *Lettre Ouverte aux Hommes*, Editions Albin Michel, Paris, 1968.

3 Janet Radcliffe Richards, *The Sceptical Feminist: A Philosophical Enquiry*, Routledge & Kegan Paul, London, Boston and Henley, 1980.

4 Alice Walker, *Living by the Word*, Harcourt Brace Jovanovich, New York and The Women's Press, 1988.

5 Jane Rule, *A Hot-Eyed Moderate*, Naiad Press, Tallahassee, Florida, 1985.

6 Joseph Hansen and Evelyn Reed, *Cosmetics, Fashions, and the Exploitation of Women*, Pathfinder Press, New York, 1986.

7 Ann Oosthuizen, *Loneliness and Other Lovers*, Sheba Feminist Publishers, 1981.

8 Anja Meulenbelt, trs. Ann Oosthuizen, *The Shame Is Over*, The Women's Press, 1980.

9 Elizabeth Wilson, *Mirror Writing: An Autobiography*, Virago, 1982.

10 Frigga Haug *et al.*, *Female Sexualization: A Collective Work of Memory*, Verso, 1986.

11 Lorraine Gamman and Shelagh Young, "Radical Cheek", *Spare Rib*, No. 190, May 1988; Sabina Spier, letter to *Spare Rib*, No. 193, August 1988.

12 Andrea Dworkin, *Letters from a War Zone: Writings 1976–1987*, Secker & Warburg, 1988.

13 Mary Scott, *Everywoman* no. 88, December 1992/January 1993.

14 Letty Cottin Pogrebin, *Getting Over Growing Older: An Intimate Journey*, Little, Brown, Boston, New York, Toronto and London, 1996.

15 Nora Scott Kinzer, *Put Down and Ripped Off: The American Woman and the Beauty Cult*, Thomas Y. Crowell, New York, 1977.

16 Raymond O'Malley and Denys Thompson, *English Five*, Heinemann, 1960.

17 Quentin Bell, *Bad Art*, Chatto & Windus, 1989; Sara Maitland, *A Big-Enough God: Artful Theology*, Mowbray, 1995.

18 Andrea Dworkin, *Pornography: Men Possessing Women*, The Women's Press, 1981.

19 Shulamith Firestone, *The Dialectic of Sex: The Case for Feminist Revolution*, Jonathan Cape, 1971.

20 Nancy Etcoff, *The Survival of the Prettiest*, Little, Brown, 1999.

21 Naomi Wolf, *The Beauty Myth*, Chatto and Windus, 1990.

22 Barbara Sichtermann, trs. John Whittam, *Femininity: The Politics of the Personal*, Polity Press, Cambridge, 1983.

23 Mary Midgley and Judith Hughes, *Women's Choices: Philosophical Problems Facing Feminism*, Weidenfeld and Nicolson, 1983.

24 Richards, *The Sceptical Feminist*.

25 Angela Neustatter, *Hyenas in Petticoats: A Look at Twenty Years of Feminism*, Harrap, 1989.

26 Sichtermann, *Femininity*.

27 Gilles Lipovetsky, trs. Catherine Porter, *The Empire of Fashion: Dressing Modern Democracy*, Princeton University Press, Princeton, New Jersey, 1994.

28 "One can be clever in Venetian point-lace and feathers, just as much as in a short wig and a plain little stock".

   "As for myself, when I go to a comedy, I only consider whether things touch me; and when I have had a good time, I don't ask myself if I was wrong, and Aristotle's rules have forbidden me to laugh."

29 Rebecca West, *The Fountain Overflows*, Macmillan, 1957.

30 Sidney Harrison, *The Young Person's Guide to Playing the Piano*, Faber and Faber, 1966.

31 Simone de Beauvoir, *Le Deuxième Sexe*, Gallimard, Paris, 1958.

32 Athena S. Leoussi, in Digby Anderson (ed.), *Gentility Recalled: 'Mere' Manners and the Making of Social Order*, Social Affairs Unit, 1996.

33 Richards, *The Sceptical Feminist*.

34 Joyce Reiser Kornblatt, *Nothing to Do With Love*, The Women's Press, 1982.

35 Phyllis Chesler, *Women and Madness*, Allen Lane, 1972; Anita Shreve, *Women Together, Women Alone: The Legacy of the Consciousness-Raising Movement*, Viking, New York, 1989.

36 Beauvoir, *Le Deuxième Sexe*.

37 Nancy Mitford, "Chic – English, French and American", *The Water Beetle*, Hamish Hamilton, 1962.

38 Mary Quant, *Quant by Quant*, Cassell, 1966.

39 Sara Halprin, *Look at My Ugly Face!*, Viking Penguin, New York, 1995.

40 Pogrebin, *Getting Over Growing Older*.

41 Brinlee Kramer in Robyn Rowland (ed.), *Women Who Do & Women Who Don't Join the Women's Movement*, Routledge Kegan Paul, 1984.

42 Rose Macaulay, *Personal Pleasures*, Gollancz, 1935.

43 Wendy Chapkis, *Beauty Secrets: Women and the Politics of Appearance*, South End Press, Boston, Massachusetts, 1986.

44 Melissa Benn, *Madonna and Child: Towards a New Politics of Motherhood*, Jonathan Cape, 1998.

45 *The Times*, 24 August 1982.

46 Helen Franks, *Goodbye Tarzan: Men After Feminism*, Allen and Unwin, 1984.

47 Shere Hite, *Women and Love: A Cultural Revolution in Progress*, Alfred A. Knopf, New York, 1987; Viking, 1988.

48 Lipovetsky, *The Empire of Fashion*.

49 Sally Cline and Dale Spender, *Reflecting Men at Twice Their Natural Size*, André Deutsch, 1987.

50 Andrea Stuart, "The Empire Line Dress", in Kirsty Dunseath (ed.), *A Second Skin: Women Write About Clothes*, The Women's Press, 1998.

51 Vance Packard, *The Hidden Persuaders*, David McKay Company Inc., New York and Longmans, Green, 1957; Penguin, Harmondsworth, 1960.

52 Lois W. Banner, *American Beauty*, Univesity of Chicago Press, Chicago and London, 1983.

53 Haug *et al.*, *Female Sexualization*.

54 Sichtermann, *Femininity*.

55 Lucy Kemnitzer and Anne Mackenzie, in Dena Taylor (ed.), *Feminist Parenting: Struggles, Triumphs & Comic Interludes*, The Crossing Press, Freedom, California, 1994.

56 Marianne Grabrucker, trs. Wendy Philipson, *There's a Good Girl: Gender Stereotyping in the First Three Years of Life. A Diary*, The Women's Press, 1988.

57 June Statham, *Daughters and Sons: Experiences of Non-Sexist Childraising*, Basil Blackwell, Oxford, 1986.

58 Susan Brownmiller, *Femininity*, Simon and Schuster, New York and Hamish Hamilton, 1984.

69 Germaine Greer, *The Female Eunuch*, McGibbon and Kee, 1970; *The Whole Woman*, Doubleday, London, 1999; *The Madwoman's Underclothes: Essays and Occasional Writings 1968–85*, Picador, 1986.

60 Elizabeth Wilson in *A Virago Keepsake to Celebrate Twenty Years of Publishing*, Virago, 1993.

61 Natasha Walter, *The New Feminism*, Little, Brown, 1998.

62 Theodore Zeldin, *The French*, Collins, 1983.

63 Janey Ironside, *Fashion as a Career*, Museum Press, 1962; *A Fashion Alphabet*, Michael Joseph, 1968.

64 Anne Scott-James, *In the Mink*, Michael Joseph, 1952.

65 Mary Tuck, "Why be beautiful?" in Susan Chitty (ed.), *The Intelligent Woman's Guide to Good Taste*, McGibbon and Kee, 1958.

66 Doris Langley Moore, *Pleasure: A Discursive Guide Book*, Cassell, 1953; Hawes, *Men Can Take It* See also Karen Hanson, "Dressing Down Dressing Up", in Hilde Hein and Carolyn Korsmeyer (eds.), *Aesthetics in Feminist Perspective*, Indiana University Press, Bloomington, Indiana, 1993, and Aileen Ribeiro, "Utopian Dress", in Juliet

Ash and Elizabeth Wilson (eds.), *Chic Thrills: A Fashion Reader*, Pandora Press, 1992.

67   Caplan, *The Myth of Women's Masochism*.

68   Chapkis, *Beauty Secrets*.

69   Susie Orbach and Luise Eichenbaum, *Bittersweet: Facing Up to Feelings of love, envy and Competition in Women's Friendships*, Century Hutchinson, 1987.

70   Sally Medora Wood, "Questions I Should Have Answered Better: A Guide to Women Who Dare to Speak Publicly", in Leslie B. Tanner (ed.), *Voices from Women's Liberation*, Mentor Books, New York, 1970.

71   Susan J. Douglas, *Where the Girls Are: Growing Up Female with the Mass Media in America*, Random House, New York, 1994; Penguin, Harmondsworth, 1995.

72   Robert Lynd, "Modern Forms of Starvation", in *In Defence of Pink*, Dent, 1937.

73   Elizabeth Wilson, "All the Rage", *New Socialist*, November/December 1983.

74   Quentin Bell, *On Human Finery*, The Hogarth Press, London, 1947; Allison & Busby, 1992.

SELECT BIBLIOGRAPHY

Paul Ableman, *The Doomed Rebellion*, Zomba Books, 1983.

Patricia Aburdene and John Naisbitt, *Megatrends for Women*, Random House, New York and London, 1993.

Carol Adams and Rae Lauriekitis, *The Gender Trap, Book 3: Messages and Images*, Virago, 1976; revised edition, 1980.

Lindsay Allason-Jones, *Women in Roman Britain*, British Museum Publications,1989.

Helen B. Andelin, *Fascinating Womanhood*, Pacific Press, Santa Barbara, California,1974.

Juliet Ash and Elizabeth Wilson (eds.), *Chic Thrills: A Fashion Reader*, Pandora Press, 1992.

Judy Attfield and Pat Kirkham (eds.), *A View from the Interior: Feminism, Women and Design,* The Women's Press, 1989.

Nancy C. Baker, *The Beauty Trap: How Every Woman Can Free Herself From It*, Judy Piatkus, 1986.

Olive M. Banks, *Faces of Feminism*, Martin Robertson, 1981.

Lois W. Banner, *American Beauty*, University of Chicago Press, Chicago and London, 1983.

Ruth Barnes and Joanne B. Eicher (eds.), *Dress and Gender: Making and Meaning* (Cross Cultural Perspectives on Women Vol. 2), Berg Publishers Inc., Rhode Island and Oxford, 1992.

Susan Bassnett, *Feminist Experiences: The Women's Movement in Four Cultures*, Allen and Unwin, 1986.

Christine Battersby, *Gender and Genius: Towards a Feminist Aesthetics*, The Women's Press, 1989.

Simone de Beauvoir, *Le Deuxième Sexe*, Gallimard, Paris, 1958.

Diane Bell and Renate Klein (eds.), *Radically Speaking: Feminism Reclaimed*, Zed Books, 1996.

Quentin Bell, *On Human Finery*, The Hogarth Press, London, 1947; Allison & Busby, 1992.

Jackie Bennett and Rosemary Forgan (eds.), *There's Something About a Convent Girl*, Virago, 1991.

Shari Benstock and Suzanne Ferriss (eds.), *On Fashion*, Rutgers University Press, New Brunswick, New Jersey, 1994.

John Berger, *Ways of Seeing*, BBC/Pelican Books, Harmondsworth, 1972.

Rosemary Betterton (ed.), *Looking On: Images of Femininity in the Visual Arts and Media*, Pandora Press, 1987.

Rosie Boycott, *A Nice Girl Like Me: A Story of the Seventies*, Chatto and Windus/Hogarth Press, 1984.

Gerd Brantenberg, *The Daughters of Egalia*, trs. Gerd Brantenberg and Louis Mackay, Journeyman Press Ltd., 1985.

Susan Brownmiller, *Femininity*, Simon and Schuster, New York and Hamish Hamilton, 1984.

Valerie Bryson, *Feminist Debates: Issues of Theory and Political Practice*, Macmillan, 1999.

"B. C." (John Scott-Waring), *The Ladies' Monitor, being a series of letters, first published in Bengal, on the subject of female apparel, tending to favour a regulated adoption of Indian costume*, 1809.

Paula J. Caplan, *The Myth of Women's Masochism*, E. P. Dutton, New York, 1985.

Jane Caputi, *The Age of Sex Crime*, The Women's Press, 1988.

Angela Carter, *Shaking a Leg: Journalism and Writings*, Vintage, 1998.

Joan Cassell, *A Group Called Women*, David McKay, New York, 1977.

"Censor" (Oliver Bell Bunce), *Don't*, Field and Tuer, 1883.

Jung Chang, *Wild Swans: Three Daughters of China*, HarperCollins, 1991.

Wendy Chapkis, *Beauty Secrets: Women and the Politics of Appearance*, South End Press, Boston, Massachusetts, 1986.

Phyllis Chesler, *Women and Madness*, Doubleday & Co. Inc., New York, 1972; Allen Lane, 1974.

Gail Chester and Julienne Dickey (eds.), *Feminism and Censorship: The Current Debate*, Prism Press, Bridport, Dorset, 1988.

Susan Chitty (ed.), *The Intelligent Woman's Guide to Good Taste*, McGibbon and Kee, 1958.

Sally Cline and Dale Spender, *Reflecting Men at Twice Their Natural Size*, André Deutsch, 1987.

Marcia Cohen, *The Sisterhood: The Inside Story of the Women's Movement and the Leaders Who Made it Happen*, Simon and Schuster, New York, 1988.

Joanne Cooke, Charlotte Bunch-Weeks and Robin Morgan (eds.), *The New Woman*, Fawcett Publications inc., Greenwich, Connecticut, 1971.

Kaz Cooke, *Real Gorgeous: The Truth About Body and Beauty*, Bloomsbury, 1995.

Anna Coote and Beatrix Campbell, *Sweet Freedom: The Struggle for Women's Liberation*, Pan Books, 1982.

Drusilla Cornell, *The Imaginary Domain: Abortion, Pornography, and Sexual Harassment*, Routledge, New York and London, 1995.

Lal Coveney, Tina Crockett, Al Garthwaite, Sheila Jeffreys and Valerie Sinclair, *Love Your Enemy? The debate between heterosexual feminism and political lesbianism*, Onlywomen Press Ltd., 1981.

Rosalind Coward, *Female Desire: Women's Sexuality Today*, Paladin Books, 1984.

——, *Our Treacherous Hearts: Why Women Let Men Get Their Way*, Faber and Faber, 1992.

Mary Daly, *Gyn/Ecology: The Metaethics of Radical Feminism*, Beacon Press, Boston, Massachusetts, 1978; The Women's Press, 1979.

Kathy Davis, *Reshaping the Female Body: The Dilemma of Cosmetic Surgery*, Routledge, New York and London, 1995.

Jill Dawson, *How Do I Look?*, Virago, 1990.

Karen DeCrow, *The Young Woman's Guide to Liberation: Alternatives to the Half-Life While the Choice Is Still Yours*, Pegasus, Indiana and New York, 1971.

Diana de Marly, *The History of Haute Couture 1850–1950*, B. T. Batsford Ltd., 1980.

——, *Fashion for Men: An Illustrated History*, Batsford, 1985.

Esmé Dodderidge, *The New Gulliver*, The Women's Press, 1988.

Susan J. Douglas, *Where the Girls Are: Growing Up Female with the Mass Media*, Times Books, New York, 1994; Penguin, Harmondsworth, 1995.

Slavenka Drakulić, *How We Survived Communism and Even Laughed*, Hutchinson, 1992.

Kirsty Dunseath (ed.), *A Second Skin: Women Write About Clothes*, The Women's Press, 1998.

Andrea Dworkin, *Woman Hating*, Plume Books, New York and London, 1974.

——, *Pornography: Men Possessing Women*, The Women's Press, 1981.

——, *Right-Wing Women*, The Women's Press, 1983.

——, *Letters from a War Zone: Writings 1976–1987*, Secker & Warburg, 1988.

——, *Life and Death: Unapologetic Writings on the Continuing War Against Women*, The Free Press, New York, 1997; Virago, 1997.

Gisela Ecker (ed.), *Feminist Aesthetics*, trs. Harriet Anderson, The Women's Press, 1985.

Barbara Ehrenreich and Deirdre English, *For Your Own Good: 150 Years of the Experts' Advice to Women*, Anchor Press/Doubleday, Garden City, New York, 1978; Pluto Press, 1979.

Barbara Ehrenreich, Elizabeth Hess and Gloria Jacobs, *Re-Making Love: The Feminization of Sex*, Anchor Press/Doubleday, Garden City, New York, 1986; Fontana Paperbacks, 1987.

Nancy Etcoff, *The Survival of the Prettiest*, Little, Brown, 1999.

Caroline Evans and Minna Thornton, *Women & Fashion: A New Look*, Quartet Books, London and New York, 1989.

Mary Evans, *A Good School: Life at a Girls' Grammar School in the 1950s*, The Women's Press, 1991.

Susan Faludi, *Backlash: The Undeclared War Against Women*, Chatto and Windus, 1992.

Ellen Fein and Sherrie Schneider, *The Rules: Ten time-Tested Secrets for Capturing the Heart of Mr Right*, Warner Books, USA, 1995; Thorsons, Wellingborough, Hampshire, 1995; *The Rules 2*, 1997.

Feminist Anthology Collective (eds.), *No Turning Back: Writings from the Women's Liberation Movement 1975–80*, The Women's Press, 1981.

Shulamith Firestone, *The Dialectic of Sex: The Case for Feminist Revolution*, Jonathan Cape, 1971.

Anna Ford, *Men*, Weidenfeld and Nicolson, 1985.

Helen Franks, *Goodbye Tarzan: Men After Feminism*, George Allen and Unwin, 1984.

Rita Freedman, *Beauty Bound: Why Women Strive for Physical Perfection*, Columbus Books, 1988.

——, *Bodylove: Learning to Like Our Looks – and Ourselves, A Practical Guide for Women*, Harper and Row, New York, 1989.

Marilyn French, *The War Against Women*, Summit Books, New York, 1992; Hamish Hamilton, 1992.

Nancy Friday, *The Power of Beauty*, HarperCollins, New York, 1996.

Betty Friedan, *The Feminine Mystique*, W. W. Norton, USA, 1963; Victor Gollancz Ltd., 1963.

——, *It Changed My Life: Writings on the Women's Movement*, Random House, New York, 1976.

Leah Fritz, *Dreamers and Dealers: An Intimate Appraisal of the Women's Movement*, Beacon Press, Boston, Massachusetts, 1979.

Marjorie Garber, *Vested Interests: Cross-Dressing and Cultural Anxiety*, Routledge, New York and London, 1992.

Leslie E. Gardiner F.I.C.S., M.R.C.S., L.R.C.P., D.L.O., *Faces, Figures and Feelings: A Cosmetic Plastic Surgeon Speaks*, Robert Hale, 1959.

Charlotte Perkins Gilman, *Herland*, 1915; The Women's Press, 1979.

Marianne Grabrucker, *There's a Good Girl: Gender Stereotyping in the First Three Years of Life. A Diary*, trs. Wendy Philipson, The Women's Press, 1988.

Francine du Plessix Gray, *Soviet Women: Walking the Tightrope*, Doubleday, New York, 1990.

Germaine Greer, *The Female Eunuch*, McGibbon and Kee, London, 1970; Paladin, 1993.

——, *The Madwoman's Underclothes: Essays and Occasional Writings 1968–85*, Picador, 1986.

——, *The Whole Woman*, Doubleday, London, New York, Toronto, Sydney and Auckland, 1999.

Susan Griffin, *Pornography and Silence*, The Women's Press, 1981.

Benoîte Groult, *Ainsi Soit-Elle*, Editions Grasset et Fasquelle, Paris, 1975.

Sara Halprin, *"Look at My Ugly Face!"*, Viking Penguin, New York, 1995.

Joseph Hansen and Evelyn Reed, *Cosmetics, Fashions, and the Exploitation of Women*, Pathfinder Press, New York, 1986.

Karen Hanson, "Dressing Down Dressing Up", in Hilde Hein and Carolyn Korsmeyer (eds.), *Aesthetics in Feminist Perspective*, Indiana University Press, Bloomington, Indiana, 1993.

Barbara Grizzuti Harrison, *Off Center*, Playboy Paperbacks, New York, 1980.

Helen Haste, *The Sexual Metaphor*, Harvester Wheatsheaf, Hemel Hempstead, Hertfordshire, 1993.

Frigga Haug *et al.*, *Female Sexualization: A Collective Work of Memory*, Verso, 1986.

Elizabeth Hawes, *Men Can Take It*, Random House, New York, 1939.

Emma Healey, *Lesbian Sex Wars*, Virago, 1996.

Susan Hemmings (ed.), *Girls Are Powerful: Young Women's Writings from Spare Rib*, Sheba Feminist Publishers, 1982.

Liz Heron, *Changes of Heart: Reflections on Women's Independence*, Pandora Press, 1986.

Shere Hite, *Women and Love*, Alfred A. Knopf, New York, 1987; Viking, 1988.

Shere Hite and Kate Colleran, *Good Guys, Bad Guys and Other Lovers*, Pandora Press, 1989.

bell hooks, *Feminism Is For Everybody: Passionate Politics*, Pluto Press, 2000.

Johan Huizinga, *The Waning of the Middle Ages: A Study of the Forms of Life, Thought, and Art in France and the Netherlands in the Fourteenth and Fifteenth Centuries*, trs. F. Hopman, 1924; Pelican, Harmondsworth, 1955.

Janey Ironside, *Fashion as a Career*, Museum Press, 1962.

——, *A Fashion Alphabet*, Michael Joseph, 1968.

Catherine Itzin (ed.) *Pornography: Women, Violence and Civil Liberties*, Oxford University Press, Oxford, 1992.

Elizabeth Janeway, *Man's World, Woman's Place: A Study in Social Mythology*, USA, 1971; Penguin, Harmondsworth, 1977.

Sheila Jeffreys, *Anticlimax: A Feminist Perspective on the Sexual Revolution*, The Women's Press, 1993.

——, *The Lesbian Heresy: A Feminist Perspective on the Lesbian Sexual Revolution*, The Women's Press, 1993.

Wendy Kaminer, *True Love Waits*, Addison-Wesley, Reading, Massachusetts, 1996.

Susanne Kappeler, *The Pornography of Representation*, Polity Press, Cambridge, 1986.

Carol Farley Kessler (ed.), *Daring to Dream: Utopian Stories by United States Women: 1836–1919*, Pandora, 1984.

Wilson Bryan Key, *Media Sexploitation*, Prentice-Hall Inc., New York, 1976.

Claudia Brush Kidwell and Valerie Steele, *Dressing the Part*, Smithsonian Press, Washington D. C., 1989.

Martin F. Kilmer, *Greek Erotica*, Duckworth, 1993.

Nora Scott Kinzer, *Put Down and Ripped Off: The American Woman and the Beauty Cult*, Thomas Y. Crowell, New York, 1977.

Francine Klagsbrun (ed.), *The First Ms. Reader*, Warner Books, New York, 1973.

David Kunzle, *Fashion and Fetishism*, Rowman and Littlefield, Totowa, New Jersey, 1982.

Robin Tolmach Lakoff and Raquel L. Scherr, *Face Value: The Politics of Beauty*, Routledge Kegan Paul, 1984.

James Laver, *Taste and Fashion from the French Revolution to the Present Day*, Harrap, 1931, revised 1945.

——, *Fashions and Fashion Plates 1800–1900*, Penguin, Harmondsworth, 1943.

——, *Style in Costume*, Oxford University Press, 1949.

——, *Children's Fashions of the XIXth Century*, Batsford, 1951.

William Leach, *True Love and Perfect Union: The Feminist Reform of Sex and Society*, Basic Books, New York, 1980.

Laura Lederer (ed.), *Take Back the Night: Women on Pornography*, William Morrow and Company, New York, 1980; Bantam Books, Toronto, New York, London and Sydney, 1982.

Carol Lee, *The Blind Side of Eden: The Sexes in Perspective*, Bloomsbury Publishing Ltd., 1989.

Margaret Leroy, *Pleasure: The Truth About Female Sexuality*, HarperCollins, 1993.

Gilles Lipovetsky, *The Empire of Fashion: Dressing Modern Democracy*, trs. Catherine Porter, Princeton University Press, Princeton, New Jersey, 1994.

Susan Lipshitz (ed.), *Tearing the Veil: Essays on Femininity*, Routledge Kegan Paul, 1978.

Catharine Lumby, *Bad Girls*, Allen and Unwin, St Leonards, Australia, 1997.

Ferdinand Lundberg and Marynia F. Farnham, M. D., *Modern Woman: The Lost Sex*, Harper and Brothers, New York and London, 1947.

Alison Lurie, *The Language of Clothes*, Heinemann, 1982.

Catharine A. Mackinnon, *Only Words*, HarperCollins, 1994.

Rhona Mahony, *Kidding Ourselves: Breadwinning, Babies and Bargaining Power*, Basic Books, New York, 1995.

Anja Meulenbelt, *The Shame Is Over: A Political Life Story*, trs. Ann Oosthuizen, The Women's Press, 1980.

Anja Meulenbelt, Johanna's Daughter, *For Ourselves*, Sheba Feminist Publishers, 1981.

Mary Midgley and Judith Hughes, *Women's Choices: Philosophical Problems Facing Feminism*, Weidenfeld and Nicolson, 1983.

Ann Monsarrat, *And the Bride Wore . . . The Story of the White Wedding*, Coronet Books, Hodder and Stoughton, 1975.

Doris Langley Moore, *The Vulgar Heart*, Cassell, 1945.

——, *Pleasure: A Discursive Guide Book*, Cassell, 1953.

Fidelis Morgan, *A Misogynist's Source Book*, Jonathan Cape, 1989.

Marabel Morgan, *The Total Woman*, Fleming Revell, Old Tappan, New Jersey, 1973.

Robin Morgan (ed.), *Sisterhood Is Powerful*, Random House, New York, 1970.

——, *Going Too Far: The Personal Chronicle of a Feminist*, Vintage Books, New York, 1978.

——, *The Anatomy of Freedom: Feminism, Physics, and Global Politics*, Anchor Press/Doubleday, New York, 1982; Martin Robertson, Oxford, 1983.

——, *The Demon Lover: On the Sexuality of Terrorism*, Methuen, 1989.

——, *The Word of a Woman: Selected Prose 1968–1992*, Virago, 1993.

Kathy Nairne and Gerrilyn Smith, *Dealing with Depression*, The Women's Press, 1984.

Angela Neustatter, *Hyenas in Petticoats: A Look at Twenty Years of Feminism*, Harrap, 1989.

Joyce Nicholson, *What Society Does to Girls*, Virago, 1977.

Virginia Novarra, *Women's Work, Men's Work: The Ambivalence of Equality*, Marion Boyars, London and Boston, Massachusetts, 1980.

Ann Oakley, *Subject Women*, Martin Robertson, Oxford, 1981.

Susie Orbach and Luise Eichenbaum, *Bittersweet: Facing Up to Feelings of Love, Envy and Competition in Women's Friendships*, Century, 1987.

Jane O'Reilly, *The Girl I Left Behind*, Collier Books, New York 1980.

Vance Packard, *The Hidden Persuaders*, David McKay Company Inc., New York, 1957; Longmans, Green, 1957; Penguin, Harmondsworth, 1960.

——, *The Waste Makers*, USA 1960; Penguin, Harmondsworth, 1963.

Gill Perry and Michael Rossington (eds.), *Femininity and Masculinity in Eighteenth-Century Art and Culture*, Manchester University Press, Manchester, 1994.

Giovanna Pezzuoli, *Prigioniera in Utopia*, Edizioni Il Formichiere, Milan, 1978.

Letty Cottin Pogrebin, *Growing Up Free: Raising Your Child in the 80s*, McGraw-Hill, New York, 1980.

——, *Getting Over Growing Older: An Intimate Journey*, Little, Brown, Boston, New York, Toronto and London, 1996.

Ted Polhemus, *Fashion and Anti-Fashion*, Thames and Hudson, 1978.

Gwen Raverat, *Period Piece: A Cambridge Childhood*, Faber and Faber, 1952.

Sue Read, *Sexual Harassment at Work*, Hamlyn Books, 1982.

Theodor Reik, *Sex in Man and Woman: The Emotional Variations*, Noonday Press, Inc., New York, 1960.

Kimberley Reynolds and Nicola Humble, *Victorian Heroines: Representations of Femininity in Nineteenth-Century Literature and Art*, Hamish Hamilton, 1993.

Dusty Rhodes and Sandra McNeil (eds.), *Women Against Violence Against Women*, Onlywomen Press, 1985.

Aileen Ribeiro, *Dress and Morality*, Batsford, 1986.

——, *The Art of Dress: Fashion in England and France from 1750 to 1820*, Yale University Press, New Haven and London, 1995.

Adrienne Rich, *On Lies, Secrets and Silence*, W. W. Norton, New York, 1979; Virago, 1980.

Janet Radcliffe Richards, *The Sceptical Feminist: A Philosophical Enquiry*, Routledge Kegan Paul, 1980.

Yvonne Roberts, *Mad About Women: Can There Ever Be Fair Play Between the Sexes?*, Virago, 1992.

Gay Robins, *Women in Ancient Egypt*, British Museum Press, London, 1993.

Hilary Robinson (ed.), *Visibly Female: Feminism and Art, An Anthology*, Camden Press, 1987.

Gillian Rodgerson and Elizabeth Wilson (eds.), *Feminism and Pornography: The Case Against Censorship*, Lawrence and Wishart, 1991.

Aline Rousselle, *Porneia: Desire and the Body in Antiquity*, trs. Felicia Pheasant, Blackwells, Oxford, 1988.

Sheila Rowbotham, *The Past Is Before Us: Feminism in Action Since the 1960s*, Pandora, 1989.

——, *A Century of Women: The History of Women in Britain and the United States*, Viking, 1997.

Marsha Rowe (ed.), *Spare Rib Reader*, Penguin, Harmondsworth, 1982.

Robyn Rowland (ed.), *Women Who Do and Women Who Don't Join the Women's Movement*, Routledge Kegan Paul, 1984.

Jane Rule, *A Hot-Eyed Moderate*, Naiad Press, Tallahassee, Florida, 1985.

Joanna Russ, *How to Suppress Women's Writing*, The Women's Press, 1984.

——, *Magic Mommas, Trembling Sisters, Puritans and Perverts*, Crossing Press, Trumansburg, New York, 1985.

Diana E. H. Russell, *Making Violence Sexy: Feminist Views on Pornography*, Open University Press, Buckingham, 1993.

Linda Tschirhart Sanford and Mary Ellen Donovan, *Women and Self-Esteem*, Anchor Press/Doubleday, New York, 1984; Penguin, Harmondsworth, 1983.

Kathie Sarachild (ed.), *Feminist Revolution*, Random House, New York, 1978.

Gill Saunders, *The Nude: A New Perspective*, The Herbert Press Ltd., 1989.

Maggie Scarf, *Unfinished Business: Pressure Points in the Lives of Women*, Doubleday, New York, 1980.

Anne Scott-James, *In the Mink*, Michael Joseph Ltd., 1952.

Amanda Sebestyen, "Sexual Assumptions in the Women's Movement", in Scarlet Friedman and Elizabeth Sarah (eds.), *On the Problem of Women*, The Women's Press, 1982.

Lynne Segal, *Is the Future Female? Troubled Thoughts on Contempoary Feminism*, Virago, 1987.

Lynne Segal and Mary McIntosh (eds.), *Sex Exposed: Women and the Pornography Debate*, Virago, 1992.

Alison Settle, *Clothes Line*, Methuen, 1937.

Simon Shepherd (ed.), *The Women's Sharp Revenge: Five Women's Pamphlets from the Renaissance*, Fourth Estate Ltd., 1985.

Anita Shreve, *Women Together, Women Alone: The Legacy of the Consciousness-Raising Movement*, Viking, New York, 1989.

Barbara Sichtermann, *Femininity: The Politics of the Personal*, trs. John Whittam, Polity Press, Cambridge, 1983.

Bonnie G. Smith, *Ladies of the Leisure Class: The Bourgeoisie of Northern France in Nineteenth Century*, Princeton University Press, Princeton, 1981.

Ann Snitow, Christine Stansell and Sharon Thompson (eds.), *Desire: The Politics of Sexuality*, Monthly Review Press, USA, 1983; Virago, 1984.

Sookie Stambler (ed.), *Women's Liberation: Blueprint for the Future*, Ace Books, New York, 1970.

June Statham, *Daughters and Sons: Experiences of Non-Sexist Childrearing*, Blackwell, Oxford, 1986.

Valerie Steele, *Paris Fashion: A Cultural History*, Oxford University Press, New York and Oxford, 1988.

Sara Stein, *Girls and Boys: The Limits of Non-Sexist Childrearing*, Chatto, 1984.

Gloria Steinem, *Outrageous Acts and Everyday Rebellions*, Henry Holt and Company, Inc., New York, 1995.

——, *Revolution from Within, A Book of Self-Esteem*, Bloomsbury, 1992.

——, *Moving Beyond Words*, Simon and Schuster, New York, 1994; Bloomsbury, 1994.

Mary Stott, *Forgetting's No Excuse*, Faber and Faber, London, 1973; revised edition, Virago, 1975.

——, *Before I Go: Reflections On My Life and Times*, Virago, London, 1985.

——, (ed.), *Women Talking*, Pandora, 1987.

Harriet Beecher Stowe, *The Chimney-Corner*, Sampson Low, Son & Marston, and Bell and Daldy, 1868.

Nadine Strossen, *Defending Pornography: Free Speech, Sex, and the Battle for Women's Rights*, Simon & Schuster, New York, 1995; Abacus, 1996.

T. DeWitt Talmage, D. D., *Marriage and Home Life*, Oliphant, Anderson and Ferrier, Edinburgh, 1892.

Leslie B. Tanner (ed.), *Voices from Women's Liberation*, Mentor Books, New York, 1970.

Dena Taylor (ed.), *Feminist Parenting: Struggles, Triumphs & Comic Interludes*, The Crossing Press, Freedom, California, 1994.

John Taylor, *It's a Small, Medium and Outsize World*, Hugh Evelyn, 1966.

David Thomas, *Not Guilty: In Defence of the Modern Man*, Weidenfeld and Nicolson, 1993.

Lisa Tickner, *The Spectacle of Women: Imagery of the Suffrage Campaign 1907–14*, Chatto and Windus, 1987.

Joyce Tyldesley, *Daughters of Isis*, Viking, New York and London, 1994.

Carole S. Vance (ed.), *Pleasure and Danger: Exploring Female Sexuality*, Pandora, 1989.

Thorstein Veblen, *The Theory of the Leisure Class*, Macmillan, New York, 1899.

Esther Vilar, *The Manipulated Man*, Farrar, Straus and Giroux, New York, 1972; Bantam, New York, 1974.

Natasha Walter, *The New Feminism*, Little, Brown, 1998.

Ralph M. Wardle, *Mary Wollstonecraft: A Critical Biography*, University of Kansas Press, Lawrence, Kansas, 1951.

Rebecca West, *The Young Rebecca: Writings of Rebecca West 1911–17*, Macmillan, 1982.

Elizabeth Wilson, *Mirror Writing: An Autobiography*, Virago, 1982.

——, "All the Rage", *New Socialist*, No. 14, November/December 1983.

——, *What Is to Be Done About Violence Against Women?*, Penguin, Harmondsworth, 1983.

——, *Adorned in Dreams: Fashion and Modernity*, Virago, 1985.

Elizabeth Wilson and Lou Taylor, *Through the Looking Glass: A History of Dress from 1860 to the Present Day*, BBC, 1987.

Naomi Wolf, *The Beauty Myth*, Chatto and Windus, 1990.

——, *Fire With Fire: The New Female Power and How It Will Change the Twenty-First Century*, Chatto and Windus, 1993.

Janet L. Wolff, *What Makes Women Buy*, McGraw-Hill, New York, Toronto and London, 1958.

Mary Wollstonecraft, *Thoughts on the Education of Daughters: with Reflections on Female Conduct, in the More Important Duties of Life*, 1787.

——, *A Vindication of the Rights of Women*, 1792; Penguin, Harmondsworth, 1975.

Women in Media, *The Packaging of Women*, 1976.

Virginia Woolf, *A Room of One's Own*, 1929; Oxford University Press, Oxford, 1992.

——, *Three Guineas*, 1938; Oxford University Press, Oxford, 1992.

Ray Wyre, *Women, Men and Rape*, Perry Publications, Oxford, 1986.

INDEX